Board Review Series

Pathology

Board Review Series

Pathology

Arthur S. Schneider, M.D.
Professor and Chairman
Department of Pathology
Chicago Medical School
North Chicago, Illinois

Philip A. Szanto, M.D.
Associate Professor of Pathology
Chicago Medical School
North Chicago, Illinois

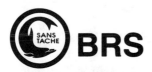 **BRS**

Board Review Series from Williams & Wilkins
Baltimore, Hong Kong, London, Sydney

Harwal Publishing Company, Malvern, Pennsylvania

Williams & Wilkins

Managing Editor: Susan E. Kelly
Manuscript Editor: Mary T. Durkin
Editorial Assistant: Kelly A. Reed
Production Supervisor: Laurie Forsyth
Production Editor: Joan M. Leary

Library of Congress Cataloging-in-Publication Data

Schneider, Arthur S.
  Pathology / Arthur S. Schneider, Philip A. Szanto.
    p.   cm.—(Board review series)
  ISBN 0-683-07608-6 (pbk. : alk. paper)
  1. Pathology—Outlines, syllabi, etc. 2. Pathology—Examinations,
questions, etc.   I. Szanto, Philip A.   II. Title.   III. Series.
  [DNLM: 1. Pathology—examination questions.   QZ 18 S358p]
RB32.S36   1992
616.07—dc20
DNLM/DLC
for Library of Congress   92-49705
                                                                      CIP

10 9 8 7 6 5 4 3 2 1

Contents

Preface

The aphorism of Hippocrates, "Life is short, and the Art long; the occasion fleeting; experience fallacious, and judgment difficult," is clearly proven true during the first years of medical school. The time that the student can devote to a single subject is very limited, and the amount of material to be covered is indeed great. Nowhere is this more true than in pathology, traditionally one of the "big courses" of the first two years. The sheer enormity of the task is problematic for students as they attempt to select significant core items that deserve special emphasis from the large amount of material presented in standard texts. The problem becomes especially acute when it is necessary to review large amounts of material when preparing for tests such as the United States Medical Licensing Examination (USMLE). This book is designed to assist students in meeting these needs.

Organization

This book is divided into 23 chapters organized parallel to most standard texts. The first 8 chapters cover general or basic pathology, presenting the major concepts of disease processes viewed as manifestations of a common set of mechanisms of injury. The succeeding 15 chapters cover systemic pathology, surveying the principal disorders of each organ system.

The text is presented in the tightly outlined format of the *Board Review Series,* which facilitates quick comprehension and review. Numerous tables supplement textual information throughout the book. Each chapter is followed by review questions and answers and explanations, and the entire text is followed by a Comprehensive Examination. All questions reflect the style and content of USMLE changes.

How To Use This Book

The book is not designed to be used as a primary text but rather as an aid to identifying key concepts during the initial period of study and as a relatively concise source of material suitable for rapid review. Following completion of a unit during the pathology course, many students will find it helpful to quickly go over the corresponding chapter and its accompanying review questions. Core items not identified will easily become apparent by this technique. To prepare for USMLE Step 1, the Comprehensive Examination can be used both as a pretest and as a post-test to help identify areas that merit further attention in the chapters or in standard texts. Special attention should be directed to the explanatory material following the Comprehensive Examination, where a large proportion of the material that has become standard on national examinations is reviewed.

Acknowledgments

We express our appreciation to our colleagues in the Department of Pathology for their comments and suggestions during the preparation of this text. Special thanks are extended to Dr. Charles McCormack of the Department of Physiology and Biophysics, who critically reviewed the chapter on endocrine disorders, and to Dr. Seymour Ehrenpreis of the Department of Pharmacology and Molecular Biology for his review of the entire manuscript. Special thanks to those who provided illustrations: Dr. Jae O. Roe, a colleague in our department; Dr. Deborah E. Powell of the University of Kentucky; Dr. Juan Rosai of the Memorial-Sloan Kettering Cancer Center; and Dr. John B. Walter of the University of Toronto. We thank our many students who used the manuscript version of this book during their pathology course and during their preparation for examinations, both in the classroom and for USMLE. They provided enthusiastic, encouraging response and constructive feedback.

It is difficult to adequately express our very special debt to Ms. Susan Grimm for her participation in the preparation of the manuscript. She worked side-by-side with us in the detailed writing of the manuscript, typed and retyped successive versions, and labored over every page for countless hours. Her diligence assured that usage was uniform from chapter to chapter, that every verb was properly single or plural, that every "which" or "that" was properly selected, that every comma or semicolon was appropriate, that every word was properly spelled and applied, and that every citation was correct. There is no way that this book could have been completed without her.

We also acknowledge the considerable efforts of the staff at Williams & Wilkins and at Harwal Publishing Company, a division of Williams & Wilkins, who were active in the production of this book. We especially thank Mr. John Gardner, who initiated the *Board Review Series;* the faculty and student reviewers who helped bring the book quality; and most of all Ms. Susan Kelly, Managing Editor of the *Board Review Series,* who, along with her talented staff, forced us (sometimes with great resistance) to do our best to produce a concise, clearly understandable book.

We also thank our respective families for their patience and forbearance during this extended period.

Arthur S. Schneider
Philip A. Szanto

1

Cellular Reaction to Injury

I. Adaptation to Environmental Stress

A. Hypertrophy

—is an **increase in the size of an organ or tissue due to an increase in the size of cells** and is further characterized by an increase in protein synthesis and an increase in size or number of intracellular organelles.

—results from cellular adaptation to increased workload exemplified by the increase in skeletal muscle mass associated with exercise and the enlargement of the left ventricle in hypertensive heart disease.

B. Hyperplasia

—is an **increase in the size of an organ or tissue due to an increase in the number of cells**.

—is exemplified by glandular proliferation in the breast during pregnancy.

—in some instances, occurs with hypertrophy. Uterine enlargement during pregnancy is caused by both hypertrophy and hyperplasia of uterine smooth muscle cells.

C. Aplasia

—is a **failure of cell production**.

1. During fetal development, aplasia results in **agenesis,** absence of an organ due to failure of production.

2. Later in life, aplasia follows permanent loss of precursor cells in proliferative tissues.

D. Hypoplasia

—is a **decrease in cell production less extreme than aplasia**.

—is seen in the partial lack of growth and maturation of gonadal structures seen in Turner's syndrome and Klinefelter's syndrome.

E. Atrophy

—is a **decrease in the size of an organ or tissue resulting from a decrease in mass of preexisting cells**.

1

—most often results from disuse, nutritional or oxygen deprivation, diminished endocrine stimulation, aging, and denervation (lack of nerve stimulation in peripheral muscles from injury to motor nerves).

—often is marked by the presence of **autophagic granules,** intracytoplasmic vacuoles containing debris from degraded organelles.

F. Metaplasia

—is the **replacement of one differentiated tissue by another**.

1. Squamous metaplasia

—is exemplified by the replacement of columnar epithelium at the squamo-columnar junction of the cervix by squamous epithelium.

—can also occur in the respiratory epithelium of the bronchus, in the endometrium, and in the pancreatic ducts.

—is associated with chronic irritation and inflammation.

—is also associated with vitamin A deficiency.

2. Osseous metaplasia

—is bone formation at sites of tissue injury. Cartilaginous metaplasia may also occur.

3. Myeloid metaplasia (extramedullary hematopoiesis)

—is proliferation of hematopoietic tissue in sites other than bone marrow, such as the liver or spleen.

II. Ischemic Cell Injury

A. Causes—ischemic cell injury

—results from cellular **anoxia** or **hypoxia,** which, in turn, results from a variety of mechanisms, including:

1. Obstruction of arterial blood flow (the most common cause)

2. Anemia, a reduction in the number of oxygen-carrying red blood cells

3. Carbon monoxide poisoning, which results in diminution in the oxygen-carrying capacity of red blood cells by chemical alteration of hemoglobin

4. Decreased perfusion of tissues by oxygen-carrying blood, as occurs in cardiac failure, hypotension, and shock

5. Poor oxygenation of blood, secondary to pulmonary disease

B. Early stage of ischemic cell injury

—affects mitochondria, with resultant decreased oxidative phosphorylation and adenosine triphosphate (ATP) synthesis. Consequences of **decreased ATP** availability include:

1. Failure of the cell membrane pump (ouabain-sensitive Na^+K^+-ATPase) results in increased intracellular Na^+ and water and decreased intracellular K^+, which cause cellular swelling and swelling of organelles.

a. Cellular swelling, or **hydropic change,** is characterized by the presence of large vacuoles in the cytoplasm.

b. Swelling of the endoplasmic reticulum is one of the first ultrastructural changes evident in reversible injury.

    c. Swelling of the mitochondria progresses from reversible, low-amplitude swelling to irreversible high-amplitude swelling, which is characterized by marked dilatation of the inner mitochondrial space.

  2. Disaggregation of ribosomes and failure of protein synthesis; ribosomal disaggregation also is promoted by membrane damage.

  3. Stimulation of phosphofructokinase activity results in increased glycolysis, lactate accumulation, and decreased intracellular pH. Acidification causes reversible clumping of nuclear chromatin.

C. Late stage of ischemic cell injury

  −results in **membrane damage** to plasma and lysosomal and other organellar membranes.

  −reversible morphologic signs of damage include the formation of:

  1. Myelin figures, whorl-like structures probably originating from damaged membranes

  2. Cell blebs, a cell surface deformity most likely caused by disorderly function of the cellular cytoskeleton

D. Cell death

  −is caused by severe or prolonged injury.

  1. The **point of no return** is marked by **irreversible damage to mitochondria and cell membranes,** leading to **massive calcium influx** and cell death. Release of aspartate aminotransferase (AST), creatine phosphokinase (CPK), and lactate dehydrogenase (LDII) into the blood is an important indicator of irreversible injury to heart muscle following interruption of myocardial blood supply by occlusion of coronary artery blood flow.

  2. The vulnerability of cells to ischemic injury varies with the tissue or cell type. Ischemic injury becomes irreversible after:

    a. 3–5 minutes for neurons. Purkinje cells of the cerebellum and neurons of the hippocampus are more susceptible to ischemic injury than other neurons.

    b. 1–2 hours for myocardial cells and hepatocytes

    c. Many hours for skeletal muscle cells

III. Free Radical Injury

A. Free radicals

  −are any molecule with a single unpaired electron in the outer orbital.

  −are exemplified by activated products of oxygen reduction, which include the superoxide (O_2^{-}) and the hydroxyl (OH•) radicals.

B. Generation of free radicals

  −occurs by the following mechanisms:

1. Normal metabolism

2. Oxygen toxicity, as in the alveolar damage that can cause adult respiratory distress syndrome and retrolental fibroplasia, an ocular disorder of premature infants

3. Ionizing radiation

4. **Drugs and chemicals,** many of which promote both proliferation of the smooth endoplasmic reticulum (SER) and induction of the P-450 system of mixed function oxidases of the SER. Proliferation and hypertrophy of the SER of the hepatocyte is a classic ultrastructural marker of barbiturate intoxication.

5. **Reperfusion after ischemic injury**

C. **Free radical degradation**

—occurs by:

1. **Intracellular enzymes,** such as glutathione peroxidase, catalase, or superoxide dismutase

2. **Endogenous substances,** such as ceruloplasmin or transferrin

3. **Spontaneous decay**

IV. Chemical Cell Injury

—is illustrated by the **model of liver cell membrane damage induced by carbon tetrachloride** (CCl_4).

A. In this model, CCl_4 is processed by the P-450 system of mixed function oxidases within the SER, producing the **highly reactive free radical CCl_3•.**

B. CCl_3• diffuses throughout the cell, initiating **lipid peroxidation of intracellular membranes**. Widespread injury results, including:

1. **Disaggregation of ribosomes,** resulting in **decreased protein synthesis**. Failure of the cell to synthesize the apoprotein moiety of lipoproteins causes accumulation of intracellular lipids (**fatty change**).

2. **Plasma membrane damage,** caused by products of lipid peroxidation, resulting in **cellular swelling** and **massive influx of calcium,** with resultant mitochondrial damage, denaturation of cell proteins, and cell death

V. Necrosis (Table 1.1)

—is the sum of the intracellular degradative reactions occurring after the death of individual cells within a living organism.

A. **General characteristics**

1. In pathologic specimens, fixed cells with well-preserved morphology are dead but not necrotic.

2. **Autolysis** refers to degradative reactions in cells caused by intracellular enzymes indigenous to the cell. **Postmortem autolysis** occurs after death of the entire organism and is not necrosis.

3. **Heterolysis** refers to cellular degradation by enzymes derived from sources extrinsic to the cell (e.g., bacteria, leukocytes).

B. **Types of necrosis**

1. **Coagulation necrosis**

—most often results from sudden cutoff of blood supply to an organ, particularly the heart and kidney.

—in early stages, is characterized by general **preservation of tissue architecture**.

Table 1.1. Types of Necrosis

Types	Mechanism	Pathologic Changes
Coagulation necrosis	Most often results from interruption of blood supply, resulting in denaturation of proteins; best seen in organs supplied by end arteries with limited collateral circulation, such as the heart and kidney	General architecture well preserved, except for nuclear changes; increased cytoplasmic binding of acidophilic dyes
Liquefaction necrosis	Enzymatic liquefaction of necrotic tissue, most often in the CNS, where it is caused by interruption of blood supply; also occurs in areas of bacterial infection	Necrotic tissue soft and liquefied
Caseous necrosis	Shares features of both coagulation and liquefaction necrosis; most commonly seen in tuberculous granulomas	Architecture not preserved but tissue not liquefied; gross appearance is soft and cheese-like; histologic appearance is amorphous, with increased affinity for acidophilic dyes
Gangrenous necrosis	Most often results from interruption of blood supply to a lower extremity or the bowel	Changes depend on tissue involved and whether or not gangrene is dry or wet
Fibrinoid necrosis	Characterized by deposition of fibrin-like proteinaceous material in walls of arteries; often observed as part of immune-mediated vasculitis	Smudgy pink appearance in vascular walls; actual necrosis may or may not be present
Fat necrosis	Liberation of pancreatic enzymes with autodigestion of pancreatic parenchyma; trauma to fat cells	Necrotic fat cells, acute inflammation, hemorrhage, calcium soap formation, clustering of lipid-laden macrophages (in the pancreas)
Apoptosis	Cell death affecting solitary cells	Nuclear and cytoplasmic condensation, as seen in Councilman body of viral hepatitis

—**increased cytoplasmic eosinophilia** occurs because of protein denaturation and loss of cytoplasmic RNA.

—is **marked by nuclear changes,** the morphologic hallmark of irreversible cell injury and necrosis. These include:

a. **Pyknosis,** chromatin clumping and shrinking with increased basophilia

b. **Karyorrhexis,** fragmentation of chromatin

c. **Karyolysis,** fading of chromatin material

d. **Disappearance of stainable nuclei**

2. **Liquefaction necrosis**

—is characterized by digestion of tissue.

—is marked by softening and liquefaction of tissue.

—characteristically results from **ischemic injury to the central nervous system (CNS).** Following the death of CNS cells, liquefaction is caused by autolysis.

—also occurs in **suppurative infections** characterized by formation of pus, liquefied tissue debris and neutrophils, by heterolytic mechanisms.

3. Caseous necrosis

—combines features of both coagulation necrosis and liquefaction necrosis.
—is marked by a cheese-like (caseous) consistency on gross examination.
—presents an **amorphous eosinophilic appearance** on histologic examination.
—occurs as **part of granulomatous inflammation,** as seen in **tuberculosis**.

4. Gangrenous necrosis

—most often affects the lower extremities or bowel and is secondary to vascular occlusion.
—is termed **wet gangrene** when complicated by infective heterolysis and consequent liquefaction necrosis.
—is termed **dry gangrene** when characterized primarily by coagulation necrosis without liquefaction.

5. Fibrinoid necrosis

—is caused by immune-mediated vascular damage.
—is marked by **deposition of fibrin-like proteinaceous material in arterial walls,** which appears smudgy and acidophilic.

6. Fat necrosis

—occurs in two forms:

a. Traumatic fat necrosis

—occurs following severe injury to tissue with high fat content, such as the breast.

b. Enzymatic fat necrosis

—is a complication of **acute hemorrhagic pancreatitis,** a severe inflammatory disorder of the pancreas.
(1) Proteolytic and lipolytic pancreatic enzymes diffuse into inflamed tissue and literally digest the parenchyma.
(2) Fatty acids liberated by the digestion form calcium salts (saponification, or **soap formation**).
(3) Vessels are eroded, with resultant hemorrhage.

7. Apoptosis

—is the death of single cells within clusters of other cells.
—is marked by shrinkage and increased acidophilic staining, with formation of small round eosinophilic masses often containing chromatin remnants.
—is exemplified by formation of Councilman bodies in viral hepatitis.
—occurs as a physiologic process for removal of cells during embryogenesis and during programmed cell cycling, as in the endometrium during menstruation.

VI. Reversible Cellular Changes and Accumulations

A. Fatty change

—is characterized by the **accumulation of intracellular parenchymal triglycerides**.

—most frequently is observed in the **liver, heart,** or **kidney**. For example, in the liver, fatty change may be secondary to alcoholism, diabetes mellitus, malnutrition, obesity, and poisonings.

—results from an imbalance between the uptake, utilization, and secretion of fat caused by the following mechanisms:

1. **Increased transport of triglycerides or fatty acids** to affected cells

2. **Decreased mobilization of fat from cells,** most often mediated by decreased production of apoproteins required for fat transport. Fatty change is thus linked to the disaggregation of ribosomes and consequent decreased protein synthesis caused by failure of ATP production in CCl_4-injured cells.

3. **Decreased use of fat by cells**

4. **Overproduction of fat in cells**

B. **Hyaline change**

—describes a characteristic (homogeneous, glassy, eosinophilic) appearance in hematoxylin and eosin sections, most often caused by nonspecific accumulations of proteinaceous material.

C. **Accumulations of exogenous pigments**

1. **Pulmonary accumulations of carbon, silica, and iron dust**

2. **Plumbism** (lead poisoning)

3. **Argyria** (silver poisoning)

—may cause a permanent gray discoloration of the skin and conjunctivae.

D. **Accumulations of endogenous pigments**

1. **Melanin**

—is **formed** from tyrosine by the action of tyrosinase, **synthesized** in melanosomes of melanocytes within the epidermis, and **transferred** by melanocytes to adjacent clusters of keratinocytes and to macrophages (melanophores) in the subjacent dermis.

a. **Increased melanin pigmentation**

—is associated with suntanning and with a wide variety of disease conditions.

b. **Decreased melanin pigmentation**

—is observed in albinism and vitiligo.

2. **Bilirubin**

—is a catabolic product of the heme moiety of hemoglobin and, to a minor extent, myoglobin.

—in various pathologic conditions, accumulates and stains the blood, sclerae, mucosae, and internal organs, producing jaundice. **Jaundice** is most often caused by:

a. **Hemolytic anemia**

—is a decrease in the number of circulating erythrocytes from increased red cell destruction.

b. **Biliary obstruction**

—is an obstruction of intrahepatic or extrahepatic bile ducts.

c. Hepatocellular disease

     –is associated with failure of conjugation of bilirubin.

3. Hemosiderin

     –is an **iron-containing pigment** derived from ferritin.

     –appears in tissues as golden brown amorphous aggregates and can be positively identified by its staining reaction (blue color) with Prussian blue dye.

     –exists normally in small amounts within tissue macrophages of the bone marrow, liver, and spleen, as physiologic iron stores.

     –pathologically accumulates in tissues in excess amounts (sometimes massive); (Table 1.2).

a. Hemosiderosis

     –occurs when accumulation of hemosiderin is primarily within tissue macrophages and is unassociated with tissue or organ damage.

b. Hemochromatosis

     –is more extensive accumulation, often within parenchymal cells, with tissue damage, scarring, and organ dysfunction.

4. Lipofuscin

     –is a yellowish, fat-soluble pigment.

     –arises from breakdown products of lipids and lipid components of cell membranes; it is referred to as wear-and-tear pigment.

     –commonly accumulates in elderly patients, in whom the pigment most often is found within hepatocytes and at the poles of nuclei of myocardial cells. The combination of lipofuscin accumulation and atrophy of organs is referred to as **brown atrophy**.

E. Pathologic calcifications

1. Metastatic calcification

     –is caused by **hypercalcemia,** most often resulting from hyperparathyroidism; osteolytic tumors, with resultant mobilization of calcium and phosphorus; hypervitaminosis D; and excess calcium intake, as in the milk–alkali syndrome.

Table 1.2. Abnormal Deposition of Hemosiderin

Type	Pathologic Features	Mechanisms
Local hemosiderosis	Local deposition of hemosiderin	Most often results from hemorrhage into tissue; hemosiderin derived from breakdown of hemoglobin
Systemic hemosiderosis	Generalized hemosiderin deposition without tissue or organ damage	May result from hemorrhage, multiple blood transfusions, hemolysis, and excessive dietary intake of iron, often accompanied by alcohol consumption
Hemochromatosis	Damage to many tissues and organs; scarring and organ dysfunction manifested as hepatic cirrhosis and fibrosis of pancreas, leading to diabetes mellitus; increased melanin pigmentation in skin	More extensive accumulation than hemosiderosis; can result from any of the causes of systemic hemosiderosis; most often a hereditary disorder characterized by increased iron absorption (idiopathic hemochromatosis)

2. Dystrophic calcification

–occurs in **previously damaged tissue,** such as areas of old trauma, tuberculosis lesions, scarred heart valves, and atherosclerotic lesions.

–is not caused by hypercalcemia; typically, the serum calcium concentration is normal.

Review Test

Directions: Each of the numbered items or incomplete statements in this section is followed by answers or by completions of the statement. Select the **one** lettered answer or completion that is **best** in each case.

1. Which of the following adaptive changes is exemplified in the illustration?

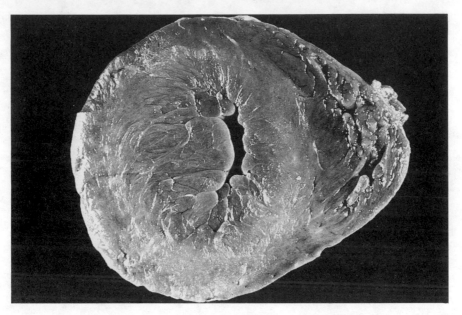

(Reprinted with permission from Golden A, Powell D, and Jennings C: *Pathology: Understanding Human Disease,* 2nd ed. Baltimore, Williams & Wilkins, 1985, p 136.)

(A) Hypertrophy
(B) Hyperplasia
(C) Atrophy
(D) Hypoplasia
(E) Aplasia

2. All of the following factors cause cellular injury through the action of free radicals EXCEPT

(A) radiation.
(B) carbon tetrachloride (CCl_4).
(C) ischemia.
(D) oxygen toxicity.
(E) enzymatic degradation by mixed function oxidases.

3. Hepatic cell injury induced by CCl_4 is characterized by all of the following changes EXCEPT

(A) lipid peroxidation.
(B) disaggregation of ribosomes.
(C) depletion of intracellular lipids.
(D) influx of calcium.
(E) mitochondrial damage.

4. Early potentially reversible changes in myocardial cells induced by anoxia include all of the following conditions EXCEPT

(A) failure of oxidative phosphorylation.
(B) depletion of ATP.
(C) inhibition of anaerobic glycolysis and glycogenolysis.
(D) decrease in cellular pH.
(E) increase in intracellular Na^+ and water and loss of intracellular K^+.

5. All of the following cause and effect associations related to CCl_4-induced hepatic cell injury are properly expressed EXCEPT

(A) processing by mixed function oxidases→ free radical formation.
(B) free radical formation→lipid peroxidation of intracellular membranes.
(C) failure of protein synthesis→disaggregation of ribosomes.
(D) decreased apolipoprotein synthesis→intracellular lipid accumulation.
(E) plasma membrane damage→mitochondrial calcification.

6. Which of the following terms is correctly defined?

(A) Heterolysis—changes induced by fixatives used in histopathologic tissue preparation
(B) Autolysis—tissue degradation by intracellular enzymes
(C) Fibrinoid necrosis—ischemic necrosis resulting from arterial occlusion by fibrin clots
(D) Apoptosis—ballooning of cell cytoplasm from lipid accumulation

7. Each type of necrosis is correctly described EXCEPT

(A) coagulation—loss of tissue architecture.
(B) liquefaction—enzymatic softening and disruption of devitalized tissue.
(C) caseous—eosinophilic, amorphous appearance.
(D) fibrinoid—deposition of fibrin-like material in arterial walls.

8. Each type of necrosis is correctly paired with its most likely site of involvement EXCEPT

(A) coagulation—heart or kidney.
(B) liquefaction—spleen or lung.
(C) caseous—granulomatous inflammatory sites.
(D) fibrinoid—arterial walls.

9. Which of the following types of necrosis is most often caused by sudden ischemia from vascular occlusion?

(A) Apoptosis
(B) Caseous necrosis
(C) Coagulation necrosis
(D) Fat necrosis
(E) Fibrinoid necrosis

10. This figure illustrates necrosis following sudden interruption of blood supply to the myocardium.

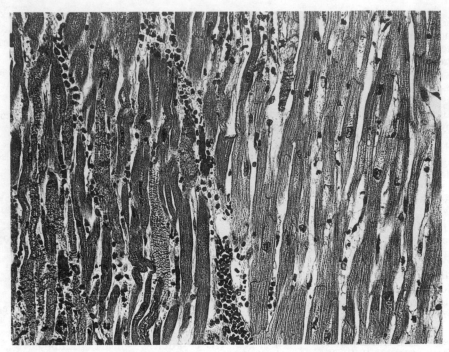

(Reprinted with permission from Golden A, Powell D, and Jennings C: *Pathology: Understanding Human Disease,* 2nd ed. Baltimore, Williams & Wilkins, 1985, p 12.)

The type of necrosis shown is best described as

(A) coagulation.
(B) liquefaction.
(C) caseous.
(D) fibrinoid.
(E) gangrenous.

11. The cellular accumulation illustrated below may result from all of the following factors EXCEPT

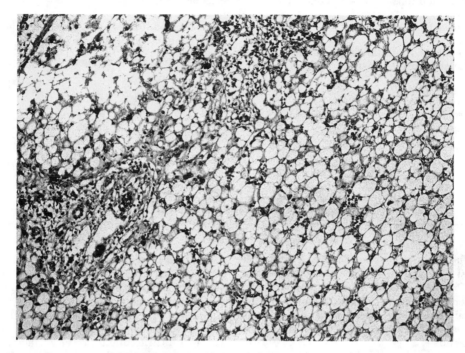

(Reprinted with permission from Golden A, Powell D, and Jennings C: *Pathology: Understanding Human Disease*, 2nd ed. Baltimore, Williams & Wilkins, 1985, p 7.)

(A) increased transport of precursor substances to cells.
(B) overproduction of accumulated material by cells.
(C) decreased mobilization of accumulated material from cells.
(D) decreased utilization of accumulated material by cells.
(E) irreversible damage to mitochondria.

12. Which one of the following cellular changes is reversible?

(A) Karyorrhexis
(B) Pyknosis
(C) Karyolysis
(D) Swelling of endoplasmic reticulum

13. All of the following abnormal clinical manifestations are correctly paired with the appropriate compound or pigment deposited EXCEPT

(A) CCl$_4$ poisoning—fat.
(B) hemolytic anemia—bilirubin.
(C) idiopathic hemochromatosis—hemosiderin.
(D) vitiligo—melanin.
(E) atrophy of hepatic and myocardial cells—lipofuscin.

14. Which of the following sites is an example of metastatic calcification?

(A) The kidney in nephrocalcinosis
(B) The mitral valve in mitral stenosis of rheumatic origin
(C) The left anterior ascending coronary artery involved by atheromatous plaques
(D) The lung involved by metastatic carcinoma of the prostate
(E) The lung in areas of old tuberculosis infection

Directions: The items in this section consist of lettered options followed by a set of numbered items. For each item, select the **one** lettered option that is most closely associated with it. Each lettered option may be selected once, more than once, or not at all.

Questions 15–16

Match each of the following cellular changes with the appropriate descriptive term.

(A) Hypertrophy
(B) Hyperplasia
(C) Atrophy
(D) Hypoplasia
(E) Aplasia

15. Increased fullness and size of breasts during pregnancy and lactation

16. Unilateral renal agenesis

Answers and Explanations

1–A. The illustration shows marked hypertrophy of the left ventricle. Hypertrophy of this extent, often seen in hypertensive heart disease, is caused by increased workload from increased ventricular pressure. This organ enlargement is the result of increase in size of the individual muscle cells.

2–C. Ischemia, with resultant tissue hypoxia, does not by itself cause free radical injury. However, reperfusion of previously ischemic tissue is a well-known cause of free radical-mediated injury. Highly reactive free radicals may be generated by ionizing radiation. CCl_4 and other drugs and chemicals can be converted to free radicals, a process mediated by the mixed function oxidases of the P-450 system within the smooth endoplasmic reticulum. Oxygen toxicity can result in the production of the cytotoxic superoxide radical, O_2^{-}, as well as other toxic oxygen species.

3–C. In CCl_4 toxicity, the free radical $CCl_3 \cdot$ initiates lipid peroxidation of intracellular membranes. Disaggregation of ribosomes, with resultant failure of protein synthesis, including synthesis of apolipoproteins, results in intracellular lipid accumulation. Increased plasma membrane permeability, apparently caused by products of lipid peroxidation, allows calcium influx with consequent mitochondrial failure.

4–C. Insufficient arterial O_2 results in failure of oxidative phosphorylation, with resultant depletion of ATP and increase in AMP and ADP. Anaerobic glycolysis and glycogenolysis are stimulated through increased phosphofructokinase and phosphorylase activities, respectively. This results in accumulation of cell lactate, with a decrease in intracellular pH and depletion of cellular glycogen stores. Decreased ATP availability also results in failure of the Na^+K^+-ATPase pump, which then leads to increased cell Na^+ and water and decreased cell K^+.

5–C. The cause is disaggregation of ribosomes; the effect is decreased protein synthesis.

6–B. Autolysis denotes the degradative reactions in dead cells caused by indigenous intracellular enzymes; heterolysis describes similar changes induced by enzymes derived from sources extrinsic to the cell. Fibrinoid necrosis is the deposition of fibrin-like material within arterial walls and is characteristic of vascular damage by immune mechanisms. Apoptosis is the death of single cells within clusters of other cells and is morphologically marked by shrinkage and increased eosinophilia of cells, often with small chromatin remnants.

7–A. Coagulation necrosis, most often observed in the heart and kidney, is characterized by general preservation of tissue architecture.

8–B. Liquefaction necrosis characteristically occurs in the brain or spinal cord but can also occur in other sites secondary to the action of neutrophilic and bacterial enzymes.

9–C. Infarction is defined as necrosis resulting from obstruction of the blood supply to the affected tissue. The type of necrosis seen depends on the organ affected and in most sites is coagulation necrosis. A notable exception is in the brain, where infarcts are usually marked by liquefaction necrosis.

10–A. The figure illustrates general preservation of myocardial architecture with some fragmentation, more intense cytoplasmic staining corresponding to increased cellular eosinophilia, and loss of nuclei, all of which are characteristic of coagulation necrosis.

11–E. The figure illustrates fatty change of the liver, which does not result from irreversible damage to mitochondria. Irreversible damage to mitochondria is associated with cell death.

12–D. Swelling of the endoplasmic reticulum from increased cell water, one of the earliest ultrastructural changes observed in injured cells, is reversible. In contrast, karyorrhexis, pyknosis, and karyolysis are all nuclear signs of cell death and represent irreversible changes.

13–D. Vitiligo is characterized by focal, patchy areas of depigmentation due to loss of melanocytes with consequent decreased melanin. CCl_4 poisoning is associated with hepatic fatty change due to impaired apolipoprotein synthesis. Hemolytic anemia leads to jaundice, accumulation of bilirubin in the blood and tissues. Idiopathic hemochromatosis is characterized by massive accumulation of hemosiderin with consequent organ damage, especially in the liver and pancreas. Lipofuscin accumulation in hepatic and myocardial cells is characteristic of the brown atrophy of these organs sometimes observed in the elderly.

14–A. Nephrocalcinosis is caused by hypercalcemia and is thus an example of metastatic calcification. The other choices are all examples of dystrophic calcification, calcification in areas of prior tissue damage.

15–B. In pregnancy and lactation there is a dramatic proliferation of glandular epithelial cells, hyperplasia, with a resultant increase in breast size.

16–E. Lack of development of a single kidney is an uncommon developmental disorder due to aplasia (failure to produce cells); often it is associated with compensatory hypertrophy of the opposite kidney.

2

Inflammation

I. Introduction—Inflammation

—is a vascular response to injury.

A. Processes

1. Exudation of fluid from vessels

2. Attraction of leukocytes to the injury; leukocytes engulf and destroy bacteria, tissue debris, and other particulate material

3. Activation of chemical mediators

4. Proteolytic degradation of extracellular debris

5. Restoration of injured tissue to its normal structure and function (this is limited by the extent of tissue destruction and the regenerative capacity of the specific tissue)

B. Cardinal signs

1. **Rubor** (redness due to dilatation of vessels)

2. **Dolor** (pain due to increased pressure exerted by the accumulation of interstitial fluid and to mediators such as bradykinin)

3. **Calor** (heat due to increased blood flow)

4. **Tumor** (swelling due to extravascular accumulation of fluid)

5. **Functio laesa** (loss of function)

C. Causes

1. Infection

2. Trauma

3. Physical injury from thermal extremes or from ionizing radiation

4. Chemical injury

5. Immunologic injury

6. Tissue death—inflammatory changes occur in viable tissue adjacent to necrotic areas

II. Acute Inflammation

A. Vasoactive changes

—begin with a brief period of vasoconstriction, followed shortly by dilation of arterioles, capillaries, and postcapillary venules. The resulting marked increase in blood flow to the affected area is clinically manifest by redness and increased warmth of the affected area.

B. Increased capillary permeability

—results in leakage of proteinaceous fluid, which causes edema.
—is caused by endothelial changes varying from contraction of endothelial cells in postcapillary venules, with widening of interendothelial gaps, to major endothelial damage involving arterioles, capillaries, and venules.

C. Cellular response of leukocytes

1. Emigration

—is the passage of inflammatory leukocytes between the endothelial cells into the adjacent interstitial tissue. Prior to emigration, circulating leukocytes from the central blood flow move toward the endothelial surface.

a. Margination

—occurs as leukocytes localize to the outer margin of the blood flow adjacent to the vascular endothelium.

b. Pavementing

—occurs as leukocytes line the endothelial surface.

c. Adhesion

—occurs as leukocytes adhere to the endothelial surface.
—is mediated by the interaction of adhesion molecules on the surfaces of both endothelial cells and leukocytes.

2. Chemotaxis

—is the process by which leukocytes are attracted to and move toward an injury.
—is mediated by diffusible chemical agents (Table 2.1); movement of leukocytes occurs along a chemical gradient.

Table 2.1. Chemotactic Factors

Factor	Description	Chemotactic For
Formylated peptides	Bacterial products of *Escherichia coli*	Neutrophils
C5a	Activated complement component	Neutrophils
HETE, LTB$_4$	Leukotrienes	Neutrophils
Kallikrein	Product of factor XIIa-mediated conversion of prekallikrein	Neutrophils
Fibrinogen	Plasma protein	Neutrophils
PAF	AGEPC; from basophils, mast cells, and other cells	Eosinophils
PDGF	From platelets and other cells	Monocytes
Fibronectin	Extracellular matrix protein	Fibroblasts and endothelial cells

PAF = platelet-activating factor
PDGF = platelet-derived growth factor
AGEPC = acetyl glycerol ether phosphocholine

−**chemotactic factors,** produced at the site of injury, include:

a. Products from bacteria

b. Complement components, especially C5a

c. Arachidonic acid metabolites, especially leukotriene B_4 (LTB_4)

3. **Phagocytosis**

−is the **ingestion** of particulate material (e.g., tissue debris, living or dead bacteria, other foreign cells) by phagocytic cells. **Neutrophils** and **monocytes–macrophages** are the most important phagocytic cells.

a. **Opsonization**

  −facilitates phagocytosis.

  −is the coating of particulate material by substances referred to as opsonins, which immobilize the particles on the surface of the phagocyte.

  (1) The most important opsonins are **immunoglobulin G (IgG) subtypes** and **C3b,** a complement component.

  (2) Fragments opsonized by IgG are bound to phagocytic cells by cell-surface receptors for the Fc portion of the IgG molecule.

  (3) Fragments opsonized by C3b bind to cellular receptors for C3b.

b. **Anatomic changes**

  −phagocytosis is morphologically characterized by internalization of the attached opsonized particle by pseudopodial extensions from the surface of the leukocyte, which enclose the foreign particle, forming an internalized vesicle, the **phagosome**.

  (1) Phagosomes fuse with cytoplasmic lysosomes, forming **phagolysosomes**.

  (2) Phagolysosome formation is associated with leukocytic degranulation.

4. **Intracellular microbial killing**

−within phagocytic cells is mediated by oxygen-dependent and oxygen-independent mechanisms.

a. **Oxygen-dependent microbial killing**

  −is the most important intracellular microbicidal process.

  (1) Phagocytosis initiates activity of the hexose monophosphate shunt, causing an oxidative burst and supplying electrons to an NADPH oxidase in the phagosomal membrane.

  (2) One of the products of the NADPH oxidase reaction is superoxide anion (O_2^-), which is further converted to hydrogen peroxide (H_2O_2) by dismutation. H_2O_2 may be further converted to the activated hydroxyl radical (OH·).

  (3) In the presence of the leukocyte enzyme myeloperoxidase and a halide ion, such as chloride, H_2O_2 oxidizes microbial proteins and disrupts cell walls. This process is referred to as the **myeloperoxidase–halide system of bacterial killing**.

b. **Oxygen-independent microbial killing**

  −is much less effective than oxygen-dependent microbial killing.

  −is mediated by proteins such as lysozyme, cationic proteins, arginase, and lactoferrin.

5. Types of inflammatory cells

a. Neutrophils are the most prominent inflammatory cells in foci of acute inflammation during the first several hours.

b. After 1–2 days, neutrophils are replaced largely by **monocytes–macrophages,** which are capable of engulfing larger particles, are longer-lived, and are capable of dividing and proliferating within the inflamed tissue.

c. Lymphocytes are the most prominent inflammatory cells in many viral infections and along with monocytes–macrophages and plasma cells are the most prominent cells in chronic inflammation.

d. Eosinophils are the predominant inflammatory cells in allergic reactions and parasitic infestations.

D. Exogenous and endogenous mediators of acute inflammation

—influence chemotaxis, vasomotor phenomena, vascular permeability, pain, and other aspects of the inflammatory process (Table 2.2).

1. Exogenous mediators

—are most often of microbial origin.

—are exemplified by the formylated peptides of *Escherichia coli,* which are chemotactic for neutrophils.

2. Endogenous mediators

—are of host origin.

a. Vasoactive amines

(1) Histamine

—mediates the increase in capillary permeability associated with contraction of endothelial cells in postcapillary venules that occurs with mild injuries.

—is liberated from **basophils, mast cells,** and **platelets**.

(a) Basophils and mast cells

—histamine is liberated by degranulation triggered by the following stimuli:

(i) Binding of specific antigen to basophil and mast cell membrane-bound **IgE** (complement is not involved)

Table 2.2. Vasoactive Mediators

Activity	Mediator
Vasoconstriction	Thromboxane A_2 (TxA_2) LTC_4, LTD_4, LTE_4 PAF
Vasodilation	PGI_2 PGD_2, PGE_2, $PGF_{2\alpha}$ Bradykinin PAF
Increased vascular permeability	Histamine Serotonin PGD_2, PGE_2, $PGF_{2\alpha}$ LTC_4, LTD_4, LTE_4 Bradykinin PAF

  (ii) Binding of complement fragments C3a and C5a, **anaphylatoxins,** to specific cell-surface receptors on basophils and mast cells (specific antigen and IgE antibodies are not involved)
  (iii) Physical stimuli such as heat and cold
  (iv) Cytokine interleukin-1 (IL-1)
  (v) Factors from neutrophils, monocytes, and platelets
(b) Platelets
  –histamine is liberated from platelets by platelet aggregation and the release reaction, which can be triggered by endothelial injury and thrombosis, or by platelet-activating factor (PAF).
  (i) PAF is derived from the granules of basophils and mast cells and from endothelial cells, macrophages, neutrophils, and eosinophils. PAF is acetyl glycerol ether phosphocholine and is also known as AGEPC.
  (ii) PAF activates and aggregates platelets, with the release of histamine and serotonin; causes vasoactive and bronchospastic effects; and activates arachidonic acid metabolism.

(2) Serotonin (5-hydroxytryptamine)
  –actions are similar to histamine.
  –is derived from platelets.
  –is liberated from platelets, along with histamine, during the release reaction.

b. Arachidonic acid metabolites
  –phospholipase A_2 stimulates the release of arachidonic acid from membrane phospholipids.
  –metabolism of arachidonic acid proceeds along two pathways:
(1) The cyclooxygenase (cyclic endoperoxide) pathway
  –is inhibited by aspirin and other anti-inflammatory drugs.
  –yields thromboxanes and prostaglandins: thromboxane A_2 (TxA_2) in platelets, prostacyclin (PGI_2) in endothelial cells, and other prostaglandins in other tissues.
  (a) Platelet TxA_2 is a powerful vasoconstrictor and platelet aggregant.
  (b) Endothelial PGI_2 is a powerful vasodilator and inhibitor of platelet aggregation.
(2) The lipoxygenase pathway
  –yields hydroperoxyeicosatetraenoic acid (**HPETE**) and its derivatives, **12-HPETE** in platelets and **5-HPETE** and **15-HPETE** in leukocytes.
  (a) 5-HPETE in turn gives rise to hydroxyeicosatetraenoic acid (HETE), a chemotactic factor for neutrophils.
  (b) It also gives rise to **leukotrienes** (LTB_4, a chemotactic factor, and LTC_4, LTD_4, and LTE_4, potent vasoconstrictors, bronchoconstrictors, and mediators of increased capillary permeability, which sometimes are jointly referred to as the **slow reacting substance of anaphylaxis,** or SRS-A).

c. **Cytokines**
   —are **soluble proteins** secreted by several types of cells, which can act as effector molecules influencing the behavior of other cells.
   —are mediators of immunologic response.
   —are also important mediators of inflammation. The cytokines **IL-1** and **tumor necrosis factor** (TNF, cachectin) are secreted by monocytes–macrophages and other cells and have several effects on inflammation.
   (1) Inducing **acute phase responses**
       (a) **Systemic effects** of inflammation, including fever and leukocytosis
       (b) **Hepatic synthesis** of acute phase proteins, such as C-reactive protein, serum amyloid-associated protein, complement components, fibrinogen, prothrombin, α-1-antitrypsin, α-2-macroglobulin, and ceruloplasmin
   (2) Reducing the thromboresistant properties of endothelium, thus promoting thrombosis

d. **The kinin system**
   —is initiated by activated Hageman factor (factor XIIa). Factor XIIa also activates the intrinsic pathway of coagulation and the plasminogen (fibrinolytic) system. Activation of this system in turn activates the complement cascade. Thus, **factor XIIa links the kinin, coagulation, plasminogen, and complement systems**.
   —converts prekallikrein to kallikrein (a chemotactic factor).
   —results in the cleavage, by kallikrein, of high-molecular-weight kininogen (HMW-K) to **bradykinin**, which is a nine-carbon peptide that mediates vascular permeability, arteriolar dilation, and pain.

e. **The complement system**
   —consists of a group of **plasma proteins** that participate in immune lysis of cells.
   —also plays a significant role in inflammation.
   (1) **C3a and C5a** (anaphylatoxins) mediate degranulation of basophils and mast cells, with the release of histamine. C5a is chemotactic, mediates the release of histamine from platelet dense granules, induces expression of leukocyte adhesion molecules, and activates the lipoxygenase pathway of arachidonic acid metabolism.
   (2) **C3b** is an opsonin.
   (3) **C5b-9,** the membrane attack complex, is a lytic agent for bacteria and other cells.

E. **Outcome of acute inflammation**
   1. **Resolution**
      —of tissue structure and function often occurs if the injurious agent is eliminated.
   2. **Tissue destruction and persistent acute inflammation**
      a. **Abscess**
         —is a cavity filled with pus (neutrophils, monocytes, and liquefied cellular debris).
         —is often walled off by fibrous tissue and is relatively inaccessible to the circulation.

−results from tissue destruction by lysosomal products and other degradative enzymes.

b. Ulcer

−is the loss of surface epithelium.

−can be caused by acute inflammation of epithelial surfaces (e.g., peptic ulcer, ulcers of the skin).

c. Fistula

−is an abnormal communication between two organs or between an organ and a surface.

d. Scar

−is the final result of tissue destruction, with resultant distortion of structure and, in some cases, altered function.

3. Conversion to chronic inflammation

−is marked by the replacement of neutrophils and monocytes with lymphocytes, plasma cells, and macrophages.

−often includes proliferation of fibroblasts and new vessels, with resultant scarring and distortion of architecture.

F. Hereditary defects that impair the acute inflammatory response

1. Deficiency of complement components

−clinically manifests as increased susceptibility to infection. Notable deficiencies of factors include C2, C3, and C5.

2. Defects in neutrophils

a. Chronic granulomatous disease of childhood

−is usually an **X-linked** disorder characterized by **deficient activity of NADPH oxidase**.

−is marked by phagocytic cells that ingest but do not kill certain microorganisms.

(1) Catalase-positive organisms are ingested but not killed. These organisms (e.g., *Staphylococcus aureus*) can destroy H_2O_2 generated by bacterial metabolism. Because enzyme-deficient neutrophils cannot produce H_2O_2 and bacterial H_2O_2 is destroyed by bacterial catalase, H_2O_2 is not available as a substrate for myeloperoxidase. Thus, the myeloperoxidase–halide system of bacterial killing fails.

(2) Catalase-negative organisms are ingested and killed. These organisms (e.g., streptococci) produce sufficient H_2O_2 to permit oxygen-dependent microbicidal mechanisms to proceed. In effect, the substrate for myeloperoxidase is produced by the bacteria, and the bacteria in a sense kill themselves.

b. Myeloperoxidase deficiency

−is sometimes associated with recurrent infections but often is of little clinical consequence.

c. Chédiak-Higashi syndrome

−is an autosomal recessive disorder.

−is characterized by neutropenia, albinism, cranial and peripheral neuropathy, and a tendency to develop repeated infections.

—is marked by the presence of abnormal white blood cells, which are characterized as follows:

(1) **Functionally,** by abnormal microtubule formation, affecting movement and membrane fusion of lysosomes

(2) **Morphologically,** by large cytoplasmic granules (representing abnormal lysosomes) in granulocytes, lymphocytes, and monocytes and by large abnormal melanosomes in melanocytes

III. Chronic Inflammation

—can occur when the inciting injury is persistent or recurring, or when the inflammatory reaction is insufficient to completely degrade the agent (e.g., bacteria, tissue debris, foreign bodies) that incites the inflammatory reaction.

—often occurs de novo, without a preceding acute inflammatory reaction.

—occurs in two major patterns.

A. Chronic nonspecific inflammation

—is characterized by a **cellular reaction** with a preponderance of mononuclear cells (macrophages, lymphocytes, and plasma cells).

—is often characterized by **proliferation of fibroblasts and new vessels**.

—often involves **scarring** and **distortion of tissue architecture**.

—is mediated by the interaction of monocytes–macrophages with lymphocytes.

1. Monocytes are recruited from the circulation by a variety of chemotactic factors.

2. Cytokines derived from monocytes–macrophages activate lymphocytes. The activated lymphocytes then are the source of cytokines that activate monocytes–macrophages.

3. B lymphocyte activation by macrophage-presented antigen results in the formation of antibody-producing plasma cells.

B. Granulomatous inflammation

—is characterized by granulomas, nodular collections of specialized macrophages referred to as **epithelioid cells**. Granulomas are usually surrounded by a rim of lymphocytes.

—involves activation of macrophages by interactions with T lymphocytes. Poorly digestible antigen is presented by macrophages to CD4+ lymphocytes. Interaction with the antigen-specific T-cell receptor of these cells triggers the release of cytokines (especially interferon γ), which mediate the transformation of monocytes and macrophages to epithelioid and giant cells.

—is sometimes characterized by **caseous necrosis,** usually central within the granuloma.

—is also characterized by the presence of **multinucleated giant cells** derived from macrophages. The **Langhans giant cell** has nuclei arranged in a horseshoe-shaped pattern about the periphery of the cell and is particularly characteristic of, but not specific for, the granulomatous inflammation of tuberculosis. The **foreign body giant cell** has scattered nuclei.

—is the characteristic form of inflammation associated with a number of diverse etiologic agents, including:

1. Infectious agents

a. *Mycobacterium tuberculosis* and *M. leprae*

b. *Blastomyces dermatitidis, Histoplasma capsulatum,* and many other fungi

c. *Treponema pallidum*

d. The bacterium of cat-scratch disease

2. Foreign bodies

3. Unknown etiology, including sarcoidosis

IV. Tissue Repair

A. Restoration of normal structure

—occurs when the connective tissue infrastructure remains relatively intact.

—also requires that the surviving affected parenchymal cells have the capacity to regenerate.

1. Labile cells

—divide actively throughout life to replace lost cells.

—are capable of regeneration following injury.

—include cells of the epidermis and gastrointestinal mucosa, cells lining the surface of the genitourinary tract, and hematopoietic cells of the bone marrow.

2. Stable cells

—characteristically undergo few divisions but are capable of division when activated.

—are also capable of regeneration following injury.

—include hepatocytes, renal tubular cells, parenchymal cells of many glands, and many mesenchymal cells (e.g., smooth muscle, cartilage, connective tissue, endothelium, osteoblasts).

3. Permanent cells

—are incapable of division and regeneration.

—include neurons and myocardial cells.

—are replaced by scar tissue (typically fibrosis; gliosis in the CNS) after irreversible injury and cell loss.

B. Cellular proliferation

—is mediated by an assemblage of growth factors.

1. Platelet-derived growth factor (PDGF)

—is synthesized by platelets and a number of other cells.

—promotes the chemotactic migration of fibroblasts and smooth muscle cells.

—is chemotactic for monocytes.

—is a **competence factor** that promotes the proliferative response of fibroblasts and smooth muscle cells upon concurrent stimulation by **progression factors** (e.g., other growth factors). Indirectly in this manner, PDGF promotes the synthesis of collagen.

—reacts with specific cell-surface receptors. Generally, growth factor receptors are transmembrane proteins that respond to ligand interaction by conformational changes that induce tyrosine kinase activity in their intracellular domains.

2. Epidermal growth factor (EGF)

 —promotes the growth of endothelial cells and fibroblasts as well as epithelial cells.

 —is a progression factor.

3. Fibroblast growth factors (FGFs)

 —promote the synthesis of extracellular matrix protein (including fibronectin) by fibroblasts, endothelial cells, monocytes, and other cells. **Fibronectin** is a glycoprotein with the following characteristics:

 a. Chemotactic for fibroblasts and endothelial cells

 b. Promotes angiogenesis (new vessel formation)

 c. Links other extracellular matrix components (e.g., collagen, proteoglycans) and macromolecules (e.g., fibrin, heparin) to cell-surface receptors called integrins. Integrins mediate interactions between cells and extracellular matrix.

4. Transforming growth factors (TGFs)

 a. TGF-α functions similarly to EGF.

 b. TGF-β is a **growth inhibitor** for many cell types and may aid in modulating the repair process.

5. Macrophage-derived growth factors (IL-1 and TNF)

 —promote the proliferation of fibroblasts, smooth muscle cells, and endothelial cells.

C. The repair process

 1. Removal of debris

  —begins in the early stages of inflammation and is initiated by liquefaction and removal of dead cellular material and other debris.

 2. Formation of granulation tissue

  —granulation tissue is highly vascular, newly formed connective tissue consisting of **capillaries** and **fibroblasts**; it fills defects created by liquefaction of cellular debris. (Granulation tissue is not related to granulomas or granulomatous inflammation.)

 3. Scarring

  —**collagen** is produced by fibroblasts. As the amount of collagen in granulation tissue progressively increases, the tissue becomes progressively less vascular and less cellular.

  —progressive **contraction of the wound** also occurs, often resulting in deformity of the original structure.

D. Factors that delay or impede repair

 1. Retention of debris

 2. Impaired circulation

 3. Persistent infection

 4. Metabolic disorders, such as diabetes mellitus (associated with both susceptibility to infection and impaired circulation)

 5. Dietary deficiency of ascorbic acid or protein, which are required for collagen formation

Review Test

Directions: Each of the numbered items or incomplete statements in this section is followed by answers or by completions of the statement. Select the **one** lettered answer or completion that is **best** in each case.

1. An infiltrate of which one of the following cells is most characteristic of the early stages of acute inflammation?

(A) Neutrophils
(B) Eosinophils
(C) Basophils
(D) Lymphocytes
(E) Monocytes

2. Each classic term describing acute inflammation is correctly matched with its cause EXCEPT

(A) rubor—vasodilatation.
(B) dolor—inflammatory cells infiltrating sensory nerves.
(C) calor—increased blood flow.
(D) tumor—exudation of fluid and cells into extravascular tissues.

3. Degranulation of basophils and mast cells is mediated by all of the following EXCEPT

(A) AGEPC.
(B) complement components.
(C) immunoglobulin E.
(D) interleukin-1.
(E) physical stimuli.

4. Each of the following phrases concerning leukotrienes is true EXCEPT they

(A) may cause vasoconstriction.
(B) may increase vascular permeability.
(C) may induce bronchoconstriction.
(D) are arachidonic acid derivatives.
(E) are products of the cyclooxygenase pathway.

5. Chronic granulomatous disease of childhood is characterized by all of the following EXCEPT

(A) increased susceptibility to infection with catalase-positive organisms.
(B) deficiency of NADPH oxidase activity.
(C) increased H_2O_2 production.
(D) effective leukocytic killing of most streptococci.
(E) X-linked inheritance.

6. All of the following are characteristic of the type of inflammation shown in the figure EXCEPT

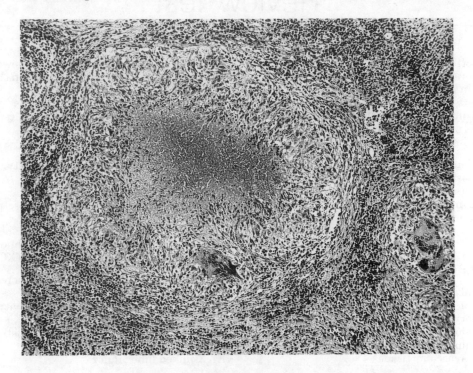

(Reprinted with permission from Golden A, Powell D, and Jennings C: *Pathology: Understanding Human Disease,* 2nd ed. Baltimore, Williams & Wilkins, 1985, p 40.)

(A) inciting cause is often mycobacteria or fungi.
(B) injurious agent is not easily removed by phagocytic cells.
(C) most characteristic cell type is derived from lymphocytes.
(D) it is often marked by caseous necrosis.
(E) it is often marked by the presence of multinucleated giant cells.

7. Each of the following terms is correctly matched with an identifying characteristic EXCEPT

(A) Langhans cell—multiple nuclei in a horseshoe pattern.
(B) fistula—an abnormal communication.
(C) abscess—neutrophils and necrotic debris.
(D) granulation tissue—modified macrophages.

8. Which of the following findings is an invariable histologic feature of granulomatous inflammation?

(A) Caseous necrosis
(B) Multinucleated giant cells
(C) Positive acid-fast staining of causative organism
(D) Epithelioid cells
(E) Surrounding cuff of lymphocytes

9. Multinucleated giant cells are a characteristic finding in each of the following diseases EXCEPT

(A) blastomycosis.
(B) cat-scratch disease.
(C) leprosy.
(D) *Streptococcus pneumoniae* infection.
(E) sarcoidosis.

10. Which of the following cells is a permanent cell?

(A) Epidermal cell
(B) Hepatocyte
(C) Intestinal mucosal cell
(D) Neuron
(E) Renal tubular cell

11. All of the following are associated with delayed repair after acute inflammation EXCEPT

(A) advanced age.
(B) ascorbic acid deficiency.
(C) diabetes mellitus.
(D) protein deficiency.
(E) retention of debris.

Directions: Each group of items in this section consists of lettered options followed by a set of numbered items. For each item, select the **one** lettered option that is most closely associated with it. Each lettered option may be selected once, more than once, or not at all.

Questions 12–15

Match each of the following actions with the appropriate mediator.

(A) Histamine
(B) Bradykinin
(C) C3a and C5a
(D) C3b

12. Endothelial cell contraction

13. Opsonization

14. Degranulation of mast cells

15. Increased vascular permeability and pain

Answers and Explanations

1–A. Neutrophils are the most characteristic cellular component of the early stages of acute inflammatory reactions.

2–B. In acute inflammation, dolor (pain) is induced by increased hydrostatic pressure in tissues and by chemical mediators such as bradykinin.

3–A. AGEPC, or platelet-activating factor (PAF), is a product of basophil and mast cell degranulation, not a mediator of degranulation. PAF induces platelet aggregation; mediates vasoconstriction, vasodilation, and increased capillary permeability; activates arachidonic acid metabolism; and causes bronchospasm.

4–E. Leukotrienes are a group of active substances derived from arachidonic acid by way of the lipoxygenase, not the cyclooxygenase, pathway. Vasoconstriction, mediation of increased capillary permeability, bronchoconstriction, and chemotaxis are the most prominent actions of leukotrienes.

5–C. H_2O_2 production is decreased, not increased, in chronic granulomatous disease of childhood. This X-linked disorder, marked by failure of the myeloperoxidase–halide system of bacterial killing, is caused by NADPH oxidase deficiency. Failure of NADPH oxidase results in a secondary deficiency of reactive oxygen metabolites, including H_2O_2, which, along with halide ions, functions as a substrate for myeloperoxidase.

6–B. The illustration shows granulomatous inflammation, a form of chronic inflammation. Epithelioid cells, which define this type of inflammation, are derived from macrophages, not lymphocytes.

7–D. Granulation tissue, formed during wound healing, consists of newly formed capillaries and young fibroblasts, and is often confused by the beginning student with granuloma formation, a form of chronic inflammatory response.

8–D. Granulomas always consist of groups of modified macrophages called epithelioid cells. Caseous necrosis and Langhans giant cells are suggestive of a tuberculous etiology. Foreign body giant cells have multiple nuclei centrally located or scattered within the cell and are present with several offending agents. Although a definitive diagnosis is facilitated by demonstration of organisms, this is not always possible. A cuff of lymphocytes often surrounds each granuloma.

9–D. Giant cells are not a feature of the acute inflammation of *Streptococcus pneumoniae* (pneumococcal pneumonia). Blastomycosis, cat-scratch disease, leprosy, and sarcoidosis are well-known causes of granulomatous inflammation, and they are often marked by the presence of multinucleated giant cells.

10–D. Permanent cells, exemplified by neurons and myocardial cells, are incapable of division and replication. Labile cells divide throughout the life of the individual. Epidermal cells and intestinal mucosal cells are examples of labile cells. Hepatocytes and renal tubular cells are examples of stable cells, which do not reproduce regularly but have the capacity to divide and reproduce as needed.

11–A. Although repair may be delayed in the elderly patient because of ancillary factors such as atherosclerosis and decreased circulation, aging in itself is not known to play a role. Both ascorbic acid deficiency and protein deficiency compromise repair because of deficient collagen formation. Diabetes mellitus is often associated with persistent infection and impaired circulation, which in turn are causes of delayed repair. Removal of debris in the early stages of inflammation initiates repair. Conversely, failure of this process impedes repair. Factors associated with delayed repair after acute inflammation are also associated with impaired healing of wounds.

12–A. In the early stages of acute inflammation, histamine mediates the contraction of endothelial cells, which widens the interendothelial gaps of postcapillary venules, increasing vascular permeability. Histamine is principally derived from the granules of basophils and mast cells and from platelets.

13–D. Complement component C3b and subtypes of IgG are the most important opsonins.

14–C. Complement components C3a and C5a (anaphylatoxins) promote degranulation of mast cells and basophils, releasing histamine, which induces increased vascular permeability.

15–B. Bradykinin causes localized pain, vasodilation, and increased capillary permeability. It is produced by the kinin system, which is activated by Hageman factor to convert prekallikrein to kallikrein. Kallikrein, in turn, produces bradykinin, a nonapeptide, from high-molecular-weight kininogen (HMW-K).

3

Hemodynamic Dysfunction

I. Hemorrhage

—is the **escape of blood** from the vasculature into surrounding tissues, a hollow organ or body cavity, or to the outside.

—is most often caused by **trauma**.

—is noted by the following terms:

A. Hematoma

—is localized hemorrhage within a tissue or organ.

B. Hemothorax, hemopericardium, hemoperitoneum, and hemarthrosis

—are hemorrhages into the pleural cavity, pericardial sac, peritoneal cavity, or a synovial space, respectively.

C. Petechial hemorrhages, petechiae, or purpura

—are small punctate hemorrhages in the skin, mucous membranes, or serosal surfaces.

D. Ecchymosis

—is diffuse hemorrhage, usually in skin and subcutaneous tissue.

II. Hyperemia

—is a **localized increase in the volume of blood** in capillaries and small vessels.

A. Active hyperemia

—results from localized arteriolar dilation (e.g., blushing, inflammation).

B. Passive congestion (passive hyperemia)

—results from obstructed venous return or increased back pressure from congestive heart failure (CHF).

1. Acute passive congestion

—occurs in shock, acute inflammation, or sudden right heart failure.

2. Chronic passive congestion

a. Chronic passive congestion of the lung is most often caused by **left heart failure** or **mitral stenosis**.

–**congestion and distention of alveolar capillaries** lead to **capillary rupture** and passage of red blood cells into the alveoli.

–phagocytosis and degradation of red blood cells result in intra-alveolar hemosiderin-laden macrophages called **heart-failure cells**.

–in long-standing congestion, fibrosis of interstitium and hemosiderin deposition result in **brown induration** of the lung.

b. Chronic passive congestion of the liver and lower extremities is most often caused by **right heart failure**.

–**nutmeg liver** may appear; this speckled, nutmeg-like appearance on cut section is produced by a combination of dilated, congested central veins and the surrounding brownish-yellow, often fatty, liver cells.

III. Infarction

–is **necrosis resulting from ischemia** caused by obstruction of the blood supply. The necrotic tissue is referred to as an **infarct**.

A. Anemic infarcts

–are **white or pale infarcts,** usually caused by arterial occlusions in the **heart, spleen, and kidney**.

B. Hemorrhagic infarcts

–are **red infarcts,** in which red blood cells ooze into the necrotic area.

–characteristically occur in the **lung and gastrointestinal tract** as the result of arterial occlusion. These sites are loose, well-vascularized tissues with redundant arterial blood supplies (in the lung, from the pulmonary and bronchial systems; in the gastrointestinal tract, from multiple anastomoses between branches of the mesenteric artery), and **hemorrhage into the infarct** occurs from the nonobstructed portion of the vasculature.

–also can be caused by **venous occlusion**.

IV. Thrombosis

–is **intravascular coagulation of blood,** often causing significant interruption of blood flow.

–is pathologically predisposed by many conditions, including venous stasis, usually from immobilization; CHF; polycythemia; sickle cell disease; visceral malignancies; and the use of oral contraceptives, especially in association with cigarette smoking.

A. Thrombogenesis

–results from the interaction of platelets, damaged endothelial cells, and the coagulation cascade.

1. Platelets

a. Platelet functions

–maintain physical integrity of vascular endothelium

–participate in endothelial repair through the contribution of platelet-derived growth factor (PDGF)

           —form platelet plugs

           —promote the coagulation cascade through activation of platelet factor 3

b. Reactions involving platelets

(1) Adhesion

    —vessel injury exposes subendothelial collagen, leading to **platelet adhesion** (adherence to the subendothelial surface).

    —interaction of specific platelet-surface **glycoprotein receptors** and subendothelial collagen is mediated by **von Willebrand's factor**.

(2) Release reaction

    —soon after adhesion, platelets release adenosine diphosphate (ADP), histamine, serotonin, PDGF, and other platelet granule constituents.

(3) Activation of coagulation cascade

    —conformational change in the platelet membrane makes platelet factor 3 available, thus activating the coagulation cascade, leading to the formation of thrombin.

(4) Arachidonic acid metabolism

    —arachidonic acid, provided by activation of platelet membrane phospholipase, proceeds through the **cyclooxygenase pathway** to the production of **thromboxane A_2** (TxA_2). Platelet TxA_2 is a potent vasoconstrictor and platelet aggregant. The inhibition of cyclooxygenase by low-dose aspirin is the basis of aspirin therapy for prevention of thrombotic disease.

(5) Platelet aggregation

    —platelets stick to each other (as contrasted to adhesion, the adherence of platelets to the underlying subendothelium).

    —additional platelets are recruited from the circulation to produce the initial hemostatic platelet plug.

    —agonists that promote aggregation include **ADP, thrombin,** and **TxA_2,** as well as **collagen, epinephrine,** and **platelet-activating factor,** derived from the granules of basophils and mast cells.

(6) Stabilization of the platelet plug

    —fibrinogen bridges bind the aggregated platelets together. The platelet mass is stabilized by fibrin.

(7) Limitation of platelet plug formation

    —prostacyclin (PGI_2), another product of the cyclooxygenase pathway, is synthesized by endothelial cells. Endothelial PGI_2 is antagonistic to platelet TxA_2 and limits further platelet aggregation. Fibrin degradation products are also inhibitors of platelet aggregation.

2. Endothelial cells

    —are resistant to the thrombogenic influence of platelets and coagulation proteins. **Intact endothelial cells** act to modulate several aspects of **hemostasis** and oppose coagulation after injury by **thromboresistance**.

    a. Produce **heparan sulfate,** an endothelial proteoglycan that activates **antithrombin III,** which neutralizes thrombin and other coagulation factors, including factors IXa, Xa, XIa, and XIIa.

b. Secrete plasminogen activators, such as **tissue plasminogen activator (TPA)**.

c. Degrade ADP.

d. Take up, inactivate, and clear **thrombin**.

e. Synthesize **thrombomodulin,** a cell-surface protein that binds thrombin and converts it to an activator of **protein C,** a vitamin K-dependent plasma protein that inhibits coagulation by the proteolysis of factors Va and VIIIa.

f. Synthesize **protein S,** a cofactor for activated protein C.

g. Synthesize and release **PGI$_2$**.

h. Synthesize and release nitric oxide, which has actions similar to those of PGI$_2$.

3. The coagulation cascade

—follows two distinct, but interconnected, pathways (Figure 3.1).

a. Intrinsic pathway of coagulation

—is initiated by **contact activation** involving factor XII (Hageman factor), factor XI, prekallikrein, and high-molecular-weight kininogen (HMW-K).

—also can be activated by **platelet factor 3,** a phospholipid that becomes available through conformational changes in the platelet membrane.

—can be evaluated by the **activated partial thromboplastin time (APTT)**.

b. Extrinsic pathway of coagulation

—is initiated by **tissue factor,** which activates **factor VII**.

—converts **prothrombin** (factor II) to **thrombin** (factor IIa). Thrombin converts **fibrinogen to fibrin**.

—can be evaluated by the **prothrombin time (PT)**.

B. Fibrinolysis (thrombus dissolution)

—is concurrent with thrombogenesis and modulates coagulation.

—restores blood flow in vessels occluded by a thrombus and facilitates healing after inflammation and injury.

1. The proenzyme **plasminogen** is converted by proteolysis to **plasmin,** the most important fibrinolytic protease.

2. Plasmin splits fibrin.

3. The fibrinolytic system interacts with the coagulation system at the level of activation of factor XII to XIIa. Factor XII to XIIa activation links the coagulation system, the complement system, and the kinin system.

C. Morphologic characteristics of thrombi and clots

1. Arterial thrombi

—are formed in areas of **active blood flow**.

—when mature, demonstrate alternate dark gray layers of platelets interspersed with lighter layers of fibrin. This layering results in the **lines of Zahn**.

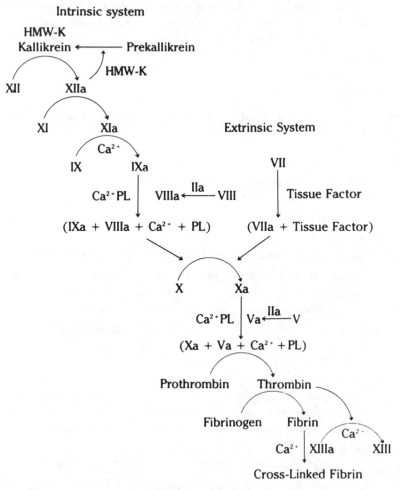

Figure 3.1. The coagulation cascade. (Reprinted with permission from Kjeldsberg C, Butler E et al: *Practical Diagnosis of Hematologic Disorders.* Chicago, ASCP Press, 1989, p 527.)

—eventually liquefy and disappear or are organized with fibrous tissue formation. Recanalization, new blood vessel formation within a thrombus, restores blood flow.

2. **Venous thrombi**

   —are formed in areas of **less active blood flow,** most often in the **veins of the legs** and in the periprostatic or other pelvic veins.
   —are predisposed by **venous stasis,** with high incidence occurring in hospitalized patients on bed rest.
   —are **dark red** with a higher concentration of red cells than arterial thrombi. Lines of Zahn are not prominent or are absent.
   —may be associated with concurrent venous inflammatory changes. Inflammation of veins with thrombus formation is referred to as **thrombophlebitis**.

3. **Postmortem clots**

   —appear soon after death and are not true thrombi.

—in contrast to true thrombi, are not attached to the vessel wall.

—settling of red cells results in a two-layered appearance: **currant jelly appearance** in the red cell-rich lower layer and a **chicken fat appearance** in the cell-poor upper layer.

V. Embolism

—is the passage and eventual trapping within the vasculature of any of a wide variety of mass objects.

A. Thromboembolism

—is embolism of fragments of **thrombi**.

—is the most frequent form of embolism.

1. Pulmonary emboli

a. An important cause of sudden death, usually occurring in **immobilized postoperative patients** and in those with **CHF**.

b. Immobilization leads to **venous thrombosis** in the lower extremities. Portions of the friable thrombus break away, travel through the venous circulation, and lodge in branches of the pulmonary artery.

c. Pulmonary emboli vary in size from **saddle emboli** obstructing the bifurcation of the pulmonary artery, which can produce sudden death, to less clinically significant small emboli.

d. Obstruction of the pulmonary artery leads to **pulmonary infarction,** a term often used interchangeably with pulmonary emobolism. **Hemorrhagic pulmonary infarcts** result. These are characteristically wedge-shaped and located just beneath the pleura.

2. Arterial emboli

a. Sites of origin

—usually arise from a **mural thrombus,** a thrombus that adheres to one wall of a heart chamber or major artery.

(1) Mural thrombi in the left atrium are associated especially with **mitral stenosis** with atrial fibrillation.

(2) Mural thrombi in the left ventricle are associated especially with **myocardial infarction** (MI).

b. Sites of arrest

(1) Branches of the carotid artery, especially the middle cerebral artery, leading to **cerebral infarction**

(2) Branches of the mesenteric artery, leading to **hemorrhagic infarction of the intestine**

(3) Branches of the renal artery, producing characteristic wedge-shaped **pale infarcts of the renal cortex**

3. Paradoxical emboli

—are left-sided emboli that originate in the venous circulation but gain access to the arterial circulation through a right-to-left shunt, most often a **patent foramen ovale** or **atrial septal defect**.

B. Other forms of embolism

1. Fat emboli

–are **particles of bone marrow and other fatty intraosseous tissue** that enter the circulation as a result of severe fractures.

–lodge in the lungs, brain, kidneys, and other organs.

–are manifest clinically by **pulmonary distress, cutaneous petechiae,** and a variety of **neurologic manifestations**.

2. Gas emboli

–result from the **introduction of air into the circulation,** most often by penetrating chest injury or as a consequence of clumsily performed criminal abortion.

–can occur as **caisson disease,** observed in deep-sea divers who return to the surface too rapidly. Bubbles of relatively insoluble nitrogen come out of solution and obstruct the circulation, producing musculoskeletal pain (**"the bends"**) and small infarcts in the central nervous system, bones, and other tissues. Because nitrogen has an affinity for adipose tissue, obese persons are at increased risk for this disorder.

3. Amniotic fluid emboli

–are caused by escape of amniotic fluid into the maternal circulation.

–can activate the coagulation process, leading to **disseminated intravascular coagulation** (DIC).

–can cause maternal death.

4. Miscellaneous sources of emboli

–include fragments of **atherosclerotic plaques,** clumps of inflamed, **infected tissue,** and **tumor fragments**.

VI. Edema

–is an abnormal accumulation of fluid in interstitial tissue spaces or body cavities.

A. Causes of edema

1. Increased hydrostatic pressure

–is exemplified by CHF.

a. Right-sided failure results in **peripheral edema**.

b. Left-sided failure results in **pulmonary edema**.

2. Increased capillary permeability

–occurs in inflammation.

3. Decreased oncotic pressure

–is from hypoalbuminemia caused by:

a. Increased loss of protein, as, for example, by renal loss in the **nephrotic syndrome**

b. Decreased production of albumin in **cirrhosis of the liver**

4. Increased sodium retention

–can occur as either a primary or secondary phenomenon.

a. Primary sodium retention, associated with **renal disorders**

   b. Secondary sodium retention, such as occurs in **CHF**
   −decreased cardiac output results in decreased renal blood flow, which activates the renin–angiotensin system.
   −in turn, this activates aldosterone production, with resultant retention of sodium and water.

   5. Blockage of lymphatics
   −results in **lymphedema**.

B. Types of edema

   1. Anasarca
   −is generalized edema.

   2. Hydrothorax
   −is accumulation of fluid in the pleural cavity.

   3. Hydropericardium
   −is abnormal accumulation of fluid in the pericardial cavity.

   4. Hydroperitoneum (ascites)
   −is abnormal accumulation of fluid in the peritoneal cavity.

   5. Transudate
   −is noninflammatory edema fluid that results from **altered intravascular hydrostatic or osmotic pressure**.
   −has a low protein content and a specific gravity less than 1.012.

   6. Exudate
   −is edema fluid from **increased vascular permeability** as a result of **inflammation**.
   −has a high protein content, a specific gravity exceeding 1.020, and characteristically contains large numbers of **inflammatory leukocytes**. Because the metabolically active leukocytes consume glucose, the glucose content is often markedly reduced.

VII. Shock

−is circulatory collapse with resultant hypoperfusion and decreased oxygenation of tissues.

A. Causes of shock

   1. Decreased cardiac output, as occurs in hemorrhage or severe left ventricular failure

   2. Widespread peripheral vasodilation, as occurs in sepsis or severe trauma, with hypotension often a prominent feature

B. Types of shock

   1. Hypovolemic shock
   −is circulatory collapse resulting from the acute reduction in circulating blood volume caused by:

   a. Severe **hemorrhage** or massive **loss of fluid** from the skin, from extensive burns or severe trauma

     b. Loss of fluid from the gastrointestinal tract, through severe **vomiting** or **diarrhea**

2. Cardiogenic shock

–is circulatory collapse resulting from pump failure of the left ventricle, most often caused by massive **MI**.

3. Septic shock

–is most characteristically associated with gram-negative infections, which cause **gram-negative endotoxemia;** also occurs with gram-positive and other infections.

    a. Initially, vasodilation may result in an overall increase in blood flow. But significant peripheral pooling of blood from peripheral vasodilation results in relative **hypovolemia** and **impaired perfusion**.

    b. Endotoxin and other bacterial products appear to induce the liberation of arachidonic acid derivatives and cytokines (e.g., interleukin-1 and tumor necrosis factor), activate complement components and the kinin system, and **cause direct toxic injury to vessels**.

    c. **Endothelial injury** can lead to **activation of the coagulation pathways** and to DIC.

4. Neurogenic shock

–is most often associated with **severe trauma** and reactive peripheral vasodilation.

C. Stages of shock

1. Nonprogressive (early) stage

–**compensatory mechanisms,** including increased heart rate and increased peripheral resistance, maintain perfusion of vital organs.

2. Progressive stage

–is characterized by tissue hypoperfusion and the onset of circulatory and metabolic imbalance, including **metabolic acidosis** from lactic acidemia. Compensatory mechanisms are no longer adequate.

3. Irreversible stage

–organ damage and metabolic disturbances are so severe that **survival is not possible**.

D. Morphologic manifestations

–a wide variety of anatomic findings are observed in shock. The most important of these is **acute tubular necrosis** of the kidney, which is potentially reversible with appropriate medical management. Other anatomic findings in shock include:

1. Areas of necrosis in the brain

2. Centrilobular necrosis of the liver

3. Fatty change in the heart or liver

4. Patchy mucosal hemorrhages in the colon

5. Depletion of lipid in the adrenal cortex

6. Pulmonary edema

Review Test

Directions: Each of the numbered items or incomplete statements in this section is followed by answers or by completions of the statement. Select the **one** lettered answer or completion that is **best** in each case.

1. Which of the following disorders is the most likely cause of the appearance seen on the illustration showing a cut section of the liver?

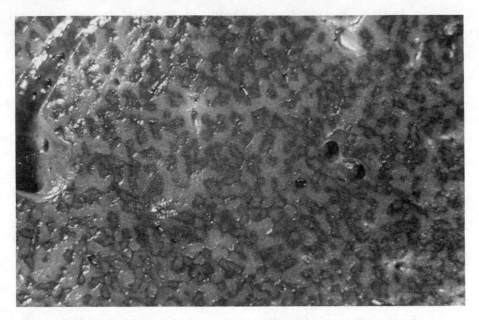

(Reprinted with permission from Golden A, Powell D, and Jennings C: *Pathology: Understanding Human Disease,* 2nd ed. Baltimore, Williams & Wilkins, 1985, p 161.)

(A) Mitral stenosis
(B) Chronic alcoholism
(C) Viral hepatitis
(D) Diabetes mellitus
(E) Niemann-Pick disease

2. All of the following terms are correctly defined EXCEPT

(A) hematoma—localized accumulation of blood within a tissue.
(B) petechiae—small, punctate hemorrhages.
(C) ecchymosis—bleeding within a body cavity.
(D) hyperemia—local increase in volume of blood within small vessels.

3. Each of the following pathologic manifestations is correctly paired with its cause EXCEPT

(A) chronic passive congestion of lung—mitral valve obstruction.
(B) chronic passive congestion of liver—right heart failure.
(C) heart-failure cells—left heart failure.
(D) active hyperemia—acute inflammation.
(E) anemic infarct—double blood supply.

40

4. Which of the following organs is a characteristic site of hemorrhagic infarction?

(A) Heart
(B) Intestine
(C) Kidney
(D) Spleen

5. All of the following substances promote production and stabilization of the platelet plug EXCEPT

(A) adenosine diphosphate (ADP).
(B) thrombin.
(C) thromboxane A_2 (TxA_2).
(D) prostacyclin (PGI_2).
(E) fibrin.

6. Which of the following factors is involved in platelet adhesion to areas of vascular injury?

(A) High-molecular-weight kininogen (HMW-K)
(B) Platelet-derived growth factor (PDGF)
(C) Thrombomodulin
(D) Platelet-surface glycoprotein receptors
(E) ADP

7. TxA_2 is a characteristic product of

(A) endothelial cells.
(B) mast cells and basophils.
(C) neutrophils.
(D) platelets.
(E) macrophages.

8. All of the following substances contribute to the thromboresistant (anticlotting) properties of the vascular endothelium EXCEPT

(A) ADP.
(B) PGI_2.
(C) heparan sulfate.
(D) thrombomodulin.
(E) protein C.

9. The rationale for low-dose aspirin prophylaxis of coronary artery disease is based on the resultant decreased synthesis of

(A) TxA_2.
(B) PGI_2.
(C) ADP.
(D) thrombin.
(E) PDGF.

10. All of the following substances involved in hemostasis are correctly paired with the appropriate activity or descriptive phrase EXCEPT

(A) factor VII—extrinsic pathway.
(B) factor XII—contact activation.
(C) plasmin—fibrinolysis.
(D) platelet factor 3—membrane phospholipid.
(E) prekallikrein—tissue factor.

11. Which of the following veins are the most frequent site of venous thrombosis?

(A) Veins of lower extremity
(B) Pelvic veins
(C) Portal vein
(D) Hepatic veins
(E) Pulmonary veins

12. All of the following hemodynamic events are correctly matched with the associated condition EXCEPT

(A) venous thrombosis—pulmonary infarct.
(B) left atrial thrombosis—cerebral infarct.
(C) fat embolism—caisson disease.
(D) amniotic fluid embolism—disseminated intravascular coagulation.
(E) gas embolism—surgery.

13. Which of the following conditions is an essential precursor to paradoxical embolism?

(A) Rheumatic endocarditis of the mitral valve
(B) Infectious endocarditis of the tricuspid valve
(C) Right-to-left vascular shunt
(D) Thrombosis of deep veins of leg

14. All of the following disorders are associated with transudates EXCEPT

(A) congestive heart failure.
(B) inflammation.
(C) nephrotic syndrome.
(D) chronic liver disease.

15. Which of the following conditions results in hypovolemic shock?

(A) Gram-negative sepsis
(B) Severe hemorrhage
(C) Head injury
(D) Massive left ventricular infarction

Answers and Explanations

1–A. The illustration reveals the nutmeg-like appearance of hepatic chronic passive congestion, a change often caused by mitral stenosis. The gross morphologic appearance is caused by congested centrilobular areas alternating with pale portal areas.

2–C. Ecchymosis is diffuse bleeding into the skin and subcutaneous tissue. In contrast, the terms for bleeding into body cavities vary with the site (i.e., hemothorax, hemopericardium, hemoperitoneum, hemarthrosis).

3–E. All of the pathologic manifestations and their causes are properly paired, with the exception of anemic infarcts, which characteristically occur in the heart, spleen, and kidney. In these organs with a single blood supply, vascular obstruction results in classic coagulation necrosis. Since necrosis results from deprivation of oxygen-containing blood, the lesions are termed anemic, white, or pale infarcts. In organs with a double blood supply, such as the lung, ischemia produces hemorrhagic, or red, infarcts.

4–B. Tissues with a redundant arterial blood supply, such as the gastrointestinal tract with its multiple anastomoses between branches of the mesenteric artery, are typical sites of hemorrhagic (red) infarcts. When a portion of the blood supply is obstructed, other portions remain patent, which can lead to hemorrhage into the infarcted area.

5–D. ADP, TxA_2, and thrombin promote platelet aggregation. The platelet mass is stabilized by fibrin. The prostaglandin PGI_2, synthesized by endothelial cells, limits platelet aggregation.

6–D. Platelet adhesion is mediated by the interaction of a specific platelet-surface glycoprotein receptor and von Willebrand's factor.

7–D. TxA_2, a product of the cyclooxygenase pathway of arachidonic acid metabolism, is synthesized in platelets.

8–A. ADP is a platelet aggregant. PGI_2 inhibits platelet aggregation. Heparan sulfate inhibits coagulation by activation of antithrombin III, which in turn inhibits thrombin and factors IXa, Xa, XIa, and XIIa. The thrombomodulin–thrombin complex activates protein C. Protein C inhibits coagulation by proteolysis of factors Va and VIIIa.

9–A. Both TxA_2 and PGI_2 are products of the cyclooxygenase pathway of arachidonic acid metabolism, and synthesis of both is inhibited by aspirin, a cyclooxygenase inhibitor. In this setting, TxA_2 inhibition is desirable since platelet aggregation is widely considered to be an important early step in atherogenesis. Inhibition of PGI_2 synthesis is an undesirable side effect of aspirin prophylaxis because PGI_2 is a potent platelet anti-aggregant.

10–E. Prekallikrein acts with factor XII (as well as factor XI and HMW-K) in contact activation, which initiates the intrinsic pathway of coagulation. The extrinsic pathway of coagulation is initiated by the activation of factor VII by tissue factor (thromboplastin). Platelet factor 3 is a platelet-membrane phospholipid that can initiate the intrinsic pathway through its action at several levels. Plasmin is a potent protease with both fibrinolytic and fibrinogenolytic activity.

11–A. Venous thrombosis most frequently occurs in the veins of the lower extremities. Since venous thrombosis is associated with impaired blood flow, it is particularly characteristic of immobility, often seen in elderly, debilitated, or chronically bedridden persons.

12–C. Caisson disease is a form of gas embolism. Gas emboli also can be introduced into the vasculature during surgical procedures. Fat emboli are characteristically associated with multiple fractures. Amniotic fluid embolism can trigger the coagulation process, leading to disseminated intravascular coagulation. Pulmonary emboli most commonly arise from venous thrombi in the lower extremities. Cerebral emboli almost always arise from arterial or atrial thrombi.

13–C. Paradoxical embolism is the phenomenon that occurs when an embolus originating in a venous thrombus enters the arterial circulation by passing through a large patent foramen ovale or other right-to-left shunt.

14–B. The edema resulting from inflammation is caused by increased capillary permeability, and the protein-rich, high-specific-gravity, glucose-poor, cell-laden edema fluid is termed an exudate. In contrast, transudates result from increased intravascular hydrostatic pressure or from altered osmotic pressure and are characterized by low protein content and low specific gravity. Congestive heart failure, nephrotic syndrome, and chronic liver disease are classic causes of generalized transudation.

15–B. The reduction in circulating blood volume, which occurs with severe hemorrhage, causes shock from reduction in cardiac output and is the classic example of hypovolemic shock. Reduced cardiac output from massive myocardial infarction causes cardiogenic shock, in which total blood volume is normal or even increased. The shock associated with gram-negative sepsis (septic shock) is marked by peripheral vasodilation and peripheral pooling, as is the neurogenic shock resulting from head injury.

4

Genetic Disorders

I. Chromosomal Disorders

A. Changes in chromosome number or structure

—normal cells are **diploid,** containing 46 chromosomes, 22 pairs of autosomes and 1 pair of sex chromosomes, XX in females or XY in males.

1. Aneuploidy

—is a chromosome number that is not a multiple of 23, the normal **haploid** number.

—is caused most often by an addition or loss of one or two chromosomes; this change may result from nondisjunction or anaphase lag.

a. Nondisjunction

—is failure of chromosomes to separate during meiosis or mitosis. **Meiotic nondisjunction** is the most common cause of aneuploidy.

—is responsible for disorders such as trisomy 21, the most common form of **Down's syndrome**.

b. Anaphase lag

—results in the **loss of a chromosome** during meiotic or mitotic division.

—in early embryonic life, can result in **mosaicism,** where an individual develops two lines of cells, one with a normal chromosome complement and another with **monosomy,** a single residual chromosome, for the affected chromosome pair.

2. Polyploidy

—is a chromosome number that is a multiple greater than two of the haploid number. Triploidy is three times the haploid number; tetraploidy is four times.

—is rarely compatible with life and usually results in **spontaneous abortion**.

3. Deletion

—is most often absence of a portion of a chromosome, although it can be loss of an entire chromosome.

–is denoted by a minus sign following the number of the chromosome and the sign for the chromosomal arm involved, *p* for the short arm and *q* for the long arm. For example, **cri du chat syndrome,** characterized by partial loss of the short arm of chromosome 5, is designated as 46XY,5p− in males or 46XX,5p− in females.

4. Inversion

–is **reunion** of a chromosome broken at two points, in which the internal fragment is reinserted in an **inverted position**.

5. Translocation

–is an **exchange** of chromosomal segments between nonhomologous chromosomes.

–is denoted by a *t* followed by the involved chromosomes in numerical order; for example, the translocation form of Down's syndrome is designated as t(14q;21q).

a. Reciprocal or balanced translocation

–is a break in two chromosomes leading to an exchange of chromosomal material. Since no genetic material is lost, balanced translocation is often **clinically silent**.

b. Robertsonian translocation

–is a variant in which the long arms of two **acrocentric chromosomes,** chromosomes in which the short arm is very short, are joined with a common centromere, and the short arms are lost.

6. Isochromosome formation

–is the result of **transverse** rather than longitudinal division of a chromosome, forming two new chromosomes, each consisting of either two long arms or two short arms. One of the two isochromosomes, usually the short-arm isochromosome, often is lost.

B. Sex chromosomes: X inactivation and Barr body formation

–**extreme karyotype deviations** in the sex chromosomes are compatible with life; this is believed to be due to the **lyonization** of X chromosomes and the scant genetic information carried by the **Y chromosome**.

1. Barr bodies

–also known as **sex chromatin,** are clumps of chromatin in the interphase nuclei of all somatic cells in females.

–according to the Lyon hypothesis, each Barr body represents one **inactivated X chromosome**.

2. Lyonization

–is the process by which all X chromosomes but one are **randomly inactivated** at an early stage of embryonic development.

–results in all normal females being **mosaics,** with two distinct cell lines, one with an active maternal X, another with an active paternal X.

–can be demonstrated if the female is heterozygous for an **X-linked gene;** if individuals demonstrate inheritable differences that distinguish the protein products of one X chromosome from the other, members of the two cell lines can be identified.

3. **Variations**
   a. **Normal females** (XX) will have one Barr body.
   b. **Normal males** (XY) or **XO individuals** will not have Barr bodies.
   c. Individuals with three X chromosomes (XXX) will have two Barr bodies; those with four X chromosomes will have three, and so on.

C. **Abnormalities of autosomal chromosomes**
   1. **Down's syndrome**
      —is the most frequently occurring chromosomal disorder.
      a. **Causes of Down's syndrome**
         (1) **Trisomy 21**
            —accounts for 95% of cases, and **incidence increases with maternal age.**
            —is produced usually by **maternal meiotic nondisjunction**. When cause is paternal nondisjunction, there is no relation to paternal age.
         (2) **Translocation**
            —leads to a **familial form** of Down's syndrome, with significant risk of the syndrome in subsequent children.
            —accounts for 3%–5% of cases and has **no relation to maternal age**.
            —is caused by parental meiotic translocation between chromosome 21 and another chromosome. The fertilized ovum will have three chromosomes bearing the chromosome 21 material, the functional equivalent of trisomy 21.
      b. **Characteristics—Down's syndrome**
         —is marked by severe **mental retardation**.
         —changes in appearance include:
         (1) Large forehead, broad nasal bridge, wide-spaced eyes, **epicanthal folds,** large protruding tongue, and small low-set ears
         (2) **Brushfield's spots,** small white spots on the periphery of the iris
         (3) Short, broad hands with curvature of the fifth finger; **simian crease,** a single palmar crease; and an unusually wide space between the first and second toes
      c. **Complications—Down's syndrome**
         (1) **Congenital heart disease,** especially ventricular septal defects
         (2) Acute **leukemia** (twenty-fold increase), most often lymphoblastic
         (3) Increased **susceptibility to infection**
         (4) In patients surviving into middle age, morphologic **changes in the brain similar to Alzheimer's disease**
   2. **Cri du chat (5p−, cry of the cat) syndrome**
      —is caused by the **deletion** of the short arm of chromosome 5.
      —is characterized by **severe mental retardation, microcephaly,** and an **unusual catlike cry**.
      —is further manifested by low birth weight, round face, **hypertelorism** (wide-set eyes), low-set ears, and epicanthal folds.

3. Edwards' syndrome (trisomy 18)

   —most frequently results from **nondisjunction** resulting in trisomy 18.

   —is marked by mental retardation, prominent occiput, **micrognathia** (small lower jaw), low-set ears, **rocker-bottom feet,** flexion deformities of the fingers (index overlapping third and fourth), and **congenital heart disease**.

4. Patau's syndrome (trisomy 13)

   —is manifested by mental retardation, microcephaly, **microphthalmia,** brain abnormalities, cleft lip and palate, polydactyly, rocker-bottom feet, and congenital heart disease.

D. Abnormalities of sex chromosomes

1. Klinefelter's syndrome

   —is a disorder that occurs when there are at least two X chromosomes and one or more Y chromosomes. The most striking clinical changes are **male hypogonadism** and its secondary effects.

   —is most often characterized by the **karyotype 47,XXY**. Variants include additional X chromosomes (e.g., XXXY) and rare mosaic forms. In the typical XXY form, a **single Barr body** is noted in buccal smear preparations.

   —is most often caused by **maternal meiotic nondisjunction,** and incidence rises with maternal age.

   —is manifested by **atrophic testes; tall stature,** because fusion of the epiphyses is delayed; and a eunuchoid appearance with **gynecomastia**.

   —is marked by **decreased testosterone production** and **increased pituitary gonadotropins** from loss of feedback inhibition.

   —is a frequent cause of male infertility.

   —is sometimes associated with **mental retardation,** which is usually mild; the extent of retardation increases with increased number of X chromosomes.

   —is usually undiagnosed before puberty.

2. XYY syndrome

   —occurs with increased frequency among criminals demonstrating **violent behavior;** the significance of this association is unknown since only about 2% of XYY individuals display overtly antisocial behavior.

   —is manifested by tallness, **severe acne,** and sometimes mild mental retardation.

3. Turner's syndrome

   —is a disorder that occurs when there is complete or partial monosomy of the X chromosome. The most striking clinical changes are **female hypogonadism** and its secondary effects.

   —is the most common cause of **primary amenorrhea**.

   —is most often characterized by an **XO karyotype** (45,X), in which **no Barr bodies** are seen on buccal smear.

   —unlike many other chromosomal disorders, is usually **not complicated by mental retardation**.

   —is characterized by:

   a. Replacement of the ovaries by **fibrous streaks**

    b. Decreased estrogen production and increased pituitary gonadotropins from loss of feedback inhibition

    c. Infantile genitalia and poor breast development

    d. Short stature, webbed neck, shield-like chest with widely spaced nipples, and wide carrying angle of the arms

    e. Lymphedema of the extremities and neck

    f. Coarctation of the aorta and other congenital malformations

4. XXX syndrome (47,XXX) and other multi-X chromosome anomalies
    –are usually unaccompanied by any clinical abnormalities.
    –may be marked by **menstrual irregularities** or **mild mental retardation**. The degree of mental retardation appears to increase with the number of additional X chromosomes.

5. Fragile X syndrome
    –is an important cause of hereditary **mental retardation second in frequency only to Down's syndrome**.
    –is caused by a cytogenetically demonstrable defect on the long arm of the X chromosome that leads to **chromosome breakage in vitro**.
    –is clinically manifest in both males and females; in males is characterized by bilateral **macro-orchidism** (enlarged testes).

II. Modes of Inheritance of Monogenic Disorders (Figure 4.1)

A. Autosomal dominant inheritance

    1. One heterozygous parent carries a gene associated with phenotypic expression of a disorder and the other parent is normal, by far the most likely case in nonconsanguineous matings.

    2. One-half of the children are expected to inherit the gene and are themselves heterozygotes who phenotypically manifest the gene.

    3. Distribution of the phenotype is the same in both sexes.

B. Autosomal recessive inheritance

    1. Both parents are heterozygotes who do not phenotypically manifest the disorder.

    2. One in four of their children will be homozygous for the trait and, in the case of disease states, will phenotypically manifest the disorder.

    3. Distribution of the disordered phenotype is the same in both sexes.

C. X-linked recessive inheritance

    1. In the most frequent disease setting, the **female parent** is a heterozygous **carrier,** and the male parent is genotypically and phenotypically unaffected.
      –the affected X chromosome will be inherited by one in two children; male children who inherit the affected X chromosome phenotypically manifest the disorder; heterozygous female children are carriers.

    2. In a variant setting, the **male parent** carries the affected gene on the X chromosome and the female parent is unaffected.

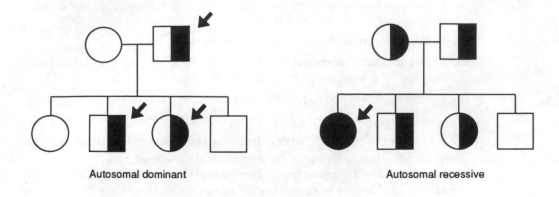

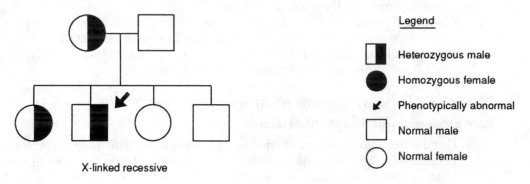

Figure 4.1. Modes of inheritance.

—all female children inherit the paternal X chromosome and become carriers; all male children are genotypically and phenotypically unaffected.

D. Other modes of inheritance

1. X-linked dominant inheritance

—is a rare variant of X-linked inheritance. Heterozygous females as well as hemizygous males phenotypically manifest the disorder.

2. Mitochondrial inheritance

—is mediated by maternally transmitted mitochondrial genes, which are **inherited exclusively by maternal transmission**.

III. Mendelian Disorders

A. Autosomal dominant disorders

1. Adult polycystic kidney disease

—is the most frequently occurring hereditary renal disorder.

—is characterized by **numerous bilateral cysts** that replace and ultimately destroy the renal parenchyma.

—becomes clinically manifest between ages 30 and 50; death usually occurs at about age 50.

2. Familial hypercholesterolemia

- —is a genetic defect characterized by anomalies of receptors for low-density lipoprotein (LDL receptors).
- —results in decreased transport of LDL cholesterol into cells, which causes hypercholesterolemia and a striking increase in incidence and in earlier onset of **atherosclerosis** and its complications.
- —is further manifest by **xanthomas,** raised yellow lesions filled with lipid-laden macrophages, in the skin and tendons.

3. Hereditary hemorrhagic telangiectasia (Osler-Weber-Rendu syndrome)

- —is a rare disorder seen with increased frequency in certain populations, such as in Mormon families of Utah.
- —is characterized by localized **telangiectases of the skin and mucous membranes** and by recurrent **hemorrhage** from these lesions.

4. Hereditary spherocytosis

- —is caused by a variety of inherited defects of erythrocyte membrane proteins.
- —is characterized by **spheroidal erythrocytes** that are sequestered and destroyed in the spleen, producing **hemolytic anemia**.

5. Huntington's disease

- —is a fatal progressive degeneration and **atrophy of the caudate nuclei,** putamen, and frontal cortex.
- —is caused by a genetic defect that has been localized to the short arm of **chromosome 4**.
- —is marked by **extrapyramidal or choreiform movements** and **progressive dementia**.
- —is characterized by **delay of clinical manifestations** until age 30 to 40.
- —can be diagnosed before onset of clinical signs by restriction fragment length polymorphism (RFLP) studies.

6. Marfan's syndrome

- —is a **defect of connective tissue** characterized by faulty scaffolding.
- —is apparently caused by deficiency of fibrillin, a glycoprotein constituent of microfibrils.
- —is characterized by defects in skeletal, visual, and cardiovascular structures.

   a. Patients are tall and thin with abnormally long legs and arms, spider-like fingers (**arachnodactyly**), and hyperextensible joints.

   b. Dislocation of the ocular lens (**ectopia lentis**) is frequent.

   c. Cardiovascular defects can lead to aortic dilatation with resultant **aneurysm of the proximal aorta,** aortic valvular insufficiency, and dissecting aneurysm of the aorta. Loss of connective tissue support may lead to **mitral valve prolapse**.

7. Neurofibromatosis (von Recklinghausen's disease)

- —is distinguished by **multiple neurofibromas** in skin and other locations, **café au lait spots,** and pigmented iris hamartomas (**Lisch nodules**). The benign neurofibromas can become malignant.

–is also marked by **skeletal disorders** such as scoliosis and bone cysts, and **increased incidence of other tumors,** especially the multiple endocrine neoplasia syndromes (MEN types IIa and IIb), pheochromocytoma, and malignancies such as Wilms' tumor, rhabdomyosarcoma, and leukemia.

8. Tuberous sclerosis

–is characterized by the presence of **glial nodules** and **distorted neurons** in the cerebral cortex.

–is marked by **seizures, mental retardation,** and adenoma sebaceum (a facial skin lesion consisting of malformed blood vessels and connective tissue).

–is associated with rhabdomyomas of the heart and with **renal angiomyolipomas,** lesions consisting of malformed blood vessels, smooth muscle, and fat cells.

9. Von Hippel-Lindau disease

–is characterized by **hemangioblastoma** or **cavernous hemangioma** of the cerebellum, brain stem, or retina; **adenomas;** and **cysts** of the liver, kidney, pancreas, and other organs.

–is associated with remarkably increased incidence of **renal cell carcinoma**. The gene for von Hippel-Lindau disease has been localized to the short arm of chromosome 3, deletion of which has been noted in many cases of sporadic renal cell carcinoma.

B. Autosomal recessive disorders

–include most **inborn errors of metabolism** (see Table 4.1).

1. Lysosomal storage diseases

–are a group of disorders characterized by **deficiency of a specific single lysosomal enzyme,** resulting in accumulation of abnormal metabolic products.

Table 4.1. Some Autosomal Recessive Disorders

Disorder	Enzyme Deficiency	Accumulation
Tay-Sachs disease	Hexosaminidase A	G_{M2} ganglioside
Gaucher's disease	Glucocerebrosidase	Glucocerebroside
Niemann-Pick disease	Sphingomyelinase	Sphingomyelin
Hurler's syndrome	α-L-Iduronidase	Heparan sulfate, dermatan sulfate
Von Gierke's disease (type I glycogenosis)	Glucose-6-phosphatase	Glycogen
Pompe's disease (type II glycogenosis)	α-1,4-glucosidase	Glycogen
Cori's disease (type III glycogenosis)	Amylo-1,6-glucosidase	Glycogen
McArdle's syndrome (type V glycogenosis)	Muscle phosphorylase	Glycogen
Galactosemia	Galactose-1-phosphate uridyl transferase	Galactose-1-phosphate
Phenylketonuria	Phenylalanine hydroxylase	Phenylalanine and its degradation products
Alkaptonuria	Homogentisic oxidase	Homogentisic acid

a. Tay-Sachs disease (amaurotic familial idiocy)

—is the most common form of gangliosidosis and occurs primarily in those of Ashkenazic Jewish descent (central European origin).

—is caused by deficiency of **hexosaminidase A,** with consequent accumulation of G_{M2} **ganglioside,** especially in neurons.

—is characterized by **central nervous system (CNS) degeneration,** severe mental and motor deterioration, **blindness** (amaurosis), a characteristic **cherry-red spot** in the macula, and death before age 4.

b. Gaucher's disease

—is a disorder of lipid metabolism caused by a deficiency of **glucocerebrosidase,** which results in accumulation of **glucocerebroside** in cells of the mononuclear phagocyte system.

—can be identified by the presence of **Gaucher's cells,** enlarged histiocytes with a distinctive "wrinkled tissue paper" cytoplasmic appearance.

—appears in three major variants:

(1) Type I, or adult Gaucher's disease, which accounts for about 80% of cases, is characterized by **hepatosplenomegaly, erosion of the femoral head and of the long bones,** and **mild anemia.** Gaucher's cells are seen in the liver, spleen, lymph nodes, and bone marrow. A normal lifespan is possible.

(2) Type II, or infantile Gaucher's disease, is marked by **severe CNS involvement** and results in **death before age 1**. There is no detectable glucocerebrosidase in tissues.

(3) Type III, or juvenile Gaucher's disease, involves both the brain and the viscera but is **less severe than type II**. Onset is usually in early childhood.

c. Niemann-Pick disease

—is most often caused by deficiency of **sphingomyelinase,** with consequent **sphingomyelin** accumulation in phagocytes.

—is characterized by **"foamy histiocytes,"** containing sphingomyelin, which proliferate in the liver, spleen, lymph nodes, and skin.

—is also marked by **hepatosplenomegaly,** anemia, fever, and, in some variants, by neurologic deterioration. About half of patients have a cherry-red spot in the macula similar to that of Tay-Sachs disease. Death occurs by age 3.

d. Hurler's syndrome

—is a mucopolysaccharidosis that is caused by deficiency of **α-L-iduronidase,** with consequent accumulations of the mucopolysaccharides **heparan sulfate** and **dermatan sulfate** in the heart, brain, liver, and other organs.

—is marked by progressive deterioration, hepatosplenomegaly, dwarfism, gargoyle-like facies, stubby fingers, corneal clouding, progressive mental retardation, and death by age 10.

—is clinically similar to, but should not be confused with, Hunter's syndrome, an X-linked recessive disorder.

2. Glycogen storage diseases

—are a group of disorders caused by defects in the synthesis or degradation of glycogen.

a. Von Gierke's disease

—is glycogen storage disease type I, or hepatorenal glycogenosis.
—is caused by deficiency of **glucose-6-phosphatase,** with consequent accumulation of glycogen, primarily in the liver and kidney.
—is characterized by hepatomegaly and hypoglycemia.

b. Pompe's disease

—is glycogen storage disease type II but also can be classified as a lysosomal storage disease.
—is due to deficiency of **α-1,4-glucosidase** (a lysosomal enzyme), with consequent accumulation of glycogen, especially in the liver, heart, and skeletal muscle.
—is characterized by cardiomegaly, muscle hypotonia, and splenomegaly; death occurs from cardiorespiratory failure before age 3.

c. Cori's disease

—is glycogen storage disease type III.
—is caused by deficiency of the **debranching enzyme, amylo-1,6-glucosidase,** leading to variable accumulation of glycogen in the liver, heart, or skeletal muscle.
—is characterized by stunted growth, hepatomegaly, and hypoglycemia.

d. McArdle's syndrome

—is glycogen storage disease type V.
—is caused by deficiency of **muscle phosphorylase,** with consequent glycogen accumulation in skeletal muscle.
—produces painful muscle cramps and muscle weakness following exercise.

3. Disorders of carbohydrate metabolism—galactosemia

a. Classic galactosemia

—is caused by deficiency of **galactose-1-phosphate uridyl transferase,** with resultant accumulation of **galactose-1-phosphate** in many tissues.
—is marked by **failure to thrive, infantile cataracts, mental retardation,** and progressive hepatic failure leading to **cirrhosis** and death. Most of these changes can be prevented by **early removal of galactose from the diet**.

b. Galactokinase-deficiency galactosemia

—is much less frequent than classic galactosemia.
—is often marked only by infantile cataracts.

4. Disorders of amino acid metabolism

a. Phenylketonuria (PKU)

—in most cases is caused by mutation of the **phenylalanine hydroxylase** gene. Phenylalanine hydroxylase deficiency results in failure of conversion of phenylalanine to tyrosine in the liver.

—results in high serum concentrations of **phenylalanine,** which are neurotoxic and cause progressive cerebral demyelination. Minor pathways of phenylalanine catabolism come into play, and metabolites such as **phenylpyruvic acid** ("phenylketone") and phenylacetic acid accumulate. These are found in large amounts in the urine of children with PKU.

—is characterized by progressive **mental deterioration,** usually pronounced by age 1; other symptoms include seizures, hyperactivity, and other neurologic abnormalities; decreased pigmentation of hair, eyes, and skin (children are characteristically **blond and blue-eyed**); and **mousy body odor** from phenylacetic acid in urine and sweat.

—can be successfully treated by a phenylalanine-free diet. Screening tests for serum phenylalanine or urinary catabolites are ordinarily performed on the third or fourth day of life. Earlier screening may result in false-negative results.

b. Alkaptonuria

—is caused by incomplete metabolism of phenylalanine and tyrosine due to deficiency of **homogentisic oxidase,** leading to accumulation and urinary excretion of **homogentisic acid**.

—is characterized by urine that turns dark and finally black on standing; **ochronosis,** dark pigmentation of fibrous tissues and cartilage; and incapacitating ochronotic arthritis. Cardiac valves also may be involved.

5. Cystic fibrosis (mucoviscidosis, fibrocystic disease of the pancreas)

—is the most common lethal genetic disease of Caucasians.

—is caused by mutations in the **cystic fibrosis transmembrane conductance regulator (CFTR) gene,** which has been localized to the midsection of the long arm of **chromosome 7**. This gene codes for a membrane protein that facilitates the movement of chloride and other ions across membranes.

—is characterized by **malfunction of exocrine glands,** resulting in **increased viscosity of mucus** and increased sodium and chloride concentrations in sweat and tears. The **sweat test** is therefore an important diagnostic procedure. Secretion by sweat glands of chloride and sodium is normal, but their reabsorption by sweat ducts is impaired.

—is manifest clinically by:

a. Chronic pulmonary disease

—is caused by retention of viscid mucus, which leads to secondary infection; severe chronic bronchitis, bronchiectasis, and lung abscess are common.

b. Pancreatic insufficiency

—is deficiency of pancreatic enzymes that leads to malabsorption and steatorrhea.

c. Meconium ileus

—is small-bowel obstruction in the newborn caused by thick, viscous meconium.

C. **X-linked recessive disorders** (Table 4.2)

1. **Hunter's syndrome**
   – is a lysosomal storage disease, a form of mucopolysaccharidosis clinically similar to, but less severe than, Hurler syndrome.
   – is caused by deficiency of L-**iduronosulfate sulfatase,** resulting in accumulations of **heparan sulfate** and **dermatan sulfate**.
   – is characterized by hepatosplenomegaly, micrognathia, retinal degeneration, joint stiffness, mild mental retardation, and cardiac lesions.

2. **Fabry's disease (angiokeratoma corporis diffusum universale)**
   – is a lysosomal storage disease caused by deficiency of α-**galactosidase A,** with resultant accumulation of **ceramide trihexoside** in body tissues.
   – is marked by characteristic **skin lesions (angiokeratomas)** over lower trunk, febrile episodes, severe burning pain in the extremities, and cardiovascular and cerebrovascular involvement.
   – results in death in early adult life from **renal failure**.

3. **Classic hemophilia (hemophilia A)**
   – is a relatively common X-linked disorder caused by mutations affecting the **F8 gene,** which has been localized to the tip of the long arm of the X chromosome.
   – is manifest as deficiency of coagulation **factor VIII**.
   – is marked by **hemorrhage** from minor wounds and trauma, bleeding from oral mucosa, hematuria, and hemarthroses. Recurrent hemarthroses can lead to progressive crippling deformities.

4. **Lesch-Nyhan syndrome**
   – is caused by deficiency of **hypoxanthine-guanine phosphoribosyl-transferase (HGPRT),** with resultant impaired purine metabolism and excess production of uric acid.
   – is characterized by **gout,** mental retardation, choreoathetosis, spasticity, **self-mutilation,** and aggressive behavior.

IV. Polygenic Disorders

– are more common than monogenic disorders.
– result from abnormalities of complex processes that are regulated by the protein products of two or more genes. Environmental factors also play an important role in the modulation of the genetic defects.

Table 4.2. Examples of X-Linked Disorders

Disorder	Enzyme Deficiency	Accumulation
Hunter's syndrome	L-Iduronosulfate sulfatase	Heparan sulfate, dermatan sulfate
Fabry's disease	α-Galactosidase A	Ceramide trihexoside
G6PD deficiency	G6PD	. . .
Classic hemophilia (hemophilia A)	Factor VIII	. . .
Lesch-Nyhan syndrome	HGPRT	Uric acid
Duchenne muscular dystrophy	Dystrophin	. . .

G6PD = glucose-6-phosphate dehydrogenase
HGPRT = hypoxanthine-guanine phosphoribosyltransferase

—is believed to underlie such common disorders as ischemic heart disease, diabetes mellitus, hypertension, gout, schizophrenia, bipolar disorder, and neural tube defects.

V. Disorders of Sexual Differentiation

—occur when genetic sex, gonadal sex, or genital sex of an individual are discordant.

A. Definitions

1. Genetic sex

—is determined by the **presence or absence of a Y chromosome**. At least one Y chromosome is necessary for male gender to be manifest.

2. Gonadal sex

—is determined by the **presence of ovaries or testes**. The gene responsible for development of the testes (H-Y gene) is localized to the Y chromosome.

3. Genital sex

—is based on the **appearance of the external genitalia**.

B. True hermaphrodite

—is very rare.

—has both ovarian and testicular tissue, with ambiguous external genitalia.

—may result from the fusion of two sperm (one X-carrying sperm and one Y-carrying sperm) with a binucleated ovum.

C. Pseudohermaphrodite

—has gonads of only one sex, but the appearance of the external genitalia does not correspond to the gonads present. Thus, a male pseudohermaphrodite has testes but the external genitalia are not clearly male. A female pseudohermaphrodite has ovaries but the external genitalia are not clearly female.

1. Male pseudohermaphrodite

—may be caused by tissue resistance to androgens (testicular feminization), defects in testosterone synthesis, or hormones administered to the mother during pregnancy.

—has also been linked to **chromosomal anomalies,** such as 46XY/45X mosaicism.

2. Female pseudohermaphrodite

—is most often caused by increased androgenic hormones from congenital adrenal hyperplasia, an androgen-secreting adrenal or ovarian tumor in the mother, or hormones administered to the mother during pregnancy.

Review Test

Directions: Each of the numbered items or incomplete statements in this section is followed by answers or by completions of the statement. Select the **one** lettered answer or completion that is **best** in each case.

1. All of the following associations are correctly paired EXCEPT

(A) fragile X—mental retardation.
(B) XXY—male infertility.
(C) XXXXX—violent criminals.
(D) trisomy—Patau's syndrome.
(E) 5p- —characteristic cry.

2. A person with an XXY karyotype would demonstrate all of the following characteristics EXCEPT

(A) atrophic testes.
(B) both testicular and ovarian tissue.
(C) male phenotype.
(D) one Barr body on buccal smear.
(E) tall stature.

3. All of the following phrases concerning Down's syndrome are correct EXCEPT

(A) most common chromosomal disorder.
(B) absence of Barr bodies in female patients.
(C) mental retardation.
(D) increased incidence of congenital heart disease and other congenital abnormalities.
(E) nondisjunction most frequent cause.

4. All of the following abnormalities may be seen in Marfan's syndrome EXCEPT

(A) ectopia lentis.
(B) dissecting aneurysm of the aorta.
(C) mitral valve prolapse.
(D) aortic valvular insufficiency.
(E) sclerodactyly.

5. Neurofibromatosis may be marked by all of the following characteristics EXCEPT

(A) café au lait spots.
(B) pigmented nodules in iris.
(C) multiple neural tumors.
(D) bone cysts.
(E) X-linked inheritance.

6. All of the following disorders are associated with autosomal dominant inheritance EXCEPT

(A) von Hippel-Lindau disease.
(B) tuberous sclerosis.
(C) familial hypercholesterolemia.
(D) Marfan's syndrome.
(E) cystic fibrosis.

7. All of the following lysosomal storage diseases are correctly paired with the stored product(s) EXCEPT

(A) Tay-Sachs disease—G_{M2} ganglioside.
(B) Gaucher's disease—glucocerebroside.
(C) Niemann-Pick disease—sphingomyelin.
(D) Hurler syndrome—heparan sulfate and dermatan sulfate.
(E) Pompe's disease—ceramide trihexoside.

8. All of the following disorders are associated with autosomal recessive inheritance EXCEPT

(A) Tay-Sachs disease.
(B) Hunter's syndrome.
(C) galactosemia.
(D) phenylketonuria.
(E) cystic fibrosis.

9. All of the following disorders are transmitted by X-linked inheritance EXCEPT

(A) Fabry's disease.
(B) Lesch-Nyhan syndrome.
(C) glucose-6-phosphate dehydrogenase deficiency.
(D) classic hemophilia (hemophilia A).
(E) von Gierke's disease.

Directions: Each group of items in this section consists of lettered options followed by a set of numbered items. For each item, select the **one** lettered option that is most closely associated with it. Each lettered option may be selected once, more than once, or not at all.

Questions 10–13

Match each chromosomal anomaly with the most likely associated condition.

(A) Deletion
(B) Polyploidy
(C) Inversion
(D) Nondisjunction

10. Edwards' syndrome

11. Cri du chat syndrome

12. Spontaneous abortion

13. Down's syndrome

Questions 14–16

Match each congenital syndrome with the associated abnormality.

(A) Partial deletion of a chromosome
(B) Ovarian fibrous streaks
(C) Gynecomastia

14. Klinefelter's syndrome

15. Turner's syndrome

16. Cri du chat syndrome

Questions 17–19

Match the related number of chromosomes with the chromosomal anomaly.

(A) Aneuploidy
(B) Mosaicism
(C) Polyploidy

17. 45

18. 47

19. 69

Questions 20 and 21

Match the statement about Down's syndrome with the chromosomal anomaly.

(A) Anaphase lag
(B) Nondisjunction
(C) Translocation

20. Most common cause of Down's syndrome

21. Hereditary form of Down's syndrome

Answers and Explanations

1–C. The multi-X syndrome is usually unaccompanied by clinical abnormalities, although minor menstrual irregularities or varying degrees of mental retardation may appear. Mental retardation is apparently related to the number of additional X chromosomes and would be expected in XXXXX individuals. There is no association with violent behavior such as that putatively seen with the XYY karyotype. The fragile X syndrome is second only to Down's syndrome as a cause of hereditary mental retardation. Klinefelter's syndrome (XXY) is a frequent cause of male infertility. Trisomy 13 results in Patau's syndrome, and the 5p– karyotype results in the cri du chat syndrome.

2–B. XXY is the most frequent karyotype leading to Klinefelter's syndrome. These patients demonstrate tall stature and atrophic testes. Ovarian tissue is not present. A single Y chromosome results in a male phenotype, and the number of Barr bodies is always one less than the number of X chromosomes.

3–B. Absence of Barr bodies in phenotypic females is characteristic of classic Turner's syndrome (XO) but has no special relationship with Down's syndrome.

4–E. Sclerodactyly refers to the claw-like fingers of progressive systemic sclerosis (scleroderma). Arachnodactyly is the term for the long, spider-like fingers of Marfan's syndrome.

5–E. Autosomal dominant inheritance characterizes neurofibromatosis, which, in addition to numerous subcutaneous neurofibromatous tumors, produces melanin-pigmented skin lesions (café au lait spots), brown nodules in the iris, and a variety of skeletal disorders, such as scoliosis and bone cysts.

6–E. Cystic fibrosis is an autosomal recessive disorder.

7–E. Glycogen storage due to deficiency of α-1,4-glucosidase, a lysosomal glucosidase, is characteristic of Pompe's disease, the only one of the glycogen storage diseases that is also a lysosomal storage disease. Ceramide trihexoside accumulation occurs in Fabry's disease.

8–B. Hunter's syndrome is an X-linked recessive disorder similar to, but generally less severe than, Hurler syndrome. Both are associated with abnormal accumulations of mucopolysaccharides such as heparan sulfate and dermatan sulfate, and both are members of the mucopolysaccharidosis subgroup of the lysosomal storage diseases. Both are associated with gargoylism, but Hunter's syndrome is associated with X-linked inheritance; Hurler's syndrome, with autosomal recessive inheritance.

9–E. Von Gierke's disease is a form of glycogen storage disease inherited as an autosomal recessive characteristic.

10–D. Edwards' syndrome (trisomy 18) is almost always caused by nondisjunction, although translocation forms also occur.

11–A. The cri du chat syndrome is due to deletion of the short arm of chromosome 5.

12–B. Polyploidy is a common finding in aborted fetuses.

13–D. The most common cause of the trisomy 21 of Down's syndrome is nondisjunction. Translocation, a less common cause of Down's syndrome, is associated with heritable Down's syndrome.

14–C. Prominent clinical manifestations of Klinefelter's syndrome include gynecomastia, tall stature, eunuchoid appearance, and small testes. Although XXY is the most common basis of Klinefelter's syndrome, additional X chromosomes may be present.

15–B. Turner's syndrome is an X-chromosomal disorder manifest by webbing of the neck, small stature, sexual infantilism, ovarian fibrous streaks, and high gonadotropin levels with low estrogen levels, as well as an increased incidence of cardiovascular defects, most notably coarctation of the aorta. Many of these patients are normal in physical appearance.

16–A. The cri du chat syndrome is caused by deletion of the short arm of chromosome 5. Clinical manifestations include mental retardation, a catlike cry, and characteristic appearance changes.

17–A. Aneuploidy is a chromosome number other than a multiple of the normal haploid number of 23 and is most often characterized by addition or loss of only one or two chromosomes. For example, Turner's syndrome is most often due to the loss of a single X chromosome, resulting in a 45,XO karyotype.

18–A. A chromosome number of 47 represents the addition of a single chromosome and is thus another example of aneuploidy.

19–C. A chromosome number of 69 (three times the haploid number of 23) is an example of triploidy, a form of polyploidy. Although rarely compatible with life, polyploidy is frequently observed in spontaneously aborted fetuses.

20–B. Trisomy 21, the most frequently occurring form of Down's syndrome, is most often caused by nondisjunction.

21–C. The hereditary form of Down's syndrome is most often caused by a translocation between chromosome 21 and a second acrocentric chromosome. If the translocated chromosome is transmitted by a gamete, the greater part of the genetic content of chromosome 21 is added to an existing chromosome 21 pair in the fertilized ovum.

5
Immune Dysfunction

I. Cells of the Immune System

A. Lymphocytes

–include B cells, T cells, and natural killer (NK) cells.

–are identified by cell-surface glycoproteins specific for both cell type and stage of differentiation.

1. B cells

–originate from stem cells in the bone marrow.

–continue their differentiation within the bone marrow and peripherally, where they cluster in the **germinal centers of lymph nodes** and in the **lymphoid follicles of the spleen**.

–are characterized by the presence of **surface immunoglobulin**.

–account for approximately 15% of circulating peripheral blood lymphocytes.

2. T cells

–originate from stem cells in the bone marrow and differentiate in the **thymus**.

–populate the **paracortical and deep medullary areas of lymph nodes** and **periarteriolar sheaths of the spleen**.

–account for approximately 70% of circulating peripheral blood lymphocytes.

–are subclassified by surface markers as follows:

a. CD4+ T cells (T4+ T cells)

–account for approximately 60% of circulating T cells.

b. CD8+ T cells (T8+ T cells)

–account for approximately 30% of circulating T cells. The normal 2:1 ratio of CD4+ to CD8+ T cells is dramatically altered in some disease states. For example, in AIDS, the ratio is often 0.5:1 or less.

3. Natural killer (NK) cells

–are also called **large granular lymphocytes (LGL)** because of their distinctive large size, pale cytoplasm, and prominent granulation.

–account for approximately 15% of circulating lymphocytes.

–kill tumor cells, fungi, and cells altered by viral infection. Neither specific sensitization nor antibody is involved in this type of cell killing.

–can also lyse cells by **antibody-dependent cell-mediated cytotoxicity (ADCC)**.

B. Macrophages

–are derivatives of peripheral blood monocytes and are members of the mononuclear phagocyte system (MPS) of cells.

–secrete a variety of cytokines, including **interleukin-1 (IL-1),** as well as other products, including acid hydrolases, neutral proteases, and prostaglandins.

–process and present antigen (along with HLA class II antigens) to CD4+ T cells.

–participate in **delayed hypersensitivity reactions**.

–may be capable of directly killing tumor cells.

C. Dendritic cells of lymphoid tissue

–are characterized by **dendritic cytoplasmic processes**.

–express large quantities of **cell surface HLA class II antigens**.

–in contrast to macrophages, are poorly phagocytic but resemble macrophages in that they are antigen-presenting cells.

D. Langerhans' cells of the skin

–are marked ultrastructurally by the presence of **Birbeck granules,** tennis racket-shaped cytoplasmic structures.

–are similar to dendritic cells of lymphoid tissue in that they express HLA class II antigens and are antigen-presenting cells.

II. Cytokines

–are soluble proteins secreted by lymphocytes (lymphokines), monocytes–macrophages (monokines), and NK cells, as well as other cell types.

–act as effector molecules influencing the behavior of B cells, T cells, NK cells, monocytes, macrophages, hematopoietic cells, and many other cell types (Table 5.1).

III. The Complement System

–consists of about 20 plasma proteins and their products, which can be activated by way of the classic or alternate pathway to form a final product—the membrane attack complex—that lyses targeted cells.

A. The classic pathway

–is initiated by reaction with **antigen–antibody complexes**. The final lytic form of activated complement is the result of a series of **enzymatic cleavages** and recombinations of cleavage products.

B. The alternate pathway

–is initiated directly by **nonimmunologic stimuli,** such as invading microorganisms, and, like the classic pathway, leads to cleavage products that cause cell lysis.

–bypasses the initial stages of the classic pathway.

Table 5.1. Cytokine Functions

Cytokine	Source	Major Functions
Interleukin-1 (IL-1)	Monocytes, macrophages, and other cells	Stimulates T-cell proliferation and IL-2 production
Interleukin-2 (IL-2)	Macrophages, T cells, and NK cells	Stimulates proliferation of T cells, B cells, and NK cells; activates monocytes
Interleukin-3 (IL-3)	T cells	Acts as growth factor for tissue mast cells and hematopoietic stem cells
Interleukin-4 (IL-4)	T cells	Promotes growth of B and T cells; enhances expression of HLA class II antigens
Interleukin-5 (IL-5)	T cells	Promotes end-stage maturation of B cells into plasma cells
Interleukin-6 (IL-6)	T cells, monocytes, and other cells	Promotes maturation of B and T cells; inhibits growth of fibroblasts
Interferon-alpha (IFN-α)	B cells and macrophages	Has antiviral activity
Interferon-beta (IFN-β)	Fibroblasts	Has antiviral activity
Interferon-gamma (IFN-γ)	T cells and NK cells	Has antiviral activity; activates macrophages; enhances expression of HLA class II antigens
Tumor necrosis factor-α (TNF-α, cachectin)	Macrophages, T cells, and NK cells	Stimulates T-cell proliferation and IL-2 production; cytotoxic to some tumor cells
Tumor necrosis factor-β (TNF-β)	T cells	Stimulates T-cell proliferation and IL-2 production; cytotoxic to some tumor cells

NK = natural killer; HLA = human leukocyte antigen.

IV. The HLA (Human Leukocyte Antigens) System

—consists of a group of related proteins referred to as **HLA antigens**. The genes that code for HLA antigens are termed **histocompatibility genes** and are localized to a region on the short arm of chromosome 6, known as the **major histocompatibility complex (MHC)**.

—is important in **organ transplantation,** where HLA typing and matching of donor and recipient are now widely used to predict tissue compatibility.

A. HLA antigens

—are divided into two major classes on the basis of structure and tissue distribution.

1. Class I antigens

—include the HLA-A, HLA-B, and HLA-C antigens, which are found on almost all human cells.

—are the principal antigens involved in **tissue graft rejection**. Serologic testing for HLA-A and HLA-B antigens is used to predict the likelihood of long-term graft survival.

—are identified by standard serologic techniques.

2. Class II antigens

—are chiefly found on immunocompetent cells, including macrophages, dendritic cells, Langerhans' cells, B cells, and some T cells.

—include the HLA-DP, HLA-DQ, and HLA-DR antigens, identifiable by standard serologic techniques or by mixed lymphocyte reactions, and HLA-D antigens, identifiable only by mixed lymphocyte reactions.

B. Association of HLA antigens with disease

—there is a significant association of certain HLA antigens with a number of specific diseases. Many HLA-associated disorders involve immunologic abnormalities, but the mechanisms for these observed associations await full explanation.

1. HLA-B27 antigen is associated with almost 90% of cases of **ankylosing spondylitis**.

2. Specific HLA antigens are also associated with insulin-dependent diabetes mellitus, rheumatoid arthritis, uveitis, and Reiter's syndrome (urethritis, conjunctivitis, and arthritis), as well as with many other entities.

V. Mechanisms of Immune Injury

—adverse reactions caused by immune mechanisms are termed **hypersensitivity reactions**. The classification of Gell and Coombs divides hypersensitivity reactions into four types (Table 5.2). Types I, II, and III require the active production of antibody by plasma cells (terminally differentiated B cells). Type IV is mediated by the interaction of T cells and macrophages.

A. Type I (anaphylactic) hypersensitivity

1. Steps in the reaction

a. Immunoglobulin E (IgE) antibody production by IgE B cells is stimulated by antigen. The IgE antibody is then bound to the Fc receptors of **basophils** and **tissue mast cells**.

b. On **subsequent exposure,** antigen (allergen) reacts with bound IgE antibody (complement is not involved), resulting in cytolysis and degranulation of basophils or tissue mast cells.

c. Degranulation results in **histamine** release, which increases vascular permeability. Various other substances are produced, many of which are vasoactive, smooth muscle spasm-inducing, or chemotactic.

2. Clinical examples

a. Allergic or **atopic** reactions, such as **seasonal rhinitis** (hay fever), allergic **asthma,** or **urticaria** (hives)

b. Systemic anaphylaxis (anaphylactic shock)

—is a potentially fatal reaction, characterized by the rapid onset of urticaria, bronchospasm, laryngeal edema, and shock after exposure to an offending antigen.

B. Type II (cytotoxic) hypersensitivity

1. Complement-fixing antibodies react directly with antigens that are integral components of the target cell. The interaction of complement with the cell surface results in cell lysis and destruction.

Table 5.2. Mechanisms of Immune Injury (Modified Gell and Coombs Classification)

Type of Hypersensitivity	Mechanism	Examples
Type I (anaphylactic)	Antigen reacts with IgE bound to surface of basophils or tissue mast cells, causing degranulation with release of histamine and other substances, many of which are vasoactive, smooth muscle spasm-inducing, or chemotactic	Hay fever; allergic asthma; hives; anaphylactic shock
Type II (cytotoxic)	Antibodies react with antigens that are intrinsic components of cell membrane or other structures, such as basement membranes, resulting in direct damage, complement-mediated increased susceptibility to phagocytosis, or antibody-dependent cell-mediated cytotoxicity; also may be caused by inactivation of cell-surface receptors by anti-receptor antibodies	Warm antibody autoimmune hemolytic anemia; hemolytic disease of the newborn; Goodpasture's syndrome; Graves' disease
Type III (immune complex)	Insoluble complement-bound aggregates of antigen–antibody complexes are deposited in vessel walls or on serosal surfaces or other extravascular sites; neutrophils are chemotactically attracted and release lysosomal enzymes, prostaglandins, kinins, and free radicals, resulting in tissue damage	Serum sickness; Arthus reaction; polyarteritis nodosa; SLE; immune complex-mediated glomerular diseases
Type IV (cell-mediated)	Delayed hypersensitivity: proliferation of antigen-specific CD4+ memory T cells, with secretion of IL-2 and other cytokines, which in turn recruit and stimulate phagocytic macrophages; may also involve cytotoxic CD8+ T lymphocyte killing of specific target cells	Tuberculin reaction; contact dermatitis; tumor cell killing; virally infected cell killing

a. The antigens involved are usually localized to tissue basement membranes or blood cell membranes.

b. Clinical examples include **warm antibody autoimmune hemolytic anemia, hemolytic transfusion reactions,** and **hemolytic disease of the newborn** (erythroblastosis fetalis), in which the antigens are components of red cell membranes; and **Goodpasture's syndrome,** in which the pulmonary alveolar and glomerular basement membranes are affected.

2. Antibody-dependent cell-mediated cytotoxicity (ADCC)

a. Antibody reacts directly with integral surface antigens of targeted cells.

   b. The free Fc portion of the antibody molecule reacts with the Fc receptor of a variety of cytotoxic leukocytes, most importantly **NK cells**. Other leukocytes, including monocytes, neutrophils, and eosinophils, also bear Fc receptors and can participate in ADCC.

   c. The target cells are killed by the Fc receptor-bound cytotoxic leukocytes. Complement is not involved.

3. **Reaction of anti-receptor antibodies with cell-surface receptor protein**

   a. This variant, sometimes classified separately as type V hypersensitivity, is exemplified by the reaction of **thyroid-stimulating immunoglobulin** with the thyroid-stimulating hormone (TSH) receptor of thyroid follicular cells in **Graves' disease**.

   b. In this disorder, the antigen–antibody reaction mimics the effect of TSH on the follicular cells and results in glandular hyperplasia and hyperproduction of thyroid hormone with clinical hyperthyroidism.

C. Type III (immune complex) hypersensitivity

1. Exogenous antibody produced in response to exposure to antigen combines with antigen, resulting in circulating **antigen–antibody complexes**.

2. Immune complexes are most often removed by cells of the mononuclear phagocyte system without adverse effect. In other instances, insoluble aggregates of immune complex are deposited in vessel walls or on serosal surfaces or other extravascular sites. This involves smaller immune complexes that are less easily removed by the mononuclear phagocyte system.

3. The immune complexes bind **complement,** which is highly chemotactic for neutrophils. The neutrophils release lysosomal enzymes, resulting in tissue damage, which can also result from other substances released by neutrophils, including prostaglandins, kinins, and free radicals.

4. **Hageman factor (factor XII)** also is activated, with further activation of the intrinsic pathway of coagulation, resulting in thrombosis in nearby small vessels, and activation of the kinin system, resulting in vasodilation and edema.

5. **Platelet aggregation** causes microthrombus formation and leads to the release of vasoactive amines from platelet-dense granules.

6. **Clinical examples**

   a. Serum sickness

   —is a systemic deposition of antigen–antibody complexes in multiple sites, especially the heart, joints, and kidneys. In the past, antibody-containing foreign serum (most often horse serum) was administered therapeutically for passive immunization against microorganisms or their toxic products. Because of the danger of serum sickness, this mode of therapy is no longer employed.

   b. The Arthus reaction

   —is a localized immune complex reaction that occurs when exogenous antigen is introduced, either by injection or by organ transplant, in the presence of an excess of preformed antibodies.

c. **Polyarteritis nodosa**

—is a generalized immune complex disease especially involving small- and medium-sized arteries.

d. **Immune complex-mediated glomerular diseases**

—include poststreptococcal glomerulonephritis, membranous glomerulonephritis, and lupus nephropathy.

D. Type IV (cell-mediated) hypersensitivity

1. Delayed hypersensitivity

—is exemplified by the **tuberculin reaction,** a localized inflammatory reaction initiated by the intracutaneous injection of tuberculin and marked by proliferation of lymphocytes, monocytes, and small numbers of neutrophils, with a tendency toward cellular accumulations about small vessels (perivascular cuffing). Induration (hardening) results from fibrin formation.

—is also exemplified by **contact dermatitis,** which may result from either delayed hypersensitivity or direct chemical injury to the skin.

—involves the interaction of the T-cell receptor of **CD4+ lymphocytes** with antigen, presented by **macrophages,** and with **HLA class II antigens** on macrophages, resulting in stimulation of antigen-specific CD4+ memory T cells.

a. On subsequent contact with antigen, the CD4+ memory T cells proliferate and secrete cytokines.

b. IL-2 and other cytokines secreted by the CD4+ T cells recruit and stimulate the phagocytic activity of macrophages.

2. Cytotoxic T lymphocyte (CTL) mediated cytotoxicity

—is direct **CD8+ T cell-mediated killing** of target cells (typically tumor cells or virus-infected cells).

a. Specific target cell antigen is recognized by the T-cell receptor of CD8+ lymphocytes.

b. Target cell **HLA class I antigens** recognized as self-antigens are also required.

c. Cytokines are not involved.

VI. Transplantation Immunology

A. General considerations

—for a successful graft, donor and recipient must be matched for ABO blood groups and, ideally, for as many HLA antigens as possible.

—adverse immune responses can be suppressed by immunosuppressant drugs, radiation, or recipient T-cell depletion. However, these processes can result in clinically significant immunodeficiency.

B. Types of transplant rejection

—three basic patterns of graft rejection are well-illustrated by rejection following kidney transplantation.

1. Hyperacute rejection

—is primarily **antibody-mediated** and occurs in the presence of preexisting antibody to donor antigens.

–most often **occurs within minutes** of transplantation.

–is a **localized Arthus reaction** marked by acute inflammation, fibrinoid necrosis of small vessels, and extensive thrombosis.

2. Acute rejection

–is caused by either **cell-mediated or antibody-mediated** mechanisms, or both.

–generally occurs **days to months after transplantation**.

–is characterized by infiltration of lymphocytes and macrophages.

–may, when antibody-mediated mechanisms are prominent, show evidence of arteritis with thrombosis and cortical necrosis.

3. Chronic rejection

–is primarily caused by **antibody-mediated vascular damage**.

–may occur **months to years after an otherwise successful transplantation**.

–is characterized histologically by marked vascular fibrointimal proliferation, often resulting in a small, scarred kidney.

–is becoming more common with the success of immunosuppression in overcoming acute rejection.

C. Graft-versus-host disease

–is a significant problem in **bone marrow transplantation** because immunocompetent cells are transplanted in this procedure.

–is characterized by the rejection of "foreign" host cells by engrafted T and B cells.

VII. Immunodeficiency Diseases

A. X-linked agammaglobulinemia of Bruton

–is an X-linked disorder that presents in male infants, but is usually not manifest clinically until after age 6 months because of the persistence of maternal antibodies.

1. Immune system defects

a. Failure of antibody synthesis caused by a block in maturation of pre-B cells to B cells; cell-mediated immunity is unaffected.

b. Absence of plasma cells in tissue, resulting in virtual **absence of serum immunoglobulins**

c. Absent or poorly defined germinal centers in lymphoid tissue

2. Effects

–propensity to **recurrent bacterial infections** with organisms such as pneumococci, streptococci, and *Haemophilus influenzae;* does not affect resistance to viral and fungal infections, or phagocytosis and killing of bacteria by neutrophils.

B. Isolated IgA deficiency

–is the most common inherited B-cell defect, occurring in approximately 1 in 700 persons.

–results from the inability of IgA B cells to mature to plasma cells. Other immunoglobulins are normal.

—is characterized by occasional anaphylactic reactions to transfused blood and infections, especially those involving mucosal surfaces.

C. Common variable immunodeficiency

—is a diverse group of disorders caused by **failure of terminal B-cell maturation,** resulting in diminution in the number of plasma cells and thus **hypogammaglobulinemia.**

—is manifest clinically by **recurrent bacterial infection**.

D. DiGeorge's syndrome (thymic hypoplasia)

—is a **congenital T-cell deficiency** resulting from aberrant embryonic development of the third and fourth branchial arches, with resultant hypoplasia of the thymus and parathyroid glands as well as abnormalities of the mandible, ear, and aortic arch.

—is characterized by failure of T-cell maturation, leading to **lymphopenia.** B cells remain unimpaired.

—is manifest clinically by **recurrent viral and fungal infections** and **tetany** from hypoparathyroidism with hypocalcemia.

E. Severe combined immunodeficiency disease (SCID)

—is also known as **Swiss-type agammaglobulinemia.**

—is characterized by marked deficiency of **both B and T cells** manifest as profound lymphopenia and severe defects in both humoral and cell-mediated immunity.

—can be caused by a wide variety of genetic defects.

—occurs in both autosomal recessive and X-linked forms. Approximately 50% of autosomal recessive cases are caused by adenosine deaminase **(ADA) deficiency,** which leads to accumulation of deoxyadenosine and deoxy-ATP, substances toxic to lymphocytes.

1. Clinical manifestations

  a. Severe infections (bacterial, viral, and fungal)

  b. High incidence of **malignancy**

  c. Failure to thrive, usually with fatal outcome in infancy

2. Anatomic manifestations

  a. Thymic hypoplasia with absent or markedly reduced thymic lymphoid component

  b. Hypoplasia of lymph nodes, tonsils, and other lymphoid tissues

3. Treatments

  a. Bone marrow or stem cell transplantation

  b. ADA gene transplantation

F. Immunodeficiency with thrombocytopenia and eczema

—is also known as **Wiskott-Aldrich syndrome.**

—is characterized by eczema, thrombocytopenia, recurrent infections, and poor antibody response to polysaccharide antigens.

—most often displays normal total immunoglobulins.

G. Acquired immunodeficiency syndrome (AIDS)

—is caused by **human immunodeficiency virus (HIV)** infection and has become a worldwide epidemic since the first clinical description in 1981. The vast majority of AIDS cases in the U.S. and Europe are caused by infection with the retrovirus **HIV-1**.

1. Mechanisms of HIV infection

a. The HIV virion expresses a cell-surface protein, **gp120,** with binding sites for the CD4 molecule on the surface of **CD4+ T cells**. The interaction of viral gp120 with cellular CD4 explains the affinity of HIV for CD4+ T cells.

b. Other CD4+ cell types that are targets for HIV infection include monocytes, macrophages, dendritic cells, Langerhans' cells, and microglial cells of the central nervous system (CNS).

(1) Monocytes and macrophages may function as reservoirs for HIV and possibly as vehicles for viral entry into the CNS.

(2) HIV may infect **neural cells** directly by way of CD4 receptors or may compete (through the gp120 protein) for neural receptor sites for neuroleukin, a neural tissue growth factor.

c. After cellular binding of gp120 to CD4 and internalization of HIV into the cell, proviral DNA is synthesized by reverse transcription from genomic viral RNA.

d. Proviral DNA is integrated into the host genome.

(1) In its proviral form, HIV may remain latent for an extended period until activation, possibly by infection with other viruses, such as cytomegalovirus or Epstein-Barr virus (EBV).

(2) Low-level virion production, with resultant infectivity, occurs even during the latent period.

2. High-risk populations

a. Homosexual or bisexual men (75% of cases)

(1) The risk is apparently greater with anal receptive intercourse.

(2) In Central Africa, the incidence in both sexes is about equal and is no higher in homosexual or bisexual men than in the general population.

b. Intravenous drug abusers (15% of cases)

—the virus is spread by sharing needles used by infected drug users.

c. Heterosexual partners of persons in high-risk groups (4% of cases)

—sexual transmission from intravenous drug abusers is the major mode of entry of HIV into the heterosexual population.

d. Patients receiving multiple blood transfusions (2% of cases)

—risk has been markedly diminished by screening donor blood for anti-HIV antibodies.

e. Hemophiliacs (1% of cases)

—most likely, the entire cohort of hemophiliacs who received factor VIII concentrates between 1981 and 1985 became infected with HIV. Since 1985, HIV screening and heat inactivation of HIV in factor VIII concentrates have become universal.

f. Infants of high-risk parents

   —infection can be transplacental or occur at the time of delivery.

3. Pathogenesis—AIDS

   —is caused by infection with HIV and resultant **depletion of CD4+ T cells**. The absolute numer of CD4+ T cells and the CD4+:CD8+ ratio are markedly reduced.

   —the loss of CD4+ (helper) T cells causes **failure in humoral and cell-mediated hypersensitivity reactions**.

   —in spite of the inability to produce specific antibodies, patients with AIDS paradoxically demonstrate **hypergammaglobulinemia** from polyclonal B-cell activation.

4. Clinical characteristics of AIDS

   a. Severe immunodeficiency manifested by **opportunistic infection** with organisms such as *Pneumocystis carinii,* **cytomegalovirus,** *Mucor* **species,** and **typical and atypical mycobacteria;** other opportunistic infections frequently found include *Candida, Cryptosporidium, Coccidioides, Cryptococcus, Toxoplasma, Histoplasma,* and *Giardia* infections.

   b. Increased incidence of malignancy, particularly multifocal **Kaposi's sarcoma,** an otherwise rare lesion that in AIDS is almost entirely confined to the homosexual male population, and B-cell **non-Hodgkin's lymphoma;** an increased incidence of Hodgkin's disease and hepatocellular carcinoma also occurs.

   c. Central and peripheral nervous system manifestations occur due to opportunistic infections, CNS tumors, or direct neural infection with HIV.

5. Stages of HIV infection

   —may be asymptomatic for many years.

   —before the fully developed syndrome, stages include an **acute illness** resembling infectious mononucleosis, persistent generalized **lymphadenopathy,** and **AIDS-related complex (ARC),** marked by chronic fever, weight loss, and diarrhea.

   —is marked by **HIV seropositivity** beginning soon after initial HIV infection. Antibodies to the proteins coded by the genes of retroviral *gag, env,* and *pol* regions can be demonstrated, especially antibodies to the gp120 and p24 proteins. HIV infection can also be demonstrated by amplification of viral genetic sequences by polymerase chain reaction (PCR) or by viral culture.

   —in the last stage, defined as **AIDS,** is marked by HIV infection complicated by specified secondary opportunistic infection or malignant neoplasms.

VIII. Autoimmunity

   —results in disease caused by immune reactions directed toward tissues of the host, with apparent inability to distinguish self from nonself.

   —is exemplified by a number of autoimmune disorders, including **autoimmune hemolytic anemia, Hashimoto's thyroiditis, idiopathic adrenal atrophy,** and a group of disorders referred to as **connective tissue diseases**.

   —may be mediated by a number of possible mechanisms.

A. Antigens

1. Host antigens may be recognized as nonself if modified by infection, inflammation, or complexing with a drug.

2. Antigens ordinarily isolated from the immune system may be exposed by trauma or inflammation and become recognized as foreign. Examples include thyroglobulin, lens protein, and spermatozoa.

3. A foreign antigen may share a common structure with a host antigen.

B. Antibodies

1. Many autoimmune disorders are characterized by the presence of **specific autoantibodies,** antibodies directed against host tissue.

2. The demonstration of autoantibodies is presumptive (but not entirely conclusive) evidence of the autoimmune nature of a disorder.

C. Disordered immunoregulation

1. **Increase in T-helper-cell function** or **decrease in T-suppressor-cell function**

2. **Nonspecific B-cell activation** by EBV may trigger polyclonal antibody formation

3. **Thymic defects or B-cell defects**

D. Genetic factors

1. **Genetic predisposition** is suggested because several autoimmune disorders, including Hashimoto's thyroiditis, pernicious anemia, insulin-dependent diabetes mellitus (IDDM), and Sjögren's syndrome, are associated with an increased incidence of other autoimmune disorders.

2. Some **HLA antigens** are associated with increased incidence of certain autoimmune disorders. For example, incidence of Hashimoto's thyroiditis is increased in HLA-DR5 and HLA-B5 positive individuals, and incidence of IDDM is increased in HLA-DR3 and HLA-DR4 positive individuals.

E. Environmental factors

1. Infection (particularly viral) or other environmental agents may initiate autoimmune reactions in genetically susceptible individuals.

2. Some viruses apparently trigger autoimmune islet cell inflammation and resultant IDDM.

IX. Connective Tissue (Collagen) Diseases

—encompass a group of loosely related conditions, most of which feature **fibrinoid change** in connective tissue.

—may be of autoimmune origin; **antinuclear antibodies (ANA)** and a wide variety of other autoantibodies are often present.

A. Systemic lupus erythematosus (SLE)

—is the prototype connective tissue disease.

—most often affects **women** (80% of patients), usually those of childbearing age.

—is marked by the presence of a spectrum of ANA and by **extensive immune complex-mediated inflammatory lesions** involving multiple organ systems, especially the joints, skin, serous membranes, lungs, and kidneys. The lesions of greatest clinical importance in SLE are those in the **kidney**.

1. **Clinical manifestations**

   a. **Fever, malaise, lymphadenopathy, and weight loss**

   b. **Joint symptoms,** including arthralgia and arthritis

   c. Skin rashes, including a **characteristic butterfly rash** over the base of the nose and malar eminences, often with associated photosensitivity

   d. **Raynaud's phenomenon,** manifested by vasospasm of small vessels, most often of the fingers

   e. **Serosal inflammation,** especially pericarditis and pleuritis

   f. **Diffuse interstitial pulmonary fibrosis,** manifest as interstitial pneumonitis or diffuse fibrosing alveolitis

   g. **Endocarditis** of the characteristic atypical verrucous (Libman-Sacks) form, in which vegetations are seen on both sides of the mitral valve leaflet. The tricuspid valve is less frequently involved.

   h. **Immune complex vasculitis** occurring in vessels of almost any organ. In the spleen, perivascular fibrosis with concentric rings of collagen around splenic arterioles results in a characteristic onion-skin appearance.

   i. **Glomerular changes** varying from minimal involvement to severe diffuse proliferative disease with marked subendothelial and mesangial immune complex deposition, endothelial proliferation, and thickening of basement membranes
      (1) Subendothelial immune complex deposition in the glomeruli is of considerable diagnostic significance. This change results in the wire-loop appearance seen by light microscopy.
      (2) Thickening of basement membranes can result in changes indistinguishable from those of membranous glomerulonephritis.

   j. **Neurologic and psychiatric manifestations**

   k. **Eye changes,** with yellowish, cotton wool-like fundal lesions (cytoid bodies)

2. **Laboratory findings**

   a. **The LE test**
      —is based on the LE phenomenon, which occurs in vitro.
      (1) In this procedure, morphologically characteristic LE cells are formed in a mixture of mechanically damaged neutrophils and autoantibody-containing patient serum.
      (2) The LE test is positive in only about 70% of cases and has now been largely replaced by more sensitive determinations.

   b. **A positive test for ANA**
      —is seen in almost all patients with SLE. ANA are also found in patients with other connective tissue diseases.

(1) The ANA test becomes almost specific for SLE when the antinuclear antibodies react with **double-stranded DNA**. When this reaction is assessed by microscopic examination of cells using immunofluorescent techniques, a characteristic peripheral nuclear staining, or **"rim" pattern,** is seen.

(2) ANA that react with **Sm (Smith) antigen,** a ribonucleoprotein, are also highly specific for SLE.

c. **Serum complement often markedly decreased,** especially in association with active renal involvement

d. **Immune complexes at dermal–epidermal junction,** demonstrable in skin biopsies

e. **Biological false-positive (BFP) tests for syphilis** in about 15% of patients. This may be the earliest laboratory abnormality in some cases of SLE.

B. Progressive systemic sclerosis (PSS, scleroderma)

–is **widespread fibrosis and degenerative changes** that affect the skin, gastrointestinal tract, heart, muscle, and other organs; they occur most frequently in young women.

–is marked by the presence of the ANA **anti-Scl-70** in one-third of patients. ANA with anti-centromere activity is characteristic of a PSS variant, the **CREST syndrome (***C*alcinosis, *R*aynaud's phenomenon, *E*sophageal dysfunction, *S*clerodactyly, and *T*elangiectasia).

–usually presents initially with skin changes, polyarthralgias, and esophageal symptoms.

–is characterized by the following:

1. **Hypertrophy of collagen fibers of the subcutaneous tissue,** leading to tightening of the facial skin and a characteristic **fixed facial appearance**

2. **Sclerodactyly** (claw-like appearance of the hand)

3. **Raynaud's phenomenon** in about 75% of patients

4. **Visceral organ involvement,** especially of the esophagus, gastrointestinal tract, kidneys, lungs, and heart

   a. The **esophagus** is frequently affected, and dysphagia is common.

   b. **Interstitial pulmonary fibrosis** is a serious complication.

   c. **Hypertension** often occurs.

C. Sjögren's syndrome

–most often affects women of late middle age.

1. **Clinical manifestations**

   a. A **triad** including **xerostomia** (dry mouth), **keratoconjunctivitis sicca** (dry eyes), and **one of several connective tissue or other autoimmune diseases,** most often rheumatoid arthritis

   (1) Other associated disorders may include SLE, PSS, polymyositis, or Hashimoto's thyroiditis.

   (2) The **sicca syndrome** is a variant characterized by xerostomia and keratoconjunctivitis alone.

   b. Bilaterally enlarged parotids diffusely infiltrated by lymphocytes and plasma cells. This cellular infiltration can partly or completely obscure the parenchyma of the parotid gland and can mimic, or in some cases lead to, malignant lymphoma.

   2. Laboratory findings

   a. Significant polyclonal **hypergammaglobulinemia** (a broad-based elevation of serum gamma globulins demonstrable by electrophoresis)

   b. ANA, including the highly specific **anti-SS-B** and somewhat less specific anti-SS-A

D. Polymyositis

   −is a **chronic inflammatory process** especially involving the proximal muscles of the extremities. When the skin is also involved, with a characteristic reddish-purple rash over exposed areas of the face and neck, the condition is called **dermatomyositis.**

   −occurs principally in women and is frequently associated with malignancy.

   −is characterized by **increased serum creatine kinase** and frequent presence of ANA.

   −can be confirmed by muscle biopsy.

E. Mixed connective tissue disease (MCTD)

   −occurs principally in women (80% of patients), with a peak incidence at age 35 to 40.

   −shares clinical features with other connective tissue disorders, but in contrast, renal involvement is uncommon in MCTD.

   −is often manifest clinically by arthralgias, Raynaud's phenomenon, esophageal hypomotility, and myositis.

   −is most uniquely characterized by **specific ANA** (high titer anti-nRNP and an immunofluorescent speckled nuclear appearance on morphologic ANA analysis).

F. Polyarteritis nodosa

   −is an **immune complex vasculitis** characterized by segmental fibrinoid necrosis in the walls of **small and medium arteries** of almost any organ.

   −occurs predominantly in **men** (in contrast to the other connective tissue diseases).

   1. Antigen

   −is usually unknown, but may be:

   a. Hepatitis B antigen is implicated in 30% of cases.

   b. Drugs, such as sulfonamides and penicillin, may form immunogenic hapten–protein complexes.

   2. Clinical manifestations

   −may include abdominal pain, hypertension, uremia, polyneuritis, allergic asthma, urticaria or rash, splenomegaly, fever, leukocytosis, and proteinuria.

   −may involve the lung, resulting in chest pain, cough, dyspnea, and hemoptysis. Severe dyspnea and eosinophilia occur in 20% of patients.

X. Amyloidosis

—is a group of disorders characterized by the deposition of amyloid, a proteinaceous material with certain physicochemical features.

A. Amyloid

1. Structure—amyloid

—is not a single substance but a group of substances that share a common physical structure that can be formed by a number of different proteins (Table 5.3).

—always has a **β-pleated sheet configuration** (demonstrable by x-ray diffraction).

2. Morphologic features—amyloid

—is characteristically **extracellular** in distribution, most often appearing as accumulations proximate to basement membranes.

—has an amorphous eosinophilic appearance in routine hematoxylin and eosin sections.

—is characteristically stained by **Congo red** dye, demonstrating apple green **birefringence** when viewed under polarized light and confirming the suspected presence of amyloid.

—can be demonstrated by a variety of other methods, including immunochemical, fluorescent, and metachromatic techniques.

B. Clinical patterns of amyloidosis

1. Primary amyloidosis (immunocytic dyscrasia amyloidosis)

—is caused by deposition of amyloid fibrils derived from **immunoglobulin light chains,** referred to as **AL (amyloid light chain) protein**.

—is most characteristically marked by amyloid deposition in tissues of mesodermal origin, such as **heart, muscle,** and **tongue**.

—**may involve the kidney,** with amyloid deposits in the glomerular mesangium as well as in the interstitial tissue between tubules.

—includes the amyloidosis frequently associated with **plasma cell disorders** such as multiple myeloma and Waldenström's macroglobulinemia.

2. Secondary amyloidosis (reactive systemic amyloidosis)

—is marked by deposition of fibrils consisting of the amyloid protein termed

Table 5.3. Associations of Various Amyloid Proteins

Type of Amyloidosis	Amyloid Protein
Systemic amyloidosis	
Primary (immunocytic dyscrasia)	AL protein derived from immunoglobulin light chains
Secondary (reactive systemic)	AA protein derived from precursor serum protein
Other amyloid-associated conditions	
Portuguese type of polyneuropathy	Transthyretin
Alzheimer's disease	A4 amyloid (or amyloid β-protein)
Familial Mediterranean fever	AA amyloid
Medullary carcinoma of the thyroid	Amyloid protein derived from calcitonin
Insulin-resistant diabetes mellitus	Amylin (islet amyloid polypeptide, IAPP)
Senile amyloidosis	Transthyretin

AL = amyloid light chain; AA = amyloid-associated.

AA protein, which is formed from a precursor, serum amyloid-associated protein (SAA). Chronic tissue destruction leads to increased SAA.

—usually involves parenchymatous organs, especially the **kidney** (nephrotic syndrome is very common), **liver, adrenals, pancreas, lymph nodes,** and **spleen**. Perifollicular involvement in the spleen results in "sago spleen," an appearance reminiscent of tapioca-like granules.

—characteristically is a complication of **chronic inflammatory disease** such as rheumatoid arthritis, tuberculosis, osteomyelitis, syphilis, or leprosy.

—also may complicate noninflammatory disorders such as renal cell carcinoma and Hodgkin's disease.

3. Other forms of amyloidosis

a. Portuguese type of polyneuropathy

—is associated with amyloid derived from a protein known as **transthyretin** (a serum protein that **trans**ports **thy**roxine and **retin**ol).

—is characterized by severe peripheral nerve involvement caused by amyloid deposits.

b. Alzheimer's disease

—is characterized by deposits of an amyloid protein referred to as **A4 amyloid,** or **amyloid β-protein,** which differs from AL, AA, and transthyretin-derived amyloid. The gene that codes for the protein precursors of A4 amyloid has been localized to **chromosome 21**.

c. Familial Mediterranean fever

—is an autosomal recessive disorder occurring in persons of eastern Mediterranean origin.

—is characterized by episodic fever and polyserositis.

—has a distribution and type of amyloid similar to that of **secondary amyloidosis** (AA amyloid).

d. Medullary carcinoma of the thyroid

—is characterized by prominent **amyloid deposits** within the tumor, apparently derived from calcitonin.

e. Diabetes mellitus

—in the insulin-resistant adult-onset form (type II) is characterized by **deposits of amyloid in islet cells**. This amyloid is thought to be derived from either insulin or glucagon, and is referred to as **amylin** or, alternatively, **islet amyloid polypeptide (IAPP)**. It is postulated that amylin interferes with insulin sensing by beta cells.

f. Senile amyloidosis

—is characterized by minor deposits of amyloid found at autopsy in the very elderly.

—may involve the heart, brain, and other organs. When senile amyloidosis occurs in the heart, the amyloid protein is derived from **transthyretin**.

Review Test

Directions: Each of the numbered items or incomplete statements in this section is followed by answers or by completions of the statement. Select the **one** lettered answer or completion that is **best** in each case.

1. A finding of diagnostic significance is the well-known association of HLA-B27 antigen with which of the following disorders?

(A) Rheumatoid arthritis
(B) Ankylosing spondylitis
(C) Felty's syndrome
(D) Systemic lupus erythematosus (SLE)
(E) Hashimoto's thyroiditis

2. The following mechanisms of immune injury are correctly paired with one of their major characteristics EXCEPT

(A) type I—bound IgE.
(B) type II—cell surface antigens.
(C) type III—antibody-dependent cell-mediated cytotoxicity (ADCC).
(D) type IV—sensitized T cells.

3. Within minutes of a bee sting, a 23-year-old woman develops generalized pruritus and hyperemia of the skin, followed shortly by swelling of the face and eyelids, dyspnea, and laryngeal edema. This reaction is mediated by

(A) antigen–antibody complexes.
(B) cytotoxic T cells.
(C) IgA antibodies.
(D) IgE antibodies.
(E) IgG antibodies.

4. Characteristics or phenomena associated with acute rejection after renal transplantation include all of the following EXCEPT

(A) occurs days to months after transplantation.
(B) antibody-mediated or cell-mediated.
(C) localized Arthus reaction.
(D) mononuclear infiltrates.
(E) arteritis with thrombosis.

5. Bruton's disease is characterized by all of the following manifestations EXCEPT

(A) absent circulating B cells.
(B) normal circulating T cells.
(C) absent plasma cells.
(D) low serum levels of immunoglobulin.
(E) impaired resistance to viral infections.

6. Each of the following disease states is matched with the correct manifestation or association EXCEPT

(A) severe combined immunodeficiency disease—adenosine deaminase deficiency.
(B) isolated IgA deficiency—reactions to blood transfusions.
(C) Wiskott-Aldrich syndrome—thrombocytopenia.
(D) DiGeorge's syndrome—autosomal dominant inheritance.
(E) AIDS—reversed CD4 + :CD8 + ratio.

7. Features of systemic lupus erythematosus include all of the following EXCEPT

(A) glomerular lesions.
(B) hepatitis B antigen frequently implicated.
(C) arthralgias and arthritis.
(D) skin manifestations.
(E) endocarditis.

8. Frequent findings in mixed connective tissue disease include all of the following EXCEPT

(A) arthralgias.
(B) renal failure.
(C) Raynaud's phenomenon.
(D) esophageal hypomotility.
(E) myositis.

9. Characteristics of Sjögren's syndrome include all of the following EXCEPT

(A) dry mouth.
(B) dry eyes.
(C) infiltration of parotids with lymphocytes and plasma cells.
(D) hypogammaglobulinemia.
(E) associated connective tissue disorders.

10. Each of the following disease entities is correctly paired with the appropriate antibody EXCEPT

(A) SLE—anti-Sm antibody.
(B) Sjögren's syndrome—anti-SS-B antibody.
(C) mixed connective tissue disease—anti-nRNP antibody.
(D) polyarteritis nodosa—antibody to double-stranded DNA.
(E) progressive systemic sclerosis—anti-Scl-70 antibody.

11. Which of the following findings is characteristic of secondary (reactive systemic) amyloidosis?

(A) Association with chronic inflammatory diseases
(B) Amino acid sequences of amyloid similar to immunoglobulin light chains
(C) Organ distribution primarily in tissues of mesodermal origin, such as heart, muscle, and tongue
(D) Frequent association with plasma cell disorders
(E) Amyloid coded by a gene localized to chromosome 21

12. All of the following diseases that predispose to amyloidosis are correctly matched with the appropriate amyloid protein EXCEPT

(A) rheumatoid arthritis—AA amyloid.
(B) multiple myeloma—AL amyloid.
(C) medullary carcinoma of the thyroid—AA amyloid.
(D) Alzheimer's disease—A4 amyloid.
(E) senile amyloidosis of the heart—transthyretin.

Directions: Each group of items in this section consists of lettered options followed by a set of numbered items. For each item, select the **one** lettered option that is most closely associated with it. Each lettered option may be selected once, more than once, or not at all.

Questions 13–16

Match the phrase with the appropriate type of cell.

(A) B cells
(B) T cells
(C) Large granular lymphocytes
(D) Macrophages

13. Antigen-presenting cell
14. Germinal centers of lymph nodes
15. Majority of peripheral blood lymphocytes
16. ADCC

Answers and Explanations

1–B. The most striking association of HLA antigens with disease is the occurrence of the HLA-B27 antigen in almost 90% of patients with ankylosing spondylitis. This association is the basis of an important clinical laboratory diagnostic procedure. The other disorders listed are widely considered to be of autoimmune origin, and an increased association with a variety of other HLA haplotypes has been noted in this general class of disorders.

2–C. Type III hypersensitivity is mediated by immune complex formation and deposition, complement binding, and resultant acute inflammation. ADCC is a variant of type II hypersensitivity in which circulating antibodies interact with cell-surface antigens on target cells. The Fc portion of the antibodies binds to natural killer (NK) cells (or other cells with Fc receptors), which then kill the target cells.

3–D. The clinical description is characteristic of systemic anaphylaxis, an IgE-mediated type I hypersensitivity reaction. In type I hypersensitivity, reaction of antigen with preformed IgE antibodies fixed by Fc receptors to the surface of basophils or tissue mast cells results in cytolysis and degranulation of these cells, with release of histamine and other mediators.

4–C. A localized Arthus reaction (localized immune complex reaction that occurs when exogenous antigen is inserted in the midst of preformed antibody) is the cause of the almost immediate phenomenon termed hyperacute rejection. In contrast, acute rejection occurs days to months after transplantation and is either antibody-mediated or cell-mediated, or both.

5–E. This disease of male children is X-linked and is descriptively termed X-linked agammaglobulinemia of Bruton. T cells are unaffected as are T-cell functions such as cell-mediated immunity and resistance to viral infections. Failure of maturation of pre-B cells is associated with absence of B lymphocytes and plasma cells, failure of antibody synthesis with resultant serum agammaglobulinemia, and recurrent bacterial infections.

6–D. DiGeorge's syndrome is a congenital developmental defect possibly caused by intrauterine infection.

7–B. Hepatitis B antigen has been implicated in about a third of patients with polyarteritis nodosa, but not in SLE. Glomerular lesions are the most universal and serious manifestations of SLE. A variety of joint manifestations are frequent. Skin manifestations include the characteristic malar butterfly rash and photosensitivity. Endocarditis with vegetations on both sides of the valve (Libman-Sacks endocarditis, atypical verrucous endocarditis) is sometimes seen.

8–B. Mixed connective tissue disease (MCTD) shares many features in common with SLE, progressive systemic sclerosis (scleroderma), and polymyositis. However, in contrast to these disorders, renal involvement is an uncommon feature of MCTD.

9–D. Dry mouth (xerostomia), dry eyes (keratoconjunctivitis sicca), and one of several possible connective tissue diseases, such as rheumatoid arthritis, make up the triad of findings of Sjögren's syndrome. Other important findings include parotid enlargement due to a diffuse infiltrate of lymphocytes and plasma cells and polyclonal hypergammaglobulinemia.

10–D. Antibodies to double-stranded DNA and to the Sm antigen are highly specific findings in SLE but not in polyarteritis nodosa.

11–A. Reactive systemic amyloidosis occurs as a secondary phenomenon to long-standing chronic inflammatory disorders such as rheumatoid arthritis, tuberculosis, and osteomyelitis. The characteristic amyloid protein is formed from a precursor, serum amyloid-associated protein (SAA). Organ distribution is primarily in parenchymatous organs.

12–C. In medullary carcinoma of the thyroid, amyloid is apparently a catabolic product of calcitonin and is not the AA amyloid associated with rheumatoid arthritis and other chronic inflammatory disorders. The AL amyloid associated with plasma cell disorders such as multiple myeloma is derived from immunoglobulin light chains. Alzheimer's disease is noted by the presence of amyloid plaques containing A4 amyloid. Senile amyloidosis, when it occurs in the heart, is characterized by amyloid deposits derived from transthyretin.

13–D. Macrophages and closely related cells (such as Langerhans' cells of the skin and dendritic cells of lymph nodes) process foreign antigens for presentation to lymphocytes.

14–A. B cells are found throughout the lymphoid system but are localized in clusters in the germinal centers of lymph nodes and in the lymphoid follicles of the spleen.

15–B. T cells account for approximately 70% of circulating peripheral blood lymphocytes.

16–C. ADCC is characteristically mediated by NK cells, which are also referred to as large granular lymphocytes (LGL). ADCC also is mediated by a variety of other leukocytes (e.g., monocytes, neutrophils, eosinophils), all of which bear Fc receptors. This mode of cytotoxicity is dependent on the reaction of antibody with antigens of the target cell, followed by further combination of the antibody with the Fc receptor of the cytotoxic leukocyte, leading to death of the target cell.

6

Neoplasia

I. General Characteristics—Neoplasia

—is the uncontrolled, disorderly proliferation of cells, resulting in a benign or malignant tumor, or neoplasm.

A. Dysplasia

—is a **reversible** change.

—often precedes malignancy.

—morphologically manifests by disorderly maturation and spatial arrangement of cells, marked variability in nuclear size and shape (pleomorphism), and increased, often abnormal, mitosis.

—is exemplified by dysplasia of squamous epithelium of the cervix, which often is a precursor of malignancy.

B. Neoplasms

—if the resemblance to tissue of origin is close, the neoplasm is termed **well-differentiated;** if little resemblance to the tissue of origin is seen, it is **poorly differentiated**.

—neoplasms grow at the expense of function and vitality of normal tissue without benefit to the host and are largely independent of host control mechanisms.

II. Classification and Nomenclature of Tumors

—neoplasms are classified as either **malignant** or **benign,** based on their behavior.

—they are also described by terms derived from the **appearance** of the neoplasm, **tissue of origin,** or degree of **differentiation**.

A. Malignant tumors (cancer)

—are capable of **invasion** (spread of the neoplasm into adjacent structures) and **metastasis** (implantation of the neoplasm into noncontiguous sites); this is the most important **defining characteristic of malignancy,** although there are some malignant tumors, such as basal cell carcinoma of the skin, that rarely metastasize.

—are usually less differentiated than benign tumors.

—are marked by **anaplasia,** in which tumor cells are very poorly differentiated and exhibit **pleomorphism, hyperchromatism** (dark-staining nuclei), an **increased nuclear–cytoplasmic ratio,** abnormal mitoses, cellular dyspolarity, and often **prominent nucleoli**. In general, highly anaplastic tumors are very aggressive, and well-differentiated tumors are less aggressive.

1. **Carcinoma**

—is a malignant tumor of **epithelial** origin and can be seen in the following variations:

a. **Squamous cell carcinoma**

—originates from stratified squamous epithelium of, for example, the skin, mouth, esophagus, and vagina, as well as from areas of squamous metaplasia, as in the bronchi or the squamocolumnar junction of the uterine cervix.

—is marked by the production of keratin.

b. **Transitional cell carcinoma**

—arises from the transitional cell epithelium of the urinary tract.

c. **Adenocarcinoma**

—is carcinoma of **glandular epithelium** and includes malignant tumors of the gastrointestinal mucosa, endometrium, and pancreas.

—is often associated with **desmoplasia,** tumor-induced proliferation of non-neoplastic fibrous connective tissue, particularly in adenocarcinoma of the **breast, pancreas,** and **prostate**.

2. **Sarcoma**

—is a malignant tumor of **mesenchymal origin**.

—is often used with a prefix that denotes the tissue of origin of the tumor, as in **osteosarcoma** (bone), **rhabdomyosarcoma** (skeletal muscle), **leiomyosarcoma** (smooth muscle), and **liposarcoma** (fatty tissue).

3. **Eponymically named tumors**

—include Burkitt's lymphoma, Hodgkin's disease, and Wilms' tumor.

4. **APUDoma**

—is a tumor characterized by **amine precursor uptake and decarboxylation** (APUD) and the resultant production of hormone-like substances.

5. **Teratoma**

—is a neoplasm derived from all **three germ cell layers,** which may contain structures such as skin, bone, cartilage, teeth, and intestinal epithelium.

—may be either malignant or benign.

—usually arises in the ovaries or testes.

B. **Benign tumors**

—are usually **well-differentiated,** closely resembling the tissue of origin.

—do not metastasize and grow slowly. They can be harmful if their growth compresses adjacent tissues. For example, benign intracranial tumors can be more lethal than some malignant skin tumors.

—tend to become **encapsulated**.

—are denoted by the suffix -oma, as in lipoma and fibroma. However, this suffix is also applied to some malignant neoplasms, such as hepatoma, melanoma, lymphoma, and mesothelioma, as well as several non-neoplastic swellings, including granuloma and hematoma.

1. Papilloma

—is a benign neoplasm most often arising from **surface epithelium** such as squamous epithelium of the skin, larynx, or tongue.

—is composed of delicate **finger-like epithelial processes** overlying a core of connective tissue stroma that contains blood vessels.

—may also develop from **transitional epithelium** of the urinary bladder, ureter, or renal pelvis.

2. Adenoma

—is a benign neoplasm of **glandular epithelium** that occurs in several variants:

a. Papillary cystadenoma

—is characterized by adenomatous papillary processes that extend into cystic spaces, as in cystadenoma of the ovary.

b. Fibroadenoma

—is marked by proliferation of connective tissue surrounding neoplastic glandular epithelium; for example, fibroadenoma of the breast.

3. Benign tumors of mesenchymal origin

—are most often named by the tissue of origin; for example, leiomyoma, rhabdomyoma, lipoma, fibroma, and chondroma.

—include the most common neoplasm of women, the uterine leiomyoma, or fibroid tumor.

4. Choristoma

—is a small non-neoplastic area of **normal tissue misplaced within another organ,** such as pancreatic tissue within the wall of the stomach.

5. Hamartoma

—is a non-neoplastic, disorganized, tumor-like overgrowth of cell types that are regularly found within the affected organ; **hemangioma,** an irregular accumulation of blood vessels.

III. Properties of Neoplasms

A. Properties of transformed cells

—include the following characteristic changes, which are observed in vitro in tissue culture. These changes may reflect the altered biology of cancer cells.

1. Loss of contact inhibition

—in contrast to nontransformed cells, transformed cells continue to grow even when touching other cells.

2. Loss of adhesion

—transformed cells tend to grow separately rather than in clusters, perhaps partly due to faulty cytoskeletal structure.

3. Loss of anchorage dependence

—transformed cells will often grow in soft agar, in contrast to most normal cells, which must be anchored to a solid surface.

4. Expression of cell-surface proteases

—this change may facilitate invasiveness.

5. Increased expression of laminin receptors

—these specific glycoprotein receptors may facilitate attachment of malignant cells to basement membranes.

6. Marked reduction of cell-surface fibronectin

—fibronectin may play a role in contact-mediated growth control in normal cells, and reduced levels may be partially responsible for the uncontrolled growth of cancer cells.

7. Increased agglutinability by lectins

8. Chromosomal aneuploidy with increased DNA content

B. Tumor-specific antigens (TSA)

—are cellular proteins characteristic of some tumors that are demonstrable immunologically.
—include the following types:

1. TSAs induced by oncogenic viruses

—often represent expression of viral proteins, and remain the same regardless of the tissue infected by the virus.

2. TSAs induced by chemical carcinogenesis

—tend to be highly variable from tissue to tissue.

3. Normal tissue proteins

—apparently become accessible to immunologic probes because of conformational changes in the cell surface.

4. Proteins normally expressed only in fetal or embryonic life

—are termed **oncofetal antigens;** their expression by neoplastic cells is considered a manifestation of these cells' lack of differentiation.
—include **carcinoembryonic antigen (CEA),** associated with colon cancer and other cancers and preneoplastic processes, and **alpha-fetoprotein,** which is associated with hepatocellular carcinoma and many germ cell tumors.

C. Monoclonality

—denotes origin from a single precursor cell.
—is a characteristic of most neoplasms.
—is assessed by a variety of approaches.

1. Glucose-6-phosphate dehydrogenase (G6PD) isoenzyme studies

—offer compelling evidence for monoclonality of tumors; because of X inactivation in early embryonic life, tissues of females heterozygous for G6PD isoenzymes consist of a mosaic of cell types with random cells expressing one or the other of the two isoenzymes.

a. Monoclonal tumors

—express only one of the isoenzymes.

b. Polyclonal cellular proliferations

—exhibit both isoenzymes.

2. Monoclonality of cells of lymphoid origin

a. Indicators of monoclonality in malignancies of B-cell origin

(1) Immunoglobulins

—are produced by B-cell malignant tumors, and are demonstrable as cytoplasmic or surface immunoglobulin or, in the case of multiple myeloma, are secreted and are demonstrable in the serum.

—if monoclonal, the resultant mix of immunoglobulin molecules will exhibit **either kappa or lambda chain specificity,** but not both, a characteristic finding in neoplastic B-cell proliferations.

—if B-cell or plasma cell proliferations are polyclonal, they result in the production of heterogeneous immunoglobulin molecules, some of which express kappa specificity and others that express lambda specificity, a characteristic finding in non-neoplastic reactive B-cell hyperplasias.

(2) Immunoglobulin gene rearrangement

—is a characteristic of B-cell maturation. The number of possible combinations achieved by rearrangement is almost countless; it can be assumed that each normal B cell is marked by a unique rearrangement pattern. **Neoplastic proliferation** results in large numbers of cells, all demonstrating the same pattern of immunoglobulin gene rearrangement denoting their common origin from a single cell.

—is assessed by molecular diagnostic techniques.

—since immunoglobulin heavy chain rearrangement is limited to B cells, this approach also demonstrates the B-cell origin of a tumor.

b. Indicators of monoclonality in malignancies of T-cell origin

(1) Surface antigens (markers)

—are demonstrable as T cells mature; they may be characteristic of either the stage of maturation or functional subclass. **Cellular proliferations** in which large numbers of T cells share surface markers in common are suggestive of monoclonality.

—include the CD4 antigen marking T helper cells and the CD8 antigen marking T suppressor and cytotoxic cells.

(2) T-cell receptor gene arrangement

—is analogous to immunoglobulin gene rearrangement and is used in a similar manner to demonstrate both the T-cell origin of a tumor and its monoclonality.

D. Invasion and metastasis

1. Invasion

—is aggressive infiltration of adjacent tissues by a malignant tumor.

—often extends into lymphatics and blood vessels, with the formation of tumor emboli that may be carried to distal sites. Not all tumor emboli result in metastatic tumor implants, and the presence of tumor cells within blood vessels or lymphatics indicates only the penetration of basement membranes and is not synonymous with metastasis.

2. Metastasis

—is implantation in distal sites.

a. Multi-step process of metastasis

(1) **Growth and vascularization** of the primary tumor

(2) **Invasiveness** and penetration of basement membranes into lymphatics or blood vessels

—may involve interaction of laminin of basement membranes with cellular laminin receptors, which are characteristically increased in transformed cells.

(3) **Transport and survival** of tumor cells in the circulation

(4) **Arrest of tumor emboli** in the target tissue and passage again across basement membranes

(5) **Overcoming of target tissue defense mechanisms**

(6) Development of **successful metastatic implants**

b. Preferential routes of metastasis

—vary with specific neoplasms. **Carcinomas** tend to metastasize via lymphatic spread, and **sarcomas** tend to invade blood vessels early, resulting in widespread blood-borne (hematogenous) dissemination. Exceptions include renal cell carcinoma, which is marked by early venous invasion and hematogenous dissemination.

c. Target organs

—are most commonly the liver, lungs, brain, adrenal glands, lymph nodes, and bone marrow.

—rarely include skeletal muscle or the spleen.

E. Other clinical manifestations of malignancy

—are mediated by mechanisms other than invasion and metastasis.

1. Cachexia and wasting

—origin is complex; it is characterized by weakness, weight loss, anorexia, anemia, infection, and hypermetabolism.

—may be mediated in part by **cachectin** (TNF-α), a product of macrophages that promotes catabolism of fatty tissue.

2. Endocrine abnormalities

—are caused by tumors of endocrine gland origin, which may actively elaborate hormones, leading to a variety of syndromes.

a. Pituitary abnormalities

(1) **Prolactinoma,** leading to amenorrhea, infertility, and sometimes galactorrhea

(2) **Somatotropic (acidophilic) adenoma,** leading to gigantism in children and acromegaly in adults

(3) **Corticotropic (most often basophilic) adenoma,** leading to Cushing's disease (adrenal hypercorticism of pituitary origin)

b. Adrenocortical abnormalities

−include adrenogenital syndrome, Conn's syndrome, and Cushing's syndrome of adrenal origin, resulting from adrenal cortex tumors.

c. Ovarian abnormalities

(1) Granulosa-theca cell tumor, leading to hyperestrinism

(2) Sertoli-Leydig cell tumor, leading to excess androgen production

d. Trophoblastic tissue abnormalities

−include hyperproduction of human chorionic gonadotropin from hydatidiform mole or choriocarcinoma.

3. Paraneoplastic syndromes

a. Endocrinopathies

−are caused by ectopic production of hormones or chemically unrelated substances inducing effects similar to those of a given hormone.

−include the following:

(1) Cushing's syndrome, caused by production of ACTH-like substances by small cell (oat cell) carcinoma of the lung

(2) Inappropriate secretion of antidiuretic hormone by a variety of tumors, most commonly small cell carcinoma of the lung

(3) Hypercalcemia caused by metastatic disease in bone, secretion of a substance similar to parathormone by squamous cell bronchogenic carcinoma, or secretion of a substance similar to osteoclast-activating factor by the malignant plasma cells of multiple myeloma

(4) Hypoglycemia caused by secretion of insulin-like substances by hepatocellular carcinomas, mesotheliomas, and some sarcomas

(5) Polycythemia caused by elaboration of erythropoietin by renal tumors and other neoplasms

(6) Hyperthyroidism caused by production of substances like thyroid-stimulating hormone by hydatidiform moles, choriocarcinomas, and some lung tumors

b. Neurologic abnormalities

−may occur in the absence of metastatic disease.

−include degenerative cerebral changes with dementia, cerebellar changes with resultant gait dysfunction, and peripheral neuropathies.

c. Skin lesions

−may be associated with visceral malignancies.

−include acanthosis nigricans and dermatomyositis.

d. Coagulation abnormalities

−include migratory thrombophlebitis associated with carcinoma of the pancreas and other visceral malignancies (Trousseau's phenomenon), and disseminated intravascular coagulation associated with a variety of neoplasms.

IV. Carcinogenesis and Etiology

−the transformation of normal to neoplastic cells is caused by both endogenous and exogenous factors, including chemical and physical agents, viruses, activation of cancer-promoting genes, and inhibition of cancer-suppressing genes.

A. Chemical carcinogenesis

1. Association between chemicals and cancer (Table 6.1)

2. Types of carcinogens

a. Direct-reacting carcinogens need not be chemically altered to act.

b. Indirect-reacting carcinogens require metabolic conversion from **procarcinogens** to active **ultimate carcinogens**. For example, a mucosal glucuronidase in the urinary bladder converts β-naphthylamine glucuronide to the carcinogen β-naphthylamine.

3. Stages of chemical carcinogenesis

a. Initiation

—is the first critical carcinogenic event, and it is usually a reaction between a carcinogen and DNA. Two or more agents (chemicals, viruses, radiation) may act together as **cocarcinogens**.

b. Promotion

—is induced by a stimulator of cell proliferation and enhances the carcinogenic process. A promoter, not carcinogenic in itself, enhances other agents' carcinogenicity. For example, phorbol esters react with membrane receptors, stimulating cell replication. This may enhance clonal selection, resulting in cells with increasingly deleterious DNA changes.

Table 6.1. Some Environmental Factors, Drugs, and Chemicals Associated with Human Cancer

Factor	Type of Malignancy
Cigarette smoking	Carcinoma of lung
Excess sun exposure	Squamous cell carcinoma and basal cell carcinoma of skin; melanoma
Alkylating agents	Acute leukemia
Asbestos	Carcinoma of lung; pleural and peritoneal mesothelioma; gastrointestinal tract cancers
Smoked foods rich in nitrosamines	Adenocarcinoma of stomach
Alcohol	Carcinoma of esophagus and squamous cell carcinoma of oral mucosa (especially in association with cigarette smoking)
	Hepatocellular carcinoma (in association with cirrhosis of liver)
Arsenic	Squamous cell and basal cell carcinoma of skin
Low-fiber diet	Adenocarcinoma of colon
High-fat diet	Breast carcinoma
Aniline dyes, aromatic amines, β-naphthylamine	Transitional cell carcinoma of bladder (caused by action of bladder mucosal glucuronidase on detoxified glucuronides of these compounds)
Aflatoxin B_1	Hepatocellular carcinoma
Benzene	Acute leukemia
Polyvinyl chloride	Hepatic hemangiosarcoma (angiosarcoma)
Diethylstilbestrol (DES)	Clear-cell adenocarcinoma of vagina (occurs in daughters of patients who received DES during pregnancy)
Nickel	Carcinoma of lung
Chromium	Carcinoma of lung
Uranium	Carcinoma of lung

B. Radiation carcinogenesis

1. Exposure to ultraviolet radiation

–in the form of sunlight, is clearly related to the frequency of such skin cancers as squamous cell and basal cell carcinomas and melanomas.

–is thought to act by inducing dimer formation between neighboring thymine pairs in DNA. In most instances, such dimers are successfully repaired by enzymatically mediated mechanisms. That skin cancer may be induced by such dimer formation is suggested by the markedly increased incidence of skin tumors seen in **xeroderma pigmentosum,** an autosomal recessive disorder characterized by failure of DNA repair mechanisms.

2. Ionizing radiation

–is a classic cause of cancer, exemplified by the increased incidence of cancers in those exposed to radiation.

a. Skin cancer and leukemia in radiologists

b. Lung cancer in uranium miners

c. Thyroid cancer in patients who have received head and neck radiation therapy

d. Acute and chronic myeloid (granulocytic) leukemia in survivors of atomic blasts

e. Osteosarcoma in radium watch-dial workers

C. Viral carcinogenesis (Table 6.2)

1. Virus types

a. DNA viruses

–integrate viral DNA into host genomes, perhaps resulting in host cell expression of viral mRNA coding for specific proteins.

–include human papillomavirus, herpes simplex virus type 2, Epstein-Barr virus, and hepatitis B virus as prominent suspects that play a role in human carcinogenesis.

b. Retroviruses

–are marked by transcription of viral genomic RNA sequences into DNA by action of viral reverse transcriptase.

Table 6.2. Viruses Associated with Human Malignancy

Virus	Neoplasm	Etiologic Role of Virus
HTLV-1	Adult T-cell leukemia/lymphoma	Definite
HPV	Genital tract neoplasms, especially pre-malignant lesions and cancers of the cervix and vulva	Almost certain
EBV	Nasopharyngeal carcinoma	Almost certain
	Burkitt's lymphoma	Stimulates proliferation of B cells; increases opportunity for translocation and oncogene activation
HBV	Hepatocellular carcinoma	Almost certain
HSV-2	Cervical carcinoma	Uncertain
HIV	Kaposi's sarcoma	Association definite; role of virus unclear

HTLV-1 = human T-lymphotropic virus type 1; HPV = human papillomavirus; EBV = Epstein-Barr virus; HBV = hepatitis B virus; HSV-2 = herpes simplex virus type 2; HIV = human immunodeficiency virus.

−in the case of retroviruses that are tumorigenic in experimental animals, are frequently characterized by substitutions of genomic sequences known as viral oncogenes.

2. Viral oncogenes (v-oncs)

−are named with a three-letter abbreviation, preceded by *v* **for viral**
(Table 6.3).

−exhibit homology for DNA sequences of man and other eukaryotic species; these eukaryotic DNA sequences are termed **proto-oncogenes,** or
cellular oncogenes (c-oncs), and are identified with the same three-
letter abbreviations preceded by *c* **for cellular**.

D. Oncogenes and cancer

−the protein products of proto-oncogenes play essential roles in DNA replication and transcription.

1. Mechanisms of action of oncogene protein products

a. Activation by binding of guanosine triphosphate (GTP)—*ras*
oncogenes

−code for proteins known as p21 proteins, which are functionally similar to G proteins, membrane-signaling proteins activated by GTP
binding, which mediate signal transduction from the cell surface.

(1) Characteristics—Ras proteins and G proteins

−are located at the plasma membrane and have GTP binding and
GTPase activities.

−activation by binding GTP can stimulate or depress adenylate cy-
clase activity, altering intracellular cAMP levels, thus affecting
cellular behavior.

−are inactivated by GTPase.

(2) Mutation of the *ras* gene

−usually occurs at codon 12.

−results in an aberrant p21 protein product with intact GTP binding but with a loss of GTPase activity. Mutant Ras proteins can be
activated by GTP binding but cannot be inactivated by GTPase activity.

Table 6.3. Examples of Retroviral Oncogenes

Oncogene	Source
v-*src*	Rous sarcoma virus of chickens
v-*abl*	Abelson murine leukemia virus
v-*sis*	Simian sarcoma virus
v-*myc*	MC29 viral isolate from chickens
v-H-*ras*	Harvey rat sarcoma virus
v-K-*ras*	Kirsten rat sarcoma virus
v-*erb*	Erythroblastosis virus of chickens
v-*fms*	Feline McDonough sarcoma virus
v-*fos*	FBJ osteosarcoma virus of mice
v-*ros*	UR2 avian sarcoma virus
v-*myb*	Avian myeloblastosis virus

b. Protein tyrosine kinase activity

—is exhibited by the following:

(1) The oncogene product of the Rous sarcoma virus (designated as pp60^{src})

(2) Other oncogene products, usually oncogenic analogs of transmembrane receptor proteins

c. Growth factor or growth factor receptor activity

—alterations in expression or structural changes in oncogene products may result in inappropriate activation of receptor proteins or their oncogenic analogs, thus mimicking the actions of growth factors.

(1) On stimulation with the appropriate growth factor, receptor proteins often demonstrate tyrosine kinase activity of their cytoplasmic domains.

(2) Significant homologies occur between several oncogenes and the genes for cellular growth factors and their receptors. For example:

(a) v-*sis* and the gene for the β chain of platelet-derived growth factor

(b) v-*erb* and the gene for the epidermal growth factor (EGF) receptor

(c) v-*fms* and the gene for the colony stimulating factor-1 receptor

(d) c-*neu* and the gene for the EGF receptor

d. Nuclear proteins

—some oncogene products, including the protein products of *myc, fos,* and *myb,* are confined to the cell nucleus.

2. Oncogenes and human cancer

—mechanisms by which c-oncs become tumorigenic include the following:

a. Promoter insertion (insertional mutagenesis)

(1) Insertion of retroviral promoter or enhancer sequences into the host genome can lead to increased expression of a nearby oncogene.

(2) This mechanism is similar to the promoter-induced hyperexpression associated with translocations characteristic of several human leukemias and lymphomas.

b. Point mutations

—are exemplified by single nucleotide changes in codon 12 of the *ras* family of genes associated with a number of human tumors.

c. Chromosomal translocation

—frequent association with malignancy seen in these genetic rearrangements has been clarified by demonstrating that important genes are situated at the sites of chromosomal breaks. For example:

(1) 8:14 translocation and Burkitt's lymphoma

—the c-*myc* proto-oncogene on chromosome 8 is transposed to a site adjacent to the immunoglobulin heavy chain locus on chromosome 14. Major regulatory sequences within the immunoglobulin gene are thought to increase the expression of c-*myc*.

(2) 14;18 translocation and follicular lymphoma
   —the immunoglobulin heavy chain locus on chromosome 14 is transposed to a site adjacent to *bcl-2,* an oncogene on chromosome 18, resulting in enhanced expression of *bcl-2*.
(3) 9;22 translocation and chronic myeloid leukemia (CML)
   —the c-*abl* proto-oncogene on chromosome 9 is transposed to a site adjacent to *bcr* (breakpoint cluster region), an oncogene on chromosome 22.
   (a) The union of *bcr* and *abl* results in a **hybrid,** or chimeric, ***bcr-abl*** fusion gene that codes for a protein with increased tyrosine kinase activity.
   (b) The altered chromosome carrying this hybrid gene, the **Philadelphia chromosome,** can be demonstrated by cytogenetic techniques in hematopoietic cells of patients with CML.

d. Gene amplification
   —is reduplication of the gene, with multiple resultant genomic DNA copies, and can sometimes result in a thousand or more copies of the amplified gene.
   —extensive amplification can result in small free chromosome-like bodies termed **double minute (DM) chromosomes** or in band-like structures within chromosomes termed **homogeneously staining regions (HSRs),** which are both demonstrable cytogenetically.
   —is demonstrable in several human neoplasms.
   (1) Neuroblastoma is an aggressive childhood tumor characterized by marked N-*myc* amplification that correlates inversely with the degree of differentiation of the neuroblastoma cells.
   (2) Some breast cancers are marked by amplification of the HER-2/*neu* oncogene. Such amplification is correlated with poor prognosis.

3. Cancer suppressor genes (anti-oncogenes)
   —in contrast to the preceding mechanisms, cancer suppressor genes promote cellular proliferation when the gene is inactivated (most often by deletion). A single residual copy of the anti-oncogene suppresses tumor formation, but homozygous inactivation (loss of function of both copies) promotes the expression of the neoplastic phenotype.
   a. The prototype is **retinoblastoma,** an intraocular childhood tumor caused by inactivation of the *rb* gene. The **"two-hit" hypothesis of Knudson** holds that two mutagenic events are required to induce alterations on both chromosomes.
   (1) In the familial forms of retinoblastoma, the gene on one chromosome in the germ line is inactivated or deleted, and the gene on the other chromosome is affected by a somatic mutation.
   (2) In sporadic nonfamilial cases of retinoblastoma, both deletions occur as somatic mutations.
   b. Inactivation of the *rb* gene is also a factor in the genesis of other tumors, especially **osteosarcoma,** which often occurs following successful surgical cure of familial retinoblastoma.
   c. An anti-oncogene (WT-1) localized to chromosome 11 is operative in **Wilms' tumor,** the most common renal neoplasm of children. Other

cancer suppressor genes (p53, NF-1, APC, and DCC) play a role in the pathogenesis of a wide variety of other tumors.

E. Epidemiology

–important epidemiologic factors include geographic and racial differences, heredity, age, sex and hormonal differences, dietary factors, environmental toxins, and infection (see Table 6.1).

V. Grading and Staging

–are clinical measures used for prognostic evaluation and planning of clinical management.

A. Grading

–is histopathologic evaluation of the lesion based on the **degree of cellular differentiation.**

B. Staging

–is clinical assessment of the **degree of localization** or spread of the tumor.

–generally correlates better with prognosis than does histopathologic grading. However, both approaches are useful.

–is exemplified by the generalized **TNM system,** which evaluates size and extent of tumor (**T**), lymph node involvement (**N**), and metastasis (**M**).

–is sometimes oriented toward specific tumors, as exemplified by the **Dukes system** for colorectal carcinoma and the **Ann Arbor system** for Hodgkin's disease and non-Hodgkin's lymphomas.

Review Test

Directions: Each of the numbered items or incomplete statements in this section is followed by answers or by completions of the statement. Select the **one** lettered answer or completion that is **best** in each case.

1. Reversible disorderly maturation with variability in size, shape, and polarity of cells is

(A) metaplasia.
(B) dysplasia.
(C) anaplasia.
(D) hyperplasia.
(E) desmoplasia.

2. Which one of the following characteristics is MOST definitive of malignancy?

(A) Lack of differentiation
(B) Metastasis
(C) Pleomorphism
(D) Abnormal mitoses
(E) Increase in nuclear–cytoplasmic ratio

3. Which of the following terms refers to a malignant tumor of mesenchymal tissue?

(A) Carcinoma
(B) Choristoma
(C) Hamartoma
(D) Sarcoma
(E) Teratoma

4. A biopsy of the stomach reveals an area of normal-appearing pancreatic tissue. This is an example of which of the following lesions?

(A) Adenoma
(B) Choristoma
(C) Hamartoma
(D) Metastatic carcinoma
(E) Teratoma

5. Properties of transformed cells in tissue culture include all of the following EXCEPT

(A) loss of adhesion.
(B) increased contact inhibition.
(C) chromosomal aneuploidy.
(D) production of surface proteases.
(E) reduced cell-surface fibronectin.

6. Clinical evidence supporting the monoclonality of tumors can be derived from evaluation of all of the following substances EXCEPT

(A) G6PD isoenzymes.
(B) immunoglobulin light chains.
(C) immunoglobulin or T-cell receptor genes.
(D) laminin receptors.
(E) serum proteins.

7. All of the following statements about carcinogenesis are true EXCEPT

(A) chemical carcinogenesis is usually a multistep phenomenon.
(B) initiators cause irreversible damage to DNA.
(C) promoters of carcinogenesis induce cell proliferation.
(D) promoters of carcinogenesis exert their effect before initiation.

8. All of the following chemical carcinogens are correctly paired with the associated tumor EXCEPT

(A) β-naphthylamine—bladder cancer.
(B) polyvinyl chloride—hepatic hemangiosarcoma.
(C) aflatoxin B_1—gastric cancer.
(D) DES in mothers—vaginal clear-cell adenocarcinoma in daughters.
(E) arsenic—skin cancer.

9. The increased incidence of skin tumors associated with xeroderma pigmentosum is caused by

(A) defective DNA repair.
(B) oncogene activation by chromosome translocation.
(C) reverse transcriptase-mediated copying of viral RNA genome.
(D) accumulation of substances toxic to DNA.
(E) failure of antigen presentation by Langerhans' cells of the skin.

10. All of the following viral agents are correctly paired with the associated tumor EXCEPT

(A) HTLV-1—adult T-cell leukemia/lymphoma.
(B) human papillomavirus (HPV)—genital condyloma.
(C) Epstein-Barr virus—carcinoma of the cervix.
(D) hepatitis B virus—hepatocellular carcinoma.

11. Which of the following neoplasms is associated with gene amplification?

(A) Burkitt's lymphoma
(B) Chronic myeloid leukemia
(C) Follicular lymphoma
(D) Neuroblastoma
(E) Retinoblastoma

12. All of the following statements about neoplasms are true EXCEPT

(A) carcinomas tend to spread by lymphatic invasion.
(B) sarcomas tend to spread hematogenously.
(C) the microscopic demonstration of tumor cells in blood vessels is not a reliable indicator of metastasis.
(D) the spleen is a common site of metastasis.
(E) skeletal muscle is an uncommon site of metastasis.

13. Which of the following characteristics is the most reliable indicator of prognosis of malignant tumors?

(A) Abnormal mitoses
(B) Degree of differentiation
(C) Degree of localization
(D) Presence of nucleoli
(E) Size of tumor

14. Clinical findings of adrenal hypercorticism in a patient without a pituitary or adrenal neoplasm are most suggestive of

(A) small cell carcinoma of the lung.
(B) adenocarcinoma of the lung.
(C) hepatocellular carcinoma.
(D) squamous cell carcinoma of the cervix.
(E) renal cell carcinoma.

15. Which one of the following malignant neoplasms is correctly paired with the appropriate paraneoplastic manifestation?

(A) Adrenal cortical carcinoma—hyperuricemia
(B) Glioblastoma multiforme—hyperglycemia
(C) Hepatocellular carcinoma—polycythemia
(D) Renal cell carcinoma—hypokalemia
(E) Squamous cell carcinoma of the lung—hypercalcemia

Answers and Explanations

1–B. Dysplasia is a reversible, sometimes premalignant tissue change characterized by pleomorphism, changes in spatial orientation of cells, and increased mitotic activity. The prototype is cervical dysplasia, where the changes ordinarily do not extend beyond the inner two-thirds of the epithelium.

2–B. Metastasis is the single most important defining characteristic of malignancy.

3–D. A sarcoma is a malignant tumor of mesenchymal origin.

4–B. An area of normal-appearing pancreatic tissue in the stomach is an example of a choristoma, which is an area of normal tissue within another organ.

5–B. Loss of contact inhibition is one of the most striking characteristics of transformed cells in tissue culture. In marked contrast to normal cells, these cells continue to grow even when touching one another. This may be mediated by reduced cell-surface fibronectin, which may have a role in contact-mediated growth control. Transformed cells demonstrate loss of adhesion, tending to grow separately rather than in clusters. Aneuploidy with increased DNA content is characteristic, as is the production of cell-surface proteases considered to possibly facilitate invasiveness.

6–D. Laminin receptors have no relationship to the monoclonality of tumors. Clinical evidence supporting the monoclonality of tumors can be derived from evaluating substances such as G6PD isoenzymes, immunoglobulin light chains, immunoglobulin or T-cell receptor genes, and serum proteins.

7–D. Carcinogenesis occurs in multiple steps. Initiation, the first carcinogenic event, is almost always a reaction between a direct-reacting, or ultimate, carcinogen and DNA. Promoters act at a later stage by stimulating increased cellular replication.

8–C. Aflatoxin B_1 toxicity, along with hepatitis B virus infection, is strongly suspected to be responsible for the prevalence of hepatocellular carcinoma in Africa and Southeast Asia.

9–A. Ultraviolet light is thought to enhance neoplastic change in the skin by dimer formation between neighboring thymine pairs in DNA. These deleterious changes in DNA are repaired by enzymatically mediated mechanisms. In xeroderma pigmentosum, specific enzyme deficiencies result in failure of such repair and in a consequent increase in the tumorigenic effect of sunlight.

10–C. Epstein-Barr virus, the etiologic agent of infectious mononucleosis, has been closely linked with both Burkitt's lymphoma and nasopharyngeal carcinoma. Cervical carcinoma has been linked somewhat less definitively with HPV and perhaps with herpes simplex virus type 2. HPV is also associated with ordinary warts, such as those which occur on the fingers, and genital warts (condylomas). HTLV-1 has a clear association with the adult T-cell leukemia/lymphoma syndrome, and the hepatitis B virus is associated with hepatocellular carcinoma.

11–D. Neuroblastoma, a frequently occurring adrenal tumor of early childhood, is associated with marked amplification of the N-*myc* oncogene. The reduplication is so marked that it can often be visualized in karyotypic preparations.

12–D. In spite of its vascularity, the spleen is a rare site of metastasis for most tumors. Skeletal muscle and the myocardium are similarly spared. In contrast, frequent sites of metastasis include the liver, lung, adrenal gland, brain, lymph nodes, and bone marrow. Although there are many exceptions, carcinomas tend to spread by way of lymphatics, and sarcomas by way of vascular invasion with distal spread. Since metastasis involves not only transport of tumor cells, but also successful implantation and growth in the new site, the presence of tumor cells within vascular channels is not in itself evidence of metastasis.

13–C. The degree of tumor localization is the basis of staging, which, in general, correlates better with prognosis than does histopathologic grading, which is based on differentiation and other morphologic changes.

14–A. The elaboration of ACTH-like substances by small cell carcinoma of the lung is the classic example of a paraneoplastic syndrome. These manifestations of some tumors are caused by ectopic production of either hormones or chemically unrelated compounds with similar hormonal effects.

15–E. Squamous cell carcinoma of the lung is often associated with secretion of parathyroid hormone-like substances, with resultant hypercalcemia.

7

Environmental Pathology

I. Physical Injury

A. Mechanical injury

–can be caused by a variety of means, such as blunt force, sharp objects, or bullets.

–can produce damage by cutting, tearing, or crushing of tissues; by severe blood loss; or by interruption of blood or air supply.

1. Terminology

a. Abrasion or scrape—a superficial tearing away of epidermal cells

b. Laceration—a jagged tear, often with stretching of the underlying tissue

c. Incision—a clean cut by a sharp object

d. Puncture—a deep tubular wound produced by a sharp, thin object

e. Contusion—a bruise caused by disruption of underlying small blood vessels; commonly involves the skin but may also involve internal organs.

2. Causes of death

a. Hemorrhage into body cavities

b. Fat embolism from bone fractures

c. Ruptured viscera

d. Secondary infection

e. Renal shutdown caused by acute tubular necrosis, especially when associated with myoglobin casts arising from crush injury of skeletal muscle

3. Blunt force injuries

a. Head injury

  (1) Brain damage, with possible skull fracture; can be the direct result of cerebral trauma or caused by intracranial hemorrhage.

    (2) Brain laceration, caused by fracture with penetrating injury by skull fragments.

    (3) Brain contusion, which may occur at the point of impact (**coup injury**) or on the opposite side of the brain (**contrecoup injury**).

b. Abdominal injury

    —may result in the following conditions:

    (1) Contusion

    (2) Rupture of the spleen or liver, sometimes with severe hemorrhage

    (3) Rupture of the intestine, which can result in **peritonitis**

c. Thoracic injury

    —may result in the following conditions:

    (1) Rib fracture, possibly with penetration into pulmonary parenchyma or thoracic wall vessels

    (2) Hemothorax, or hemorrhage in the pleural cavity

    (3) Pneumothorax, or air in the pleural cavity

4. Knife and stab wounds

—can be incisions or puncture wounds.

—result in highly variable consequences, depending on the site of the injury.

5. Gunshot wounds

—are characterized by the following:

a. The entrance wound is usually smaller and rounder than the exit wound (and in some instances even smaller than the bullet) in through-and-through gunshot injuries. In contact wounds overlying unyielding bony surfaces such as the skull, the reverse is often true because of tearing and disruption of the skin due to expanding gases.

b. Tattooing and discoloration of the skin from gunpowder and heat characterize wounds from guns fired at distances of 20 inches or less.

B. Thermal injury

1. Burns

a. Classification

    (1) First-degree burns (partial-thickness burns)

    —are characterized by hyperemia without significant epidermal damage; they generally heal without intervention.

    (2) Second-degree burns (partial-thickness burns)

    —are characterized by blistering and destruction of epidermis with slight damage to underlying dermis; they generally heal without intervention.

    (3) Third-degree burns (full-thickness burns)

    —are characterized by damage to the epidermis, dermis, and dermal appendages; skin and underlying tissue often are charred and blackened; these burns often require skin grafting.

b. Complications

    (1) Inhalation of smoke or toxic fumes, resulting in pulmonary or systemic damage

(2) **Hypovolemia,** which results from fluid and electrolyte loss

(3) **Infection,** most often with *Pseudomonas aeruginosa*

(4) **Curling's ulcer** (acute gastric ulcer associated with severe burns)

2. Freezing (hypothermia)

—may be generalized, resulting in **death**.

—may be localized, resulting in **frostbite;** usually affects exposed areas such as fingers, toes, earlobes, or nose.

—severe, prolonged frostbite may result in **intracellular ice crystals, intravascular thrombosis,** and sometimes local **gangrene**.

C. Electrical injury

—occurs when electric current passes through an individual, thus completing an electric circuit. Fatal electrical injury is usually caused by current passing through the brain or heart.

—may cause **respiratory or cardiac arrest** or **cardiac arrhythmias**.

—may result in small **cutaneous burns** at the point of entry or exit of the electric current. At times thermal injury may be severe.

D. Radiation injury

1. Ultraviolet light (sunlight)

—causes **sunburn,** which is characterized by erythema, often with superficial desquamation and, in severe cases, blister formation.

—is associated with premalignant cutaneous lesions (**actinic keratosis**) and malignant cutaneous lesions such as **squamous and basal cell carcinomas and melanoma**.

2. Ionizing radiation

—is from x-ray, radioactive waste, nuclear disasters, and so on.

—damages cells by forming toxic free radicals, affecting vital cell components such as DNA and intracellular membranes.

a. Localized radiation results in the following conditions:

(1) **Skin changes** such as dermatitis, ulceration, and skin malignancies

(2) **Pulmonary changes,** including acute changes similar to those of adult respiratory distress syndrome; and chronic changes, such as septal fibrosis, bronchiolar metaplasia, and hyaline thickening of blood vessel walls

(3) **Gastrointestinal inflammation and ulceration**

(4) **Hematopoietic alterations,** including bone marrow depression or leukemia

b. Severe and generalized radiation

(1) Occurs in whole body irradiation such as that seen in nuclear disasters

(2) **Severe central nervous system (CNS) injury** primarily caused by capillary damage

(3) **Gastrointestinal mucosal denudation**

(4) **Acute bone marrow failure**

3. Radiosensitivity of specialized cells
—see Table 7.1 for cell types and characteristics.

II. Chemical Abuse

A. Alcohol abuse
—is an important cause of death and disability from a number of causes ranging from automobile accidents to homicides.

—is characterized by a constellation of changes that are collectively grouped as **chronic alcoholism**. Common pathologic findings include:

1. Alcoholic hepatitis and cirrhosis

2. Pancreatitis

3. Gastritis

4. Oral and esophageal carcinoma

5. Alcoholic cardiomyopathy

6. Aspiration pneumonia

7. Peripheral neuropathy

8. Cerebral dysfunction, such as thiamine deficiency–mediated Wernicke-Korsakoff syndrome, sometimes referred to as alcoholic encephalopathy

B. Drug abuse

1. Cocaine
—can result in the following effects and complications:

a. Mood elevation, sometimes followed by irritability, anxiety, and depression, which may lead to suicide

b. Increased myocardial irritability, which can lead to fatal arrhythmias

c. Hypertension, which can predispose to cerebral hemorrhage

d. Nasal congestion, ulceration, or septal perforation, from intranasal use

e. Burn injury, due to volatile inflammable substances used in cocaine free-base preparation

Table 7.1. Radiosensitivity of Specialized Cells

Degree of Sensitivity	Types	Characteristics
Radiosensitive	Lymphoid, hematopoietic, germ, gastrointestinal mucosal, rapidly dividing tumor cells	Regularly actively divide, especially those cells undergoing mitosis
Intermediate radiosensitivity	Fibroblasts; cells of endothelium, elastic tissue, salivary glands, eye	. . .
Radioresistant	Cells of bone, cartilage, muscle, central nervous system, kidney, liver, and most endocrine glands	Cease division shortly after fetal development is complete

    f. Viral (HIV or hepatitis B) or **bacterial** (infective endocarditis) **infection** (from intravenous use). Infective endocarditis due to intravenous drug abuse often involves valves of the right side of the heart.

    g. Epileptic seizures, respiratory arrest, myocardial infarction, and, in newborns of addicted mothers, multiple small cerebral infarcts

2. Heroin

  —is usually administered intravenously and can result in the following effects and complications:

    a. Physical dependence, with severe withdrawal symptoms

    b. Infections, such as HIV, hepatitis B, and infective endocarditis

    c. Adult respiratory distress syndrome

    d. Death from respiratory or cardiac arrest or from pulmonary edema

III. Environmental Chemical Injuries (Table 7.2)

A. Methyl alcohol (methanol)

  —is converted to the cellular toxins formaldehyde and formic acid, resulting in transient metabolic acidosis.

  —damages the cells of the retina, optic nerve, and CNS, resulting in **blindness**.

B. Carbon monoxide (CO)

  —inhibits the capacity of hemoglobin to function as an oxygen carrier because hemoglobin has an affinity for CO that is 200 times greater than its affinity for oxygen.

  —can result in severe **hypoxic injury,** often leading to death; neurons of the brain are most vulnerable. Foci of neuronal necrosis in the basal ganglia, lenticular nuclei, and cortical gray areas are characteristic.

  —when fatal, causes a **cherry-red color of the skin, blood, viscera, and muscles**.

C. Carbon tetrachloride (CCl₄)

  —induces **centrilobular necrosis and fatty change** in the liver.

Table 7.2. Some Environmental Toxins and Their Effects

Toxin	Predominant Adverse Effects
Methyl alcohol	Blindness
Carbon monoxide	Severe hypoxic injury caused by displacement of oxyhemoglobin by carboxyhemoglobin
Carbon tetrachloride	Hepatic centrilobular necrosis and fatty change
Cyanide	Cessation of intracellular oxidation because of cytochrome oxidase inhibition
Lead	Anemia; basophilic stippling of erythrocytes; encephalopathy; neuropathy; lead line; Fanconi's syndrome
Mercuric chloride	Gastrointestinal ulcerations; calcification and necrosis of renal convoluted tubules

D. Cyanide

–**inhibits intracellular cytochrome oxidase** by binding with ferric iron, thereby preventing cellular oxidation. **Death** results within minutes.

–generalized petechial hemorrhages and a scent of bitter almonds are noted at autopsy.

E. Lead

–may be **ingested,** particularly from lead in paint, or may be **inspired,** particularly from automotive emissions.

–when ingested or inhaled in toxic amounts, is manifested clinically by:

1. Red cell changes

a. Basophilic stippling

b. Hypochromic microcytic anemia

–is caused by deficient heme synthesis mediated by the inhibition of **delta-aminolevulinic acid (ALA) dehydratase** and by decreased incorporation of iron into heme.

–defects result in accumulation of both ALA and erythrocyte protoporphyrin, leading to increased urinary excretion of ALA and coproporphyrin.

2. Encephalopathy, characterized by irritability and sometimes by seizures and coma

3. Neuropathy, characterized by wristdrop and footdrop

4. Fanconi's syndrome, characterized by impaired proximal renal tubular reabsorption of phosphate, glucose, and amino acids

5. Lead line, characterized by mucosal deposits of lead sulfide at the junction of the teeth and gums

6. Increased radiodensity of the epiphyses of the long bones

F. Mercuric chloride

–when ingested, results in **focal gastrointestinal ulceration and severe renal damage** with widespread necrosis and calcification of the convoluted tubules.

G. Polychlorinated biphenyls (PCBs)

–are nonbiodegradable **environmental pollutants** that were used in the manufacture of a variety of products such as adhesives and plasticizers. Because of their toxicity, their production is now outlawed.

–exposure produces a syndrome of chloracne, impotence, and visual changes.

IV. Adverse Effects of Therapeutic Drugs

–can be manifest by a wide variety of clinically significant abnormalities. For example:

A. Antibiotics

1. Development of drug-resistant organisms

–are often mediated by plasmids carrying specific drug-resistant genes.

2. Fatal aplastic anemia

–can occur as a result of an idiosyncratic reaction to chloramphenicol.

B. **Sulfonamides**

1. **Immune complex disease,** such as polyarteritis nodosa, which can develop when sulfonamides, acting as haptens, stimulate antibody production

2. **Crystallization of sulfonamides within the renal collecting system,** causing calculi with obstruction, infection, or both

3. **Bone marrow failure**

4. **Acute, self-limited hemolytic anemia**
   —may be induced in individuals with erythrocyte glucose-6-phosphate dehydrogenase (G6PD) deficiency.

C. **Analgesics**

1. **Aspirin**

   a. **Gastroduodenal bleeding**
      —may be caused by aspirin-induced gastritis or peptic ulcer or by inhibition of platelet cyclooxygenase with resultant thromboxane A_2 deficiency and impaired platelet plug formation.

   b. **Reye's syndrome**
      —occurs in children following an acute febrile viral illness, almost always in association with aspirin intake.
      —is characterized by microvesicular fatty change in the liver and encephalopathy.

   c. **Allergic reactions,** including urticaria, asthma, nasal polyps, and angioneurotic edema

2. **Phenacetin**

   a. **Chronic analgesic nephritis and renal papillary necrosis** (the drug has been withdrawn from the U.S. market)

   b. **Urothelial neoplasms,** especially transitional cell carcinoma of the renal pelvis

   c. **Acute hemolysis** in G6PD-deficient individuals

D. **Cancer chemotherapeutic drugs**

1. **Toxic effects,** including hair loss, gastrointestinal erosions and ulcerations, and, most significantly, bone marrow failure

2. **Acute leukemia or other malignancies**

Review Test

Directions: Each of the numbered items or incomplete statements in this section is followed by answers or by completions of the statement. Select the **one** lettered answer or completion that is **best** in each case.

1. Each of the following associations of an injury and a consequence is correct EXCEPT

(A) head trauma—contrecoup injury.
(B) contact gunshot wound to skull—exit wound larger than entry wound.
(C) multiple fractures—fat embolism.
(D) crush injury of skeletal muscle—acute tubular necrosis.
(E) severe burns—acute gastric ulcer.

2. All of the following cell types are radiosensitive EXCEPT

(A) muscle cells.
(B) lymphoid cells.
(C) hematopoietic cells.
(D) gastrointestinal mucosal cells.
(E) germ cells.

3. Each of the following clinical manifestations is correctly paired with the drug most likely associated with it EXCEPT

(A) arrhythmia—cocaine.
(B) gastroduodenal bleeding—aspirin.
(C) AIDS—heroin.
(D) peripheral neuropathy—chloramphenicol.
(E) immune complex disease—sulfonamides.

4. Each of the following environmental chemical agents is correctly matched with the appropriate manifestation EXCEPT

(A) carbon monoxide—cherry-red color of skin.
(B) carbon tetrachloride—hepatocellular damage.
(C) mercuric chloride—odor of bitter almonds.
(D) methyl alcohol—blindness.
(E) lead—basophilic stippling of red cells.

Answers and Explanations

1–B. In contact gunshot wounds overlying unyielding bony surfaces such as the skull, the entry wound is often larger than the exit wound, due to the effect of expanding gases under the skin. This is in contrast to through-and-through gunshot wounds, where the reverse is true. Brain contusion in head injuries can occur at the point of impact (coup injury) or on the opposite side of the brain (contrecoup injury). Multiple fractures can be complicated by fat emboli. Skeletal muscle crush injury can result in acute tubular necrosis with myoglobin casts. Severe burns may be associated with acute ulceration of the gastric mucosa referred to as Curling's ulcer.

2–A. Muscle cells are radioresistant. In contrast, lymphoid cells, hematopoietic cells, gastrointestinal mucosal cells, and germ cells are radiosensitive.

3–D. Peripheral neuropathy is one of the common pathologic findings associated with chronic alcoholism. Fatal aplastic anemia can result from an idiosyncratic reaction to chloramphenicol.

4–C. Mercuric chloride poisoning is characterized by severe renal tubular necrosis and calcification and gastrointestinal ulceration. The odor of bitter almonds is a manifestation of cyanide poisoning.

8

Nutritional Disorders

I. Malnutrition

A. In affluent countries, malnutrition is found in children living below the poverty level, the elderly, alcoholics, persons on fad diets and with anorexia nervosa, and patients with severe wasting diseases.

B. In developing countries, protein–calorie malnutrition occurs in two forms, marasmus and kwashiorkor.

1. Marasmus

—is caused by widespread **deficiency of almost all nutrients,** notably protein and calories.

—often coexists with vitamin deficiencies.

—typically occurs in children under 1 year of age who are deprived of breast-feeding and do not have an adequate intake of substitute nutrients.

—is clinically characterized by retarded growth and loss of muscle and other protein-containing tissue, as well as subcutaneous fat ("wasting away").

2. Kwashiorkor

—is caused by **protein deficiency** but with adequate caloric intake.

—usually affects children over 1 year of age who are no longer breast-fed and receive a starch-rich, protein-poor diet.

—is clinically characterized by retarded growth and muscle wasting, caused by inadequate protein intake, but with preservation of subcutaneous fat.

—is distinguished from marasmus by the presence of the following abnormalities:

a. Fatty liver

b. Severe edema

c. Anemia

d. Malabsorption due to atrophy of the small intestinal villi

II. Vitamins

A. Water-soluble vitamins (Table 8.1)

–include the **B complex vitamins:** B_1 (thiamine), B_2 (riboflavin), B_3 (niacin), B_6 (pyridoxine), and B_{12} (cobalamin); folic acid; and vitamin C (ascorbic acid).

–are not stored in the body; thus, regular intake is essential, except for vitamin B_{12}. Vitamin B_{12} is stored in the liver in quantities sufficiently large so that deprivation for months or years is necessary for a deficiency to develop.

–rarely cause toxicity from excessive intake since excess vitamin is excreted in the urine.

Table 8.1 Water-Soluble Vitamins

Vitamin	Metabolic Functions	Clinical Manifestations of Deficiency
Vitamin B_1 (thiamine)	Coenzyme thiamine pyrophosphate plays a key role in carbohydrate and amino acid intermediary metabolism	Wet beriberi; dry beriberi; Wernicke-Korsakoff syndrome
Vitamin B_2 (riboflavin)	Component of FAD and FMN and is essential in a variety of oxidation-reduction processes	Cheilosis; corneal vascularization; glossitis; dermatitis
Vitamin B_3 (niacin, nicotinic acid)	Component of NAD and NADP, essential to glycolysis, citric acid cycle, and to a variety of oxidations (can be synthesized from tryptophan); deficiency requires diet lacking both niacin and tryptophan	Pellagra
Vitamin B_6 (pyridoxine)	Required for transamination, porphyrin synthesis, synthesis of niacin from tryptophan	Cheilosis; glossitis; anemia; convulsions in infants; neurologic dysfunction
Vitamin B_{12} (cyanocobalamin)	1-carbon transfers required for folate synthesis and activation of FH_4; $N^{5,10}$-methylene FH_4 is required for conversion of dUMP to dTMP in DNA synthesis	Megaloblastic anemia; neurologic dysfunction
Folic acid	1-carbon transfers in a number of metabolic reactions; $N^{5,10}$-methylene FH_4 required for DNA synthesis	Megaloblastic anemia; neurologic dysfunction is not a feature (as it is in vitamin B_{12} deficiency)
Vitamin C (ascorbic acid)	Required for hydroxylation of proline and lysine, which are essential for collagen synthesis; hydroxylation of dopamine in synthesis of norepinephrine; enhances maintenance of reduced state of other metabolically active agents, such as iron and FH_4	Scurvy, defective formation of mesenchymal tissue and osteoid matrix; defective wound healing; hemorrhagic phenomena

FAD = flavin adenine dinucleotide; FMN = flavin mononucleotide; NAD = nicotinamide adenine dinucleotide; NADP = nicotinamide adenine dinucleotide phosphate; FH_4 = tetrahydrofolate; $N^{5,10}$-methylene FH_4 = activated tetrahydrofolate.

1. **Dietary sources**

   a. **B complex vitamins** (except vitamin B_{12}): whole grain cereals, green leafy vegetables, fish, meat, and dairy foods

   b. **Vitamin B_{12}:** foods of animal origin only (vitamin B_{12} is synthesized by intestinal bacteria in animals)

   c. **Folic acid:** leafy vegetables, cereals, fruits, and a number of animal products

   d. **Vitamin C:** fruits (especially citrus fruits and tomatoes), vegetables, a variety of meats, and milk

2. **Deficiencies**

   —result in a shared group of clinical manifestations.

   —in B complex vitamins are often marked by glossitis, dermatitis, and diarrhea.

   —are manifested clinically most strikingly in tissues with active metabolism because these vitamins are involved in the release and storage of energy.

   a. **Vitamin B_1 (thiamine) deficiency**

      —is most often associated with severe malnutrition. (In Western countries, it is usually associated with alcoholism and with fad diets.)

      —results in three distinct syndromes:

      (1) **Dry beriberi**

         —is characterized by **peripheral neuropathy** with resultant atrophy of the muscles of the extremities.

      (2) **Wet beriberi**

         —is marked by **high output cardiac failure**.

         —results from peripheral dilatation of arterioles and capillaries, leading to increased arteriovenous shunting, hypervolemia, and cardiac dilation.

      (3) **Wernicke-Korsakoff syndrome**

         —results from degenerative changes in the brain stem and diencephalon, with involvement of cortical and bilateral **paramedian masses of gray matter** and the **mamillary bodies**.

         —is characterized by **confusion, ataxia,** and **ophthalmoplegia** (Wernicke's triad) and by marked memory loss and **confabulation**.

   b. **Vitamin B_2 (riboflavin) deficiency**

      —is rare in the United States since riboflavin is almost always added to commercially prepared bread and cereals.

      —occurs in chronic alcoholics, fad dieters, the elderly, and in persons with chronic debilitating diseases.

      —manifests clinically by **cheilosis** (skin fissures at the angles of the mouth), **glossitis, corneal vascularization,** and **seborrheic dermatitis** of the face, the scrotum, or the vulva.

   c. **Vitamin B_3 (niacin) deficiency**

      —develops only when the diet lacks both niacin and tryptophan (niacin can be synthesized from the essential amino acid tryptophan). Niacin is a component of the nicotinamide adenine dinucleotides (NAD and NADPH) and as such is essential to glycolysis, the citric acid cycle, and other metabolic processes.

—is manifest clinically as **pellagra,** which is characterized by the "three Ds": **dementia, dermatitis,** and **diarrhea.** Dermatitis affects exposed areas, such as the face and neck and the dorsa of the hands and feet.

d. Vitamin B₆ (pyridoxine) deficiency

—may cause convulsions in infants, due to increased activity of pyridoxal-dependent glutamate decarboxylase, which leads to deficient production of γ-aminobutyric acid (GABA), a neurotransmitter.

—results in clinical manifestations similar to those of vitamin B₂ (riboflavin) deficiency.

—is uncommon but occurs in the following conditions:

(1) Chronic alcoholism

(2) Association with therapeutic drugs, such as isonicotinic acid hydrazide (INH, an antituberculous agent), which react as competitive inhibitors for pyridoxine binding sites

(3) A variety of syndromes characterized by an increased need for pyridoxine, including:

    (a) Homocystinuria, an inborn error of metabolism

    (b) Pyridoxine-responsive anemia, a microcytic anemia characterized by reduced heme synthesis

e. Vitamin B₁₂ (cobalamin) deficiency

—results in a marked reduction in DNA replication and cell division.

—is manifest clinically by **megaloblastic anemia** with prominent neurologic dysfunction.

—is almost always caused by malabsorption, but may occur in strict vegetarians.

(1) The most common malabsorption disease is **pernicious anemia,** in which there is a lack of gastric intrinsic factor, a carrier protein essential to vitamin B₁₂ absorption in the terminal small bowel.

(2) Less commonly, malabsorption can result from a number of diverse causes, including Crohn's disease (which often affects the terminal ileum), blind loop syndrome, and *Diphyllobothrium latum* (giant fish tapeworm) infestation.

f. Folic acid deficiency

—is most commonly of dietary origin, often occurring in alcoholics and fad dieters.

—can be secondary to intestinal malabsorption.

—can occur, without gross dietary deprivation, as a relative deficiency because of increased demand for folate (e.g., in pregnancy and in hemolytic anemia, which is due to shortening of red blood cell life span).

—is sometimes secondary to cancer chemotherapy containing folic acid antagonists.

—results in **megaloblastic anemia**.

g. Vitamin C (ascorbic acid) deficiency

—is characterized by defective formation of mesenchymal tissue and osteoid matrix due to **impaired synthesis of hydroxyproline and hydroxylysine,** for which vitamin C is a cofactor. Poor collagen formation contributes to **impaired wound healing**. Defective connective tissue also leads to fragile capillaries, resulting in **abnormal bleeding**.

—results in **scurvy,** characterized by muscle, joint, and bone pain; swollen, bleeding gums; subperiosteal hemorrhage; and perifollicular petechial hemorrhages. Bone changes in scurvy are secondary to **defective osteoid matrix formation**.

B. Fat-soluble vitamins (Table 8.2)

—include **vitamins A, D, E, and K**.

—deficiency may result from malnutrition and intestinal **malabsorption syndromes, pancreatic exocrine insufficiency,** or **biliary obstruction,** all of which are associated with poor absorption of fats.

—excess intake (i.e., **hypervitaminosis**), with resultant toxicity, may occur, especially with vitamins A and D.

1. Vitamin A

—is a term for a group of compounds (retinoids) with similar activities that are provided by animal products, such as liver, egg yolk, and butter. Also, a variety of vegetables (e.g., carrots and green leafy vegetables) supply beta-carotene, a vitamin A precursor.

—is essential to the maintenance of mucus-secreting epithelium. A derivative, retinol, is a component of the visual pigment rhodopsin.

Table 8.2. Fat-Soluble Vitamins

Vitamin	Metabolic Functions	Clinical Manifestations of Deficiency
Vitamin A	Precursor in rhodopsin synthesis; important in glycoprotein synthesis; regulator of epithelial differentiation	Night blindness; squamous metaplasia in many tissues, most importantly in eyes where blindness may result
Vitamin D (calciferol)	Active form calcitriol (1,25-$(OH)_2D_3$) promotes intestinal calcium and phosphorus absorption and stimulates parathyroid hormone-mediated renal tubular reabsorption of calcium; thus maintains physiologic concentration of serum calcium; enhances calcification of bone	Rickets in children; osteomalacia in adults
Vitamin E (alpha tocopherol)	Antioxidant; maintenance of cell membranes probably by modulation of lipid peroxidation	Possible neurologic dysfunction
Vitamin K	Glutamyl carboxylation required for synthesis of γ-carboxyglutamyl residues of active serine proteases (e.g., clotting factors II, VII, IX, and X)	Hemorrhagic diatheses such as hemorrhagic disease of the newborn

a. Vitamin A deficiency
 −can be caused by dietary deficiency or fat malabsorption.
 −is manifest clinically by:
 (1) Night blindness, due to insufficient retinal rhodopsin
 (2) Squamous metaplasia of the trachea, bronchi, renal pelvis (often associated with renal calculi), conjunctivae, and tear ducts. Ocular abnormalities can result in **xerophthalmia** (dry eyes) and **blindness** or in **keratomalacia** (corneal softening).

b. Hypervitaminosis A
 −is most often due to excessive intake of vitamin A preparations.
 −is manifest by **alopecia, hepatocellular damage,** and **bone changes**.

2. Vitamin D
 −is synthesized in the skin by ultraviolet light from the precursor 7-dehydrocholesterol; exposure to sunlight is required for this biosynthesis.
 −is also provided by foods such as milk, butter, and eggs.
 −promotes intestinal calcium absorption mediated by a specific calcium-binding intestinal transport protein as well as intestinal phosphorus absorption.
 −enhances bone calcification, apparently through its role in intestinal calcium absorption.

a. Vitamin D deficiency
 −manifests clinically as **rickets** in children and as **osteomalacia** in adults, both due to **deficient calcification of osteoid matrix**.
 −can be caused by the following factors:
 (1) Malnutrition
 (2) Intestinal malabsorption
 (3) Inadequate exposure to sunlight
 (4) Liver disease, with impaired hepatic conversion of vitamin D to the 25-hydroxyl form, a precursor of active vitamin D, calcitriol $(1,25\text{-}(OH)_2D_3)$
 (5) Renal disease, with incomplete synthesis of active vitamin D

b. Hypervitaminosis D
 −is manifest in children by **growth retardation**.
 −is manifest in adults by **hypercalciuria, nephrocalcinosis,** and **renal calculi**.

3. Vitamin E deficiency
 −is rare but is thought to result in neurologic dysfunction.

4. Vitamin K
 −is essential for carboxylation of glutamyl residues in the synthesis of the γ-carboxyglutamyl forms (active forms) of **clotting factors II, VII, IX, and X,** and of **protein C**.
 −is provided by green and yellow vegetables and by dairy products.
 −is synthesized by intestinal microorganisms.

a. Vitamin K deficiency

—results from fat malabsorption or alterations in the intestinal flora caused by antibiotics.

—is characterized by a **hemorrhagic diathesis** (abnormal bleeding) marked by prolongation of the prothrombin and activated partial thromboplastin times.

—is the cause of **hemorrhagic disease of the newborn,** which may result from a variety of causes, including deficient intake combined with inadequate intestinal bacterial colonization.

b. There are no known clinical manifestations of excess vitamin K.

Review Test

Directions: Each of the numbered items or incomplete statements in this section is followed by answers or by completions of the statement. Select the **one** lettered answer or completion that is **best** in each case.

1. Each of the following is a characteristic of kwashiorkor EXCEPT

(A) severe edema.
(B) scant subcutaneous fat.
(C) muscle wasting.
(D) growth retardation.
(E) fatty liver.

2. High output cardiac failure suggests deficiency of which vitamin?

(A) Riboflavin
(B) Thiamine
(C) Niacin
(D) Folic acid
(E) Ascorbic acid

3. Confabulation is sometimes a manifestation of deficiency of which vitamin?

(A) Riboflavin
(B) Thiamine
(C) Niacin
(D) Folic acid
(E) Ascorbic acid

4. Glossitis, corneal vascularization, cheilosis, and seborrheic dermatitis are manifestations of dietary deficiency of

(A) riboflavin.
(B) thiamine.
(C) niacin.
(D) folic acid.
(E) ascorbic acid.

5. Diarrhea, dermatitis, and dementia are characteristics of deficiency of

(A) riboflavin.
(B) thiamine.
(C) niacin.
(D) folic acid.
(E) ascorbic acid.

6. Which one of the following statements names a characteristic of both vitamin B_{12} and folic acid?

(A) They are provided in foods of animal origin only.
(B) Copious storage occurs in the liver.
(C) Deficiency is associated with neurologic abnormalities.
(D) Deficiency is manifest by megaloblastic anemia.
(E) Deficiency occurs in patients who lack gastric intrinsic factor, a carrier protein synthesized in gastric mucosa.

7. Bleeding gums, subperiosteal hemorrhage, and cutaneous perifollicular petechial hemorrhages are all characteristics of

(A) beriberi.
(B) keratomalacia.
(C) pellagra.
(D) rickets.
(E) scurvy.

8. Intestinal malabsorption syndromes may result in deficiency of any of the following vitamins EXCEPT

(A) A.
(B) C.
(C) D.
(D) E.
(E) K.

9. All of the following clinical manifestations are correctly matched with the appropriate vitamin deficiency EXCEPT

(A) night blindness—vitamin A.
(B) hemorrhagic phenomena—vitamin K.
(C) impaired wound healing—vitamin C.
(D) osteomalacia—vitamin D.
(E) cheilosis—vitamin E.

Answers and Explanations

1–B. Kwashiorkor is the result of severe protein deprivation in the face of adequate caloric intake. Subcutaneous fat tissue is generally unaffected because sufficient calories are supplied for fat synthesis. Protein deficiency results in edema (largely secondary to hypoproteinemia; it also is caused by decreased cardiac output and renal blood flow with compensatory activation of the angiotensin-aldosterone system), muscle wasting, growth retardation, and fatty liver (due to failure of apoprotein synthesis).

2–B. High output cardiac failure is the cardinal manifestation of wet beriberi, which is caused by thiamine deficiency. Apparently, the primary event in this condition is peripheral dilatation of arterioles and capillaries, leading to functional arteriovenous shunting and hypervolemia. Cardiac dilatation and congestive heart failure follow.

3–B. Confabulation can occur in patients with Wernicke-Korsakoff syndrome, which can result from thiamine deficiency. Other characteristics of this syndrome are apathy, loss of orientation in space and time, loss of recent memory, loss of eye control, and hallucinations.

4–A. Glossitis and dermatitis are manifestations common to deficiencies of the B complex group of water-soluble vitamins. Cheilosis and corneal vascularization are especially suggestive of riboflavin deficiency.

5–C. Diarrhea, dermatitis, and dementia (the "three Ds") are the classic triad of pellagra (clinical niacin deficiency). The dermatitis tends to involve areas exposed to sunlight.

6–D. Both vitamin B_{12} and folic acid deficiencies result in megaloblastic anemia.

7–E. Scurvy is characterized by muscle, joint, and bone pain; swollen, bleeding gums; and subperiosteal and perifollicular petechial hemorrhages. Failure of ascorbate-mediated synthesis of hydroxyproline and hydroxylysine results in defective formation of mesenchymal tissue, including support tissues surrounding small vessels.

8–B. Malabsorption syndromes or secondary malabsorption due to biliary obstruction interfere with fat absorption and can lead to deficiency of any of the fat-soluble vitamins including A, D, E, or K. Water-soluble vitamin C absorption is unimpaired by fat malabsorption.

9–E. Neurologic dysfunction has been linked to inadequate vitamin E intake. Cheilosis is a manifestation of riboflavin deficiency.

9

Vascular System

I. Arterial Disorders

A. Arteriosclerosis

—is a general term for three types of vascular disease, all characterized by rigidity (sclerosis), and often thickening, of blood vessels.

1. Mönckeberg's arteriosclerosis (medial calcific sclerosis)

—involves the **media** of medium-sized muscular arteries, most typically the **radial and ulnar arteries,** and usually affects persons over age 50.
—is characterized by **ring-like calcifications** in the media of the arteries.
—**does not obstruct arterial flow** because the intima is not involved.
—results in stiff, calcific **"pipestem" arteries**.
—may coexist with atherosclerosis but is distinct from and unrelated to it.

2. Arteriolosclerosis

—is characterized by hyaline thickening or proliferative changes of **small arteries and arterioles,** especially in the kidneys.
—is usually associated with **hypertension** or **diabetes mellitus**.
—occurs in two variants:

a. Hyaline arteriolosclerosis

—is characterized by **hyaline thickening** of arteriolar walls.
—in the kidneys, is termed **benign nephrosclerosis** and is associated with hypertension.

b. Hyperplastic arteriolosclerosis

—is marked by **concentric, laminated, "onionskin" thickening of arteriolar walls**.
—may be characterized by **necrotizing arteriolitis,** intramural deposition of fibrinoid material in arterioles with vascular necrosis and inflammation.
—in the kidneys, is termed **malignant nephrosclerosis** and is associated with malignant hypertension.

3. Atherosclerosis

—is the most frequent cause of significant morbidity caused by vascular disease.

—is seen worldwide, but highest incidence occurs in Finland, Great Britain, other northern European countries, the United States, and Canada. The incidence is more than tenfold greater in Finland than in Japan.

a. Characteristics—atherosclerosis

—is characterized by fibrous plaques, or **atheromas,** within the intima of arteries, most frequently the proximal portions of the coronary arteries, the larger branches of the carotid arteries, the circle of Willis, the large vessels of the lower extremities, and the renal and mesenteric arteries.

(1) The plaques have a **central core** of cholesterol and cholesterol esters; lipid-laden macrophages, or foam cells; calcium; and necrotic debris.

(2) The core is covered by a subendothelial **fibrous cap,** made up of smooth muscle cells, foam cells, fibrin and other coagulation proteins, as well as extracellular matrix material, such as collagen, elastin, glycosaminoglycans, and proteoglycans.

(3) The plaques may be complicated by:

(a) Ulceration, hemorrhage into the plaque, or **calcification of the plaque**

(b) Thrombus formation at the site of the plaque, producing obstructive disease

(c) Embolization of the plaque material or overlying thrombus

(4) The atheromas can develop from the **fatty streak,** a lesion characterized by focal accumulations in the intima of lipid-laden foam cells that may appear as early as the first year of life and is present in the aorta of most older children.

b. Consequences of atherosclerosis

(1) The most significant consequence is **ischemic heart disease and myocardial infarction,** the most common cause of death in the United States.

(2) Other significant complications include **stroke** from cerebral ischemia and infarction, **ischemic bowel disease, peripheral vascular occlusive disease** with findings varying from claudication to ischemic necrosis and gangrene, and **renal arterial ischemia** with secondary hypertension.

(3) Weakening of the vessel wall may lead to **aneurysm** formation.

c. Risk factors for atherosclerosis

(1) Incidence increases with **age**.

(2) Sex plays a role.

—is **more common in men** in all age groups, although the incidence increases in **postmenopausal women**.

(3) Considerable evidence links **hypercholesterolemia** with atherosclerosis.

(a) Serum cholesterol may be of **dietary,** or exogenous, origin or of **biosynthetic, endogenous** origin. Cholesterol and dietary fats associate with apolipoprotein molecules and circulate as **lipoproteins**. Figure 9.1 briefly summarizes lipoprotein transport and metabolism.

(b) Relative concentrations of lipoprotein fractions are used as **clinical predictors of atherogenesis;** ideally, the ratio between low-density lipoprotein (LDL) and high-density lipoprotein (HDL) cholesterol should be 4:1.

(c) Serum concentrations of **LDL,** also known as "bad" cholesterol, are directly related to the risk of atherosclerosis, as is the total cholesterol concentration.

(d) An inverse relationship exists between the HDL concentration and the risk of atherosclerosis. **HDL,** also known as the "good" cholesterol, appears to exert its protective effect by **removing cholesterol** from tissues and from atherosclerotic plaques.

(4) Hypertension is a major risk factor for and is associated with premature atherosclerosis.

(5) Diabetes mellitus is associated with premature atherosclerosis. **Peripheral vascular occlusive disease,** often leading to gangrene of the lower extremities, is common in diabetic patients.

(6) Cigarette smoking is also a well-established risk factor.

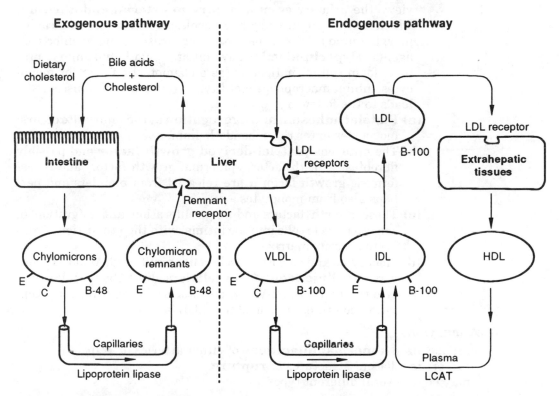

Figure 9.1. Lipoprotein transport and metabolism. HDL = high-density lipoprotein; LCAT = lecithin:cholesterol acetyltransferase; LDL = low-density lipoprotein; IDL = intermediate-density lipoprotein; VLDL = very-low-density lipoprotein. (Reprinted with permission from Goldstein J, Kita T, and Brown M: Defective lipoprotein receptors and atherosclerosis, *New England Journal of Medicine* 309:288, 1983.)

(7) Less firmly established are **obesity, physical inactivity, "Type A" personality** with stress factors in life-style, **hyperuricemia,** and use of **oral contraceptive drugs,** especially in association with cigarette smoking.

d. Pathogenesis of atherosclerosis—hypotheses and theories

(1) Insudation hypothesis

−holds that the **infiltration of the intima with lipid and protein** is the primary atherogenic event, a process accelerated by hypercholesterolemia.

(2) Encrustation or thrombogenic hypothesis

−proposes that **organization of repeated mural thrombi on the intimal surface** leads to buildup of plaques filled with lipid derived from the breakdown of platelets and leukocytes.

(3) Monoclonal hypothesis

−suggests that **smooth muscle migration and proliferation** is analogous to tumor growth and is a primary rather than a secondary event. Smooth muscle proliferations within atheromas are often monoclonal—that is, like neoplasms, they are derived from single cell precursors. This hypothesis holds that stimuli such as **hyperlipidemia may incite the proliferation**.

(4) Reaction to injury theory

−views the primary event as **injury to arterial endothelium,** which may be produced by hypercholesterolemia, mechanical injury, immune mechanisms, toxins, or viruses or other infectious agents. **Hyperlipidemia** may initiate endothelial injury, promote foam cell formation, act as a chemotactic factor for monocytes, inhibit macrophage motility, or injure smooth muscle cells.

−leads to the following:

(a) **Platelet adhesion and aggregation** at the injury site occurs; monocytes enter the subendothelium.

(b) The mitogens **platelet-derived growth factor** and possibly fibroblast growth factor, epidermal growth factor, and transforming growth factor-α are released from platelets and perhaps also from monocytes.

(c) These growth factors induce proliferation and migration of smooth muscle cells into the intima, with the production of connective tissue matrix.

(d) Monocytes and smooth muscle cells engulf lipid. Monocyte conversion to **lipid-laden foam cells** is mediated by specific monocyte receptors, the β-VLDL receptor and the scavenger receptor, which recognizes modified LDL.

B. Aneurysms

−are localized **abnormal dilatations** of either arteries or veins.

−can erode adjacent structures or **rupture**.

−may be of several different types.

1. Atherosclerotic aneurysm

−most frequently occurs in the **descending, especially the abdominal, aorta**.

2. Syphilitic (luetic) aneurysm

—is a manifestation of **tertiary syphilis,** which has become extremely rare with better treatment and control of the disease.

—is caused by **syphilitic aortitis,** which is characterized by obliterative endarteritis of the vasa vasorum and necrosis of the media.

—in contrast to atherosclerotic aneurysm, characteristically involves the **ascending aorta**. Dilatation of the ascending aorta may widen the aortic commissures, leading to **aortic valve insufficiency.**

3. Berry aneurysms

—are small, saccular lesions most often seen in the smaller arteries of the brain, especially the **circle of Willis**.

—are not present at birth but develop at sites of congenital medial weakness at **bifurcations of cerebral arteries**.

—can result in **hemorrhage into the subarachnoid space**.

4. Dissecting aneurysm (dissecting hematoma)

—is a **longitudinal intraluminal tear,** usually in the wall of the ascending aorta, forming a second arterial lumen within the media.

—is clinically dominated by severe, tearing chest pain.

—characteristically results in **aortic rupture,** most often into the pericardial sac, causing fatal cardiac tamponade.

—is typically associated with **hypertension** and with **cystic medial necrosis,** which is characterized by degenerative changes in the media with destruction of elastic and muscular tissue.

5. Arteriovenous fistula (aneurysm)

—is an **abnormal communication between an artery and a vein**.

—can be **secondary to trauma** or other pathologic processes that mechanically penetrate the walls of both vessels.

—may result in **ischemic changes** from the diversion of blood, ballooning and **aneurysm formation** from increased venous pressure, and **high output cardiac failure** from hypervolemia.

II. Venous Disorders

A. Venous thrombosis

—arises most frequently in the **deep veins of the lower extremities**.

—is predisposed by **venous circulatory stasis** or partially obstructed venous return such as occurs with cardiac failure, pregnancy, prolonged bed rest, or varicose veins.

—may give rise to **embolism** with resultant pulmonary infarction.

—occurs in two variants, depending on the presence of inflammation; **thrombophlebitis** is associated with acute inflammation of the affected vein, **phlebothrombosis** is not.

B. Varicose veins

—are abnormally **dilated and tortuous veins,** most often superficial veins of the lower extremities.

—are predisposed by **increased venous pressure** such as occurs with pregnancy, obesity, or thrombophlebitis, and in persons whose occupations require prolonged standing.

III. Tumors of Blood Vessels

A. Benign vascular tumors

—are usually not true neoplasms but are better characterized as malformations or hamartomas, and include:

1. Spider telangiectasia

—is a dilated small vessel surrounded by radiating fine channels.

—is associated with **hyperestrinism,** as seen in chronic liver disease or pregnancy.

2. Hereditary hemorrhagic telangiectasia (Osler-Weber-Rendu syndrome)

—is an autosomal dominant condition characterized by localized dilatation and convolution of venules and capillaries of the skin and mucous membranes, often complicated by epistaxis or gastrointestinal bleeding.

3. Hemangioma (angioma)

—is a malformation of a larger vessel composed of masses of channels filled with blood.

—is the most common tumor of infancy and is responsible for **port-wine stain birthmarks**.

—includes the following types:

a. Capillary hemangioma

—consists of a tangle of closely packed capillary-like channels that may occur in the skin, subcutaneous tissues, lips, liver, spleen, or kidneys.

b. Cavernous hemangioma

—consists of large cavernous vascular spaces in the skin and mucosal surfaces and in internal organs such as the liver, pancreas, spleen, and brain.

—can occur in **von Hippel-Lindau disease,** an autosomal dominant disorder that is also marked by hemangioblastomas of the cerebellum, brain stem, and retina, as well as by adenomas and cysts of the liver, kidneys, pancreas, and other organs, and by an increased incidence of renal cell carcinoma.

4. Glomangioma (glomus tumor)

—is a small, purplish, painful subungual nodule in a finger or toe.

5. Cystic hygroma

—is a cavernous **lymphangioma** that occurs most frequently in the neck or axilla.

B. Malignant vascular tumors

—are uncommon and include the following:

1. Hemangioendothelioma

—is intermediate in behavior between a benign and a malignant tumor.

2. Hemangiopericytoma

—arises from **pericytes** and varies in behavior from benign to malignant.

3. Angiosarcoma (hemangiosarcoma)

—is a rare malignant vascular tumor occurring in the skin, musculoskeletal system, breast, or liver.

−is associated with toxic exposures to **arsenic** or the **radioactive diagnostic agent thorium dioxide (Thorotrast)**. **Polyvinyl chloride** is specifically associated with angiosarcoma of the liver.

4. Kaposi's sarcoma

−is a malignant vascular tumor that most often occurs as a component of **AIDS,** especially in the homosexual male risk group.

−may be of **viral origin;** appears related to cytomegalovirus infection in AIDS patients.

−is endemic in parts of Africa; accounts for up to 10% of all cancers in Africa.

IV. Vasculitis Syndromes (Vasculitides)

−are **inflammatory and often necrotizing vascular lesions** that occur in almost any organ.

−are usually mediated by immune mechanisms.

A. Polyarteritis nodosa

−is characterized by **necrotizing immune complex inflammation** of small- and medium-sized arteries.

−is marked by destruction of arterial media and internal elastic lamella, resulting in **aneurysmal nodules**.

−is associated with **hepatitis B viral infection** in 30% of patients.

−is often manifest clinically by fever, weight loss, malaise, abdominal pain, headache, myalgia, and hypertension.

−is seen in the following sites:

1. Kidneys, with immune complex **vasculitis in the arterioles and glomeruli;** renal lesions and hypertension cause most deaths from polyarteritis nodosa.

2. Coronary arteries, resulting in **ischemic heart disease**

3. Musculoskeletal system, resulting in **myalgia, arthralgia,** or **arthritis**

4. Gastrointestinal tract, manifesting as nausea, vomiting, or **abdominal pain**

5. Central nervous system (CNS) or peripheral nervous system, the eye, or skin

B. Hypersensitivity (leukocytoclastic) vasculitis

−is a group of **immunc complex-mediated vasculitides** characterized by acute inflammation of small blood vessels (arterioles, capillaries, venules); the multiple lesions tend to be of the same age. These are in contrast to the findings in polyarteritis nodosa.

−is manifest by **palpable purpura** when the skin is involved.

−may be precipitated by **exogenous antigens** such as drugs, foods, or infectious organisms; also may occur as a **complication of systemic illnesses** such as connective tissue disorders or malignancies.

−presents clinically in distinctive syndromes, including:

1. Henoch-Schönlein purpura

−is characterized by **hemorrhagic urticaria** with fever, arthralgias, and gastrointestinal and renal involvement.

—is associated with antecedent **upper respiratory infections,** suggesting that infectious agents may be the inciting antigens; other antigens may include drugs or foods.

2. Serum sickness

—is seen in the experimental model in which rabbits, after serial injections of bovine serum albumin, develop **generalized deposition of antigen–antibody complexes** in the heart, joints, and kidneys.

—is now rare in humans, but in the past was caused by therapeutic administration of horse serum (e.g., tetanus antitoxin).

C. Wegener's granulomatosis

—is a disease of unknown etiology characterized by **necrotizing granulomatous vasculitis** of the vessels of the respiratory tract, kidneys, and other organs.

—is dominated clinically by **respiratory tract signs and symptoms,** especially of the paranasal sinuses and lungs, and **necrotizing glomerulonephritis**.

—is manifest by **fibrinoid necrosis** of small arteries and veins, **early infiltration by neutrophils,** subsequent mononuclear cell infiltration, and fibrosis. **Granuloma formation** with giant cells is prominent.

D. Giant cell arteritides

—are seen in medium- to large-sized arteries and are characterized by granuloma formation with giant cells as well as by infiltrates of mononuclear cells, neutrophils, and eosinophils.

—include two distinct clinical syndromes:

1. Temporal arteritis

—is a **systemic vasculitis** occurring most often in elderly persons.

—usually affects **branches of the carotid artery,** particularly the temporal artery.

—may be manifest clinically by:

a. Malaise and fatigue

b. Headache or claudication of the jaw

c. Tenderness, absent pulse, and **palpable nodules** along the course of the involved artery

d. Visual impairment, especially with involvement of the ophthalmic artery

e. Polymyalgia rheumatica, a complex of symptoms including proximal muscle pain, periarticular pain, and morning stiffness

f. Markedly elevated erythrocyte sedimentation rate

2. Takayasu's arteritis (pulseless disease)

—is characterized by inflammation and stenosis of medium- and large-sized arteries with frequent involvement of the aortic arch and its branches, producing **aortic arch syndrome**.

—is manifest clinically by:

a. Absent pulses in carotid, radial, or ulnar arteries

b. Nonspecific findings such as fever, night sweats, malaise, myalgia, arthritis and arthralgia, eye problems, and painful skin nodules

E. Mucocutaneous lymph node syndrome (Kawasaki disease)

—is an acute, self-limited illness of infants and young children characterized by **acute necrotizing vasculitis** of small- and medium-sized vessels.

—is manifest clinically by fever, congested conjunctivae, changes in the lips and oral mucosa, and lymphadenitis.

F. Thromboangiitis obliterans (Buerger's disease)

—is an **acute inflammation** involving small- to medium-sized arteries of the extremities, extending to adjacent veins and nerves.

—results in **painful ischemic disease,** often leading to gangrene.

—is clearly associated with heavy **cigarette smoking**.

—occurs with greater frequency in Jewish populations and is most common in young men.

G. Lymphomatoid granulomatosis

—is a rare granulomatous vasculitis characterized by **infiltration by atypical lymphocytoid and plasmacytoid cells**.

—may progress from a chronic inflammatory condition to a fully developed lymphoproliferative neoplasm, most often a **T-cell non-Hodgkin's lymphoma**.

V. Functional Vascular Disorders

A. Raynaud's disease

—is manifest by **recurrent vasospasm** of small arteries and arterioles, with resultant pallor or cyanosis, most often in the fingers and toes.

—is most often precipitated by **chilling**.

—most commonly occurs in young, healthy women.

B. Raynaud's phenomenon

—is clinically similar to Raynaud's disease but is always secondary to an underlying disorder, most characteristically systemic lupus erythematosus or progressive systemic sclerosis (scleroderma).

VI. Hypertension (Table 9.1)

A. Essential hypertension

—is hypertension of unknown etiology, accounting for the majority of cases.

—represents an interaction of predisposing determinants with a number of exogenous factors.

1. Determinants of essential hypertension

a. Genetic factors

(1) Family history of hypertensive disease is seen in three of four patients with the disorder.

(2) It is more common and usually more severe in **blacks**.

b. Environmental factors

(1) Evidence linking levels of **dietary sodium intake** with hypertension prevalence in population groups is impressive, although not everyone with excessive salt intake develops hypertension.

Table 9.1. Types of Hypertension

Type or Cause	Comments
Primary (essential) hypertension	Unknown etiology; accounts for 90%–95% of cases
Secondary hypertension	
Renal parenchymal diseases, such as postinfectious glomerulonephritis, diabetic nephropathy, adult polycystic disease	Stimulation of renin–angiotensin system
Renovascular disease	Stimulation of renin–angiotensin system
Hyperparathyroidism	. . .
Cushing's syndrome, of pituitary or adrenal origin	Excessive production of cortisol
Primary aldosteronism	Increased aldosterone secretion; sodium and water retention, often with hypokalemic acidosis
Congenital adrenal hyperplasia	Occurs in several forms; hypervolemia mediated by increased production of mineralocorticoids in 17-hydroxylase deficiency and 11-hydroxylase deficiency
Pheochromocytoma	Secretion of epinephrine and norepinephrine, resulting in sustained or paroxysmal hypertension, which may be cured by resection of the tumor
Oral contraceptive use	Hypertension an infrequent effect
Coarctation of aorta	Upper extremity hypertension only, with increased collateral circulation in the intercostal arteries, resulting in notching of ribs
Toxemia of pregnancy	Hypertension usually ceases after delivery
Increased intracranial pressure	From brain tumors or other expanding intracranial lesions
Toxic hypertension	Poisoning by lead, cadmium, and other agents

> **(2) Stress,** probably mediated by neurogenic vasoconstriction, is a factor in the development of hypertension.
>
> **(3)** Other factors include **obesity, cigarette smoking,** and **physical inactivity**.

2. Results of essential hypertension

–if untreated, can eventually lead to retinal changes, left ventricular hypertrophy and cardiac failure, and benign nephrosclerosis.

–can predispose to **ischemic heart disease** or stroke.

B. Secondary hypertension

–is secondary to known causes, including:

1. Renal disease

–is by far the most common cause of secondary hypertension.

a. Causes of renal hypertension

(1) Disorders of the renal parenchyma

(2) Unilateral renal artery stenosis

–can be caused by atherosclerosis or unilateral fibromuscular dysplasia.

–is marked by atrophy of the affected kidney and may be corrected surgically.

    b. Mechanism of renal hypertension

        —occurs through **stimulation of the renin–angiotensin system**.

        (1) Juxtaglomerular cells respond to decreased vascular tone by secreting **renin,** which facilitates the conversion of angiotensinogen to angiotensin I, which is further converted to angiotensin II.

        (2) Angiotensin II promotes hypertension by acting both as a vasoconstrictor and as an activator of aldosterone secretion.

        (3) Aldosterone promotes sodium and water retention.

2. Endocrine disorders

    a. Primary aldosteronism, or Conn's syndrome, which is usually associated with an adrenocortical adenoma or bilateral adrenal hyperplasia

    b. Acromegaly, Cushing's syndrome of pituitary or adrenocortical origin, **pheochromocytoma,** and **hyperthyroidism**

3. Other causes

    —include **coarctation of the aorta** and other congenital anomalies; **toxemia** of pregnancy; **CNS disorders,** especially brain tumors; and **drugs and chemicals,** notably amphetamines and steroids.

C. Malignant hypertension

    —can be a complication of either essential (primary) or secondary hypertension.

    —follows an **accelerated** clinical course.

    —is characterized by a marked increase in diastolic blood pressure, focal retinal hemorrhages and papilledema, left ventricular hypertrophy, and left ventricular failure.

    —most often results in **early death** from congestive heart failure, cerebrovascular accident, or renal failure.

    —produces the renal changes of **malignant nephrosclerosis:** arterioles or glomerular capillaries rupture, resulting in **"flea-bitten" kidney,** multiple pinpoint petechial hemorrhages on the kidney surface; large, swollen kidneys; necrotizing vasculitis with fibrinoid necrosis; and hyperplastic arteriolosclerosis, affecting both the glomeruli and arterioles.

    —occurs in less than 5% of patients with elevated blood pressure, most often in **young black males**.

Review Test

Directions: Each of the numbered items or incomplete statements in this section is followed by answers or by completions of the statement. Select the **one** lettered answer or completion that is **best** in each case.

1. Mönckeberg's arteriosclerosis is marked by all of the following characteristics EXCEPT

(A) it occurs most often in elderly patients.
(B) calcifications occur in the arterial media.
(C) is predominantly seen in radial and ulnar arteries.
(D) significant vascular obstruction occurs.

2. All of the following terms and phrases concerning the pathogenesis of atherosclerosis are correctly matched EXCEPT

(A) insudation hypothesis—intimal lipid infiltration.
(B) encrustation hypothesis—repeated surface thrombosis.
(C) reaction to injury theory—endothelial damage and secondary platelet deposition.
(D) monoclonal hypothesis—atherogenic antibodies.

3. The lesion shown in the illustration below is associated with which one of the following disorders?

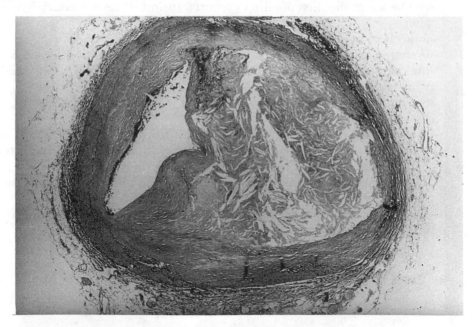

(Reprinted with permission from Golden A, Powell D, and Jennings C: *Pathology: Understanding Human Disease,* 2nd ed. Baltimore, Williams & Wilkins, 1985, p 189.)

(A) Congenital vascular muscle weakness
(B) Medial calcification
(C) Cystic medial necrosis
(D) Syphilis
(E) Hypercholesterolemia

4. Which of the following descriptions best applies to atherosclerotic plaques?

(A) Cholesterol infiltration of thickened vascular intima and media
(B) Cholesterol infiltration of thickened vascular media
(C) Cystic degeneration and necrosis of vascular media
(D) Intimal lesion consisting of fibrous cap overlying necrotic lipid-laden core
(E) Organized old thrombotic residues overlying atrophic vascular intima

5. An increased incidence of atherosclerosis has been correlated with all of the following associations EXCEPT

(A) hypertension.
(B) diabetes mellitus.
(C) hyperuricemia.
(D) increased serum high-density lipoprotein (HDL) concentration.
(E) use of oral contraceptives.

6. Dissecting aortic aneurysm is associated with all of the following characteristics EXCEPT

(A) death from hemopericardium.
(B) degenerative changes of aortic media.
(C) hypertension.
(D) severe, tearing chest pain.
(E) severe atherosclerosis.

7. The most important complication of venous thrombosis is

(A) pulmonary embolism with resultant infarction.
(B) peripheral vascular insufficiency with gangrene.
(C) arteriovenous fistula with hypervolemia.
(D) thrombophlebitis.
(E) varicose veins.

8. All of the following vascular lesions are correctly matched with the appropriate clinical association EXCEPT

(A) angiosarcoma—administration of Thorotrast.
(B) cystic hygroma—cervical and axillary masses.
(C) glomus tumor—painful subungual nodule.
(D) hereditary hemorrhagic telangiectasia—X-linked inheritance.
(E) Kaposi's sarcoma—AIDS.

9. Hepatitis B virus is frequently associated with which of the following diseases?

(A) Lymphomatoid granulomatosis
(B) Temporal arteritis
(C) Thromboangiitis obliterans
(D) Polyarteritis nodosa
(E) Takayasu's arteritis

10. A child with fever, arthralgias, gastrointestinal and renal involvement, and hemorrhagic urticaria-like lesions of the skin most likely is exhibiting

(A) Takayasu's arteritis.
(B) Henoch-Schönlein purpura.
(C) polyarteritis nodosa.
(D) temporal arteritis.
(E) Wegener's granulomatosis.

11. All of the following vasculitis syndromes and their associations are correctly matched EXCEPT

(A) Buerger's disease—high-fat diet.
(B) Kawasaki disease—lymphadenitis and involvement of conjunctivae, lips, and oral mucosa.
(C) Takayasu's arteritis—aortic arch.
(D) Wegener's granulomatosis—upper and lower respiratory tract.
(E) temporal arteritis—branches of carotid artery.

12. Chronic renal disease, pheochromocytoma, Conn's syndrome, coarctation of the aorta, and acromegaly are all conditions that may lead to

(A) hypersensitivity vasculitis.
(B) Wegener's granulomatosis.
(C) venous thrombosis.
(D) hypertension.
(E) thromboangiitis obliterans.

Directions: Each group of items in this section consists of lettered options followed by a set of numbered items. For each item, select the **one** lettered option that is most closely associated with it. Each lettered option may be selected once, more than once, or not at all.

Questions 13–16

Match the complication with its most likely cause.

(A) Congenital vascular muscle weakness
(B) Atherosclerosis
(C) Syphilis
(D) Hypertension
(E) Penetrating wounds

13. Aortic valvular insufficiency
14. Aneurysm of abdominal aorta
15. High output cardiac failure
16. Dissecting aortic aneurysm

Answers and Explanations

1–D. Mönckeberg's arteriosclerosis is ordinarily a nonobstructing lesion because the arterial intima is not involved. The condition is often seen in elderly persons in whom medium-sized muscular arteries, typically the radial and ulnar arteries, become stiffened by calcification within the media, resulting in so-called "pipestem" arteries.

2–D. The smooth muscle proliferation in atherosclerotic lesions is often monoclonal—that is, derived from a single precursor cell. The significance of this observation has led to a number of speculative concepts collectively referred to as the monoclonal hypothesis. The insudation hypothesis holds that the primary atherogenic event is intimal lipid infiltration, and in this regard it is noteworthy that the fatty streak (focal accumulations of intimal lipid-laden foam cells) is considered to be the earliest atherosclerotic change. The encrustation hypothesis considers repeated surface mural thrombosis to be the primary event in atherogenesis, whereas the widely held reaction to injury theory considers arterial endothelial damage, followed by platelet deposition and release of mitogenic factors, to be primary.

3–E. The incidence of atherosclerosis is strongly associated with hypercholesterolemia. The figure shows a large atheromatous plaque narrowing the lumen of an artery. The plaque consists of a mixture of fibrous tissue and cleft-like spaces indicating the presence of cholesterol crystals.

4–D. Atherosclerotic plaques are intimal lesions consisting of a surface fibrous cap of connective tissue with abundant collagen and smooth muscle cells overlying a necrotic core of debris, old fibrin, and pools of lipid, lipid-laden macrophages, and cholesterol.

5–D. Increased serum HDL concentration is associated with a decreased risk of atherosclerosis. This cholesterol-containing lipoprotein, the so-called "good" cholesterol, is postulated to play a scavenger role, moving excess cholesterol away from peripheral cells and atherosclerotic plaques. Hypertension, diabetes mellitus, hyperuricemia, and the use of oral contraceptives are all associated with an increased risk of atherosclerosis.

6–E. Dissecting aneurysm is unrelated to atherosclerosis. It is predisposed by cystic medial necrosis and is almost always associated with severe hypertension. The presenting symptom is often severe, tearing chest pain. Most deaths result from hemorrhage into the pericardial sac.

7–A. The most serious complication of venous thrombosis (most often of the lower extremities) is pulmonary embolism with resultant pulmonary infarction.

8–D. Hereditary hemorrhagic telangiectasia is an important autosomal dominant condition often presenting as bleeding of obscure origin.

9–D. Polyarteritis nodosa is an immune complex disease. The antigen is most often unknown. Hepatitis B surface antigen is found in approximately 30% of cases and may well be the antigen involved in the immune complexes.

10–B. The hemorrhagic urticaria-like lesions (palpable purpura) place this disorder within the hypersensitivity vasculitis group. Associated gastrointestinal and renal abnormalities are particularly characteristic of Henoch-Schönlein purpura.

11–A. Buerger's disease, or thromboangiitis obliterans, is an obstructive inflammatory arterial disorder clearly related to cigarette smoking.

12–D. Chronic renal disease, pheochromocytoma, Conn's syndrome, coarctation of the aorta, and acromegaly are all prominent causes of secondary hypertension. Renal disease is the most frequent cause. Endocrine disorders, such as pheochromocytoma, Conn's syndrome, and acromegaly, represent the next most common cause. Coarctation of the aorta is a frequent cause of hypertension limited to the upper extremities.

13–C. Syphilitic aortitis characteristically involves the proximal thoracic aorta, resulting in dilatation, often with aneurysm formation. Dilatation of the adjacent aortic valve results in aortic insufficiency. Although once the most common cause of these lesions, syphilis rarely causes this now because of treatment and control.

14–B. Atherosclerosis is the most common cause of aortic aneurysm, and the abdominal aorta is the most frequent site of involvement.

15–E. Penetrating wounds can result in arteriovenous fistula formation, which in turn is associated with hypervolemia and high output cardiac failure.

16–D. Hypertension predisposes to dissecting aneurysm, as does cystic medial necrosis.

10

The Heart

I. Ischemic Heart Disease (IHD)

—is caused by partial or complete interruption of arterial blood flow to the myocardium.

—in the majority of cases, is caused by **atherosclerotic narrowing of the coronary arteries,** sometimes acutely aggravated by superimposed thrombosis or vasospasm.

—may be clinically silent or manifest as angina pectoris, myocardial infarction (MI), or chronic ischemic heart disease.

A. Angina pectoris

—is episodic chest pain caused by inadequate oxygenation of the myocardium.

1. Stable angina

—is the most common form of angina.

—is **pain that is precipitated by exertion** and is relieved by rest or by vasodilators, such as nitroglycerin.

—results from severe narrowing of atherosclerotic coronary vessels, which are thus unable to supply sufficient oxygenated blood to support the increased myocardial demands of exertion.

2. Unstable angina

—is **prolonged or recurrent pain at rest**.

—is often indicative of imminent myocardial infarction.

3. Prinzmetal's angina

—is **intermittent chest pain at rest**.

—is generally considered to be caused by vasospasm.

B. Myocardial infarction

1. General characteristics—myocardial infarction

—is the most important cause of morbidity from ischemic heart disease and is one of the leading causes of death in the Western world.

−is marked by a series of progressive changes involving gross and microscopic appearance of the heart and release of myocardial enzymes into the bloodstream (Table 10.1).

−is characterized by two distinct patterns of myocardial ischemic necrosis.

a. Transmural infarction

−is myocardial necrosis that traverses the entire ventricular wall from the endocardium to the epicardium.

b. Subendocardial infarction

−is myocardial necrosis that is limited to the interior one-third of the wall of the left ventricle.

2. Complications of myocardial infarction

a. Arrhythmia

−is the most common cause of death in the first several hours following infarction.

b. Myocardial rupture

−is a catastrophic complication that usually occurs within the first 4–10 days and may result in death from **cardiac tamponade,** compression of the heart by hemorrhage into the pericardial space.

c. Ruptured papillary muscle

d. Mural thrombosis

−is thrombus formation on the endocardium overlying the infarct; may lead to systemic embolism.

e. Ventricular aneurysm

II. Rheumatic Fever

A. Definition—rheumatic fever

−is a **multisystem inflammatory disorder** with major cardiac manifestations and sequelae, most often affecting children between the ages of 5 and 15 years.

−usually occurs 1 to 4 weeks after an episode of tonsillitis or other infection caused by **group A β-hemolytic streptococci.**

B. Etiology—rheumatic fever

−is apparently of **immunologic origin** rather than a result of direct bacterial involvement; however, the precise nature of the immune mechanisms of injury remains unclear.

−is postulated to occur as a result of **streptococcal antigens** that elicit an antibody response reactive to streptococcal organisms as well as to human antigens in the heart and other tissues.

−has been remarkably reduced in incidence in the Western world in recent years.

C. Aschoff body

−is the classic lesion of rheumatic fever.

−is an area of **focal interstitial myocardial inflammation** that is characterized by fragmented collagen and fibrinoid material, by large cells (Anitschkow myocytes), and by occasional multinucleated giant cells (Aschoff cells).

Table 10.1. Progressive Changes in Acute Myocardial Infarction

Stage	Gross Changes	Microscopic Changes	Serum Enzymes or Clinical Correlations
0–6 hours	None	Vascular congestion at perimeter of lesion after first few hours	Beginning increase in serum CPK; arrhythmia most common cause of death in early hours
After 12 hours	None	First appearance of neutrophils in viable tissue adjacent to lesion	Continuing increase in serum CPK; beginning increase in serum AST
12–24 hours	Slight swelling and change of color	Cytoplasm displays increasing affinity for acidophilic dyes, and striations are lost; nuclei disappear; neutrophils infiltrate lesion	Serum CPK and AST continue to increase
By 24 hours	Pale or reddish brown infarct with surrounding hyperemia	Well-developed changes of coagulation necrosis; progressive infiltration by neutrophils	Serum CPK peaks; serum AST continues to increase
24–48 hours	...	...	Serum AST peaks; serum CPK decreases; serum LDH begins to rise and peaks by 2–3 days
By third day	Increasingly yellow color of infarct	Replacement of neutrophils by macrophages; phagocytosis of debris begins	Serum CPK normal; serum AST returns to normal by 3–5 days
From 7 days	Yellow infarcted area surrounded by congested red border	Beginning of growth of young fibroblasts and newly formed vessels into lesion; replacement of neutrophils by macrophages and phagocytosis of debris continue	LDH elevation persists until 7th day; risk for myocardial rupture greatest within first 4–10 days
From 10 days	Red, newly formed vascular connective tissue encircles and gradually replaces yellow necrotic tissue	Growth of fibrovascular tissue continues; replacement of neutrophils by macrophages and phagocytosis of debris are almost complete	Serum enzymes normal
Between second and fourth week	...	Progressive synthesis of collagen and other intracellular matrix proteins	...
From fifth week	Increasing pallor of infarct because of progressive fibrosis	Progressive fibrosis	...
Within 3–6 months	Well-developed gray-white scar	Mature fibrous tissue replaces area of infarction	Ventricular aneurysm may occur in scarred area

CPK = creatine phosphokinase; AST = aspartate aminotransferase; LDH = lactate dehydrogenase.

D. Other anatomic changes—rheumatic fever

–is characterized by **pancarditis,** inflammation of the pericardium, myocardium, and endocardium.

1. Pericarditis

–may result in pericardial, pleural, or other serous effusions.

2. Myocarditis

–may lead to cardiac failure, and is the cause of most deaths occurring during the early stages of acute rheumatic fever.

3. Endocarditis

–leads to valvular damage.

a. Rheumatic endocarditis usually occurs in areas subject to greatest hemodynamic stress, such as the points of valve closure and MacCallum's area of the posterior wall of the left atrium. The mitral and aortic valves, which are subjected to much greater pressure and turbulence, are more likely to be affected than are the tricuspid and pulmonary valves.

b. In the early stage, the valve leaflets are red and swollen, and tiny, wart-like, rubbery vegetations (verrucae) form along the lines of closure of the valve leaflet. The small, firm verrucae of acute rheumatic fever are nonfriable and are not a source of peripheral emboli.

c. As a consequence of fibrotic healing, the valves become thickened, fibrotic, and deformed, often with prominent calcification. These late sequelae, often occurring many years after the episode of rheumatic fever, are grouped under the term **rheumatic heart disease (RHD).**

(1) Mitral valve
–is the valve most frequently involved in rheumatic heart disease.
–is the only valve affected in almost 50% of cases.
–can be affected by stenosis, insufficiency, or a combination of both.

(2) Aortic valve
–most often is affected along with the mitral valve.
–can be affected by stenosis or insufficiency.

(3) Tricuspid valve
–is affected along with the mitral valve and aortic valves (trivalvular involvement) in approximately 5% of cases of rheumatic heart disease.

(4) Pulmonary valve
–is rarely involved.

E. Noncardiac manifestations of acute rheumatic fever

1. Fever, malaise, and increased erythrocyte sedimentation rate

2. Joint involvement

a. Arthralgia—joint pain without clinically evident inflammation

b. Arthritis—overt joint inflammation presenting as painful, red, swollen, hot joints, usually involving larger joints, especially the knees, ankles, wrists, and elbows

c. Migratory polyarthritis—sequential involvement of multiple joints

3. **Skin lesions,** including **subcutaneous nodules,** small painless swellings usually over bony prominences, and **erythema marginatum,** a distinctive skin rash characteristic of rheumatic fever, often involving the trunk and extremities

4. **Central nervous system involvement,** including **chorea,** that is, involuntary, purposeless muscular movements, and bizarre grimaces, as well as emotional lability

III. Other Forms of Endocarditis

A. Infective endocarditis

—is a **bacterial, or sometimes fungal, infection of the endocardium,** with prominent involvement of the valvular surfaces.

—is characterized by large, soft, friable, easily detached **vegetations** consisting of fibrin and intermeshed inflammatory cells and bacteria.

—may be complicated by **ulceration,** often with perforation, of the valve cusps or rupture of one of the chordae tendineae.

1. Classification

a. Acute endocarditis

—is caused by pathogens such as *Staphylococcus aureus* (50% of cases).

—is often secondary to infection occurring elsewhere in the body.

b. Subacute (bacterial) endocarditis

—is caused by less virulent organisms such as *Streptococcus viridans* (more than 50% of cases).

—tends to occur in patients with congenital heart disease or preexisting valvular heart disease, often of rheumatic origin.

2. Clinical features

a. Valvular involvement

(1) The **mitral valve** is most frequently involved.

(2) The **mitral valve along with the aortic valve** is involved in about 40% of cases.

(3) The **tricuspid valve** is involved in more than 50% of cases of endocarditis of intravenous drug users.

b. Complications

(1) **Distal embolization** occurs when vegetations fragment.

(2) Embolization can occur almost anywhere in the body and can result in **septic infarcts** in the brain or in other organs.

(3) The **renal glomeruli** may be the site of focal glomerulonephritis (focal necrotizing glomerulitis) caused by immune complex disease.

B. Nonbacterial thrombotic endocarditis (marantic endocarditis)

—is associated with debilitating disorders, such as metastatic cancer and other wasting conditions.

—is characterized by small, sterile fibrin deposits randomly arranged along the line of closure of the valve leaflets.

—can result in **peripheral embolization** but, unlike in infective endocarditis, the emboli are sterile.

C. Libman-Sacks endocarditis

—occurs in **systemic lupus erythematosus (SLE)**.

—is characterized by **small vegetations on either or both surfaces of the valve leaflets**.

D. Endocarditis of the carcinoid syndrome

—is caused by the **secretory products of carcinoid tumors** (vasoactive peptides and amines, especially serotonin [5-hydroxytryptamine]).

—results in thickened **endocardial plaques** characteristically involving the mural endocardium or the valvular cusps of the right side of the heart.

—rarely involves valves on the left side of the heart because serotonin and other carcinoid secretory products are detoxified in the lung.

IV. Valvular Heart Disease

—occurs often as a late result of **rheumatic fever**.

—may be secondary to a variety of other inflammatory processes.

—may be congenital.

A. Mitral valve

1. Prolapse

—is the **most frequent valvular lesion,** occurring in approximately 7% of the population, most often in young women.

—is characterized by myxoid degeneration of the ground substance of the valve (rarely in conjunction with Marfan's syndrome).

—results in stretching of the posterior mitral valve leaflet, producing a "floppy" cusp with prolapse into the atrium during systole. These changes produce a characteristic **systolic murmur with a midsystolic click**.

—is usually benign and asymptomatic but can result in **mitral insufficiency**.

—is often associated with a variety of **arrhythmias**.

—predisposes to **infective endocarditis**.

2. Stenosis

—is almost always due to rheumatic heart disease.

3. Insufficiency

—is usually a result of rheumatic heart disease.

—can also result from **mitral valve prolapse, infective endocarditis,** or **damage to a papillary muscle from myocardial infarction**.

—can be secondary to left ventricular dilatation, with stretching of the mitral valve ring.

B. Aortic valve

—is frequently involved, along with the mitral valve, in rheumatic heart disease and in infective endocarditis.

1. Stenosis

—often presents as **calcific aortic stenosis** caused by calcification of:

a. A congenital bicuspid aortic valve

b. An otherwise normal aortic valve as an age-related degenerative change

c. A valve affected by rheumatic heart disease

2. Insufficiency

−can be caused by:

a. Rheumatic heart disease, usually with mitral valve disease

b. Syphilitic (luetic) aortitis with dilatation of the aortic valve ring

c. Nondissecting aortic aneurysm resulting from cystic medial necrosis

C. Tricuspid valve

−is rarely involved alone in rheumatic heart disease but may be involved together with the mitral and aortic valves. This trivalvular involvement accounts for approximately 5% of cases of rheumatic heart disease.

−may be involved in **the carcinoid syndrome**.

D. Pulmonary valve

−is most commonly affected by **congenital malformations,** occurring either alone or along with other congenital defects, such as in the tetralogy of Fallot.

−is rarely involved in rheumatic heart disease.

−may be involved in **the carcinoid syndrome**.

V. Congenital Heart Disease (Table 10.2)

A. Causes and associations

1. The etiology is usually undetermined.

2. Chromosomal abnormalities such as Down's syndrome, some of the other trisomies, and Turner's syndrome are often complicated by congenital heart disease.

3. There is an apparent increase in the incidence of **patent ductus arteriosus** in patients living at high altitudes, suggesting an association with fetal oxygen deprivation.

4. Rubella (German measles) infection is a prominent cause of congenital heart disease.

a. There is strong evidence of a link between maternal rubella during the first trimester of pregnancy and a constellation of fetal defects, known as **congenital rubella syndrome,** which includes cataracts, cardiovascular defects, mental retardation and deafness.

b. Cardiac malformations are especially frequent and commonly include patent ductus arteriosus, aortic stenosis, ventricular septal defect, and pulmonary infundibular or valvular stenosis, sometimes occurring as part of the tetralogy of Fallot.

c. Other congenital abnormalities may be seen, including microcephaly and fetal and postnatal growth retardation.

d. Before or during pregnancy, it is often important to determine a woman's immune status to rubella. Demonstration of anti-rubella **antibodies** of the **IgM class indicates recent primary infection,** whereas demonstration of **IgG antibodies** indicates either recent primary infection, past infection, or reinfection.

Table 10.2. Frequently Occurring Forms of Congenital Heart Disease

Disorder	Anatomic Changes	Comments
Atrial septal defects	Patent foramen ovale, usually clinically insignificant Septum primum, affects lower part of septum; if large, may be associated with deformities of atrioventricular valves Septum secundum, defect in fossa ovalis Sinus venosus, affects upper part of septum near entrance of superior vena cava Lutembacher's syndrome, atrial septal defect with mitral stenosis	Clinical manifestations often delayed until adult life; pulmonary hypertension and reversal of flow with resultant cyanosis are late complications; can lead to paradoxical embolism Mitral stenosis is often of rheumatic origin
Ventricular septal defects	Vary greatly in size	Small defects may close spontaneously; larger defects may lead to pulmonary hypertension and eventual right-sided heart failure; reversal of flow and late cyanosis also occur
Tetralogy of Fallot	Pulmonary infundibular or valvular stenosis; ventricular septal defect; overriding aorta; right ventricular hypertrophy	Cyanosis from birth; tendency of patients to assume squatting position, presumably because of lessening of right-to-left shunting
Patent ductus arteriosus	Failure of closure of fetal ductus arteriosus	Patency maintained during fetal life by combined effects of low oxygen tension and prostaglandin synthesis; can be closed surgically or pharmacologically treated with indomethacin; if not closed, eventually leads to pulmonary hypertension, right ventricular hypertrophy, reversal of blood flow, and late cyanosis
Coarctation of aorta	Narrowing of aorta, usually distal to origin of subclavian arteries; extensive development of collateral circulation with dilatation of intercostal arteries	Hypertension limited to upper extremities and cerebral vessels; notching of ribs seen on X-ray
Transposition of great vessels	Aorta arises from right ventricle, and pulmonary artery arises from left ventricle	Compensatory anomaly such as patent ductus arteriosus necessary for survival

B. Functional abnormalities of congenital heart disease

—can be classified according to the presence or absence of **cyanosis**.

1. Noncyanotic diseases include those with no shunt (e.g., aortic stenosis, coarctation of the aorta) and those with a left-to-right shunt (e.g., patent ductus arteriosus, atrial or ventricular septal defect).

2. Cyanotic diseases include transposition of the great vessels, malformations with a right-to-left shunt (e.g., the tetralogy of Fallot), and disorders in which a left-to-right shunt reverses to right-to-left because of increased pulmonary arterial pressure (e.g., late cyanosis, cyanosis tardive).

VI. Diseases of the Myocardium

A. Cardiomyopathy

—refers to diseases of the heart muscle that are noninflammatory and are not associated with hypertension, congenital heart disease, valvular disease, or coronary artery disease.

—is usually characterized by otherwise unexplained **ventricular dysfunction** (heart failure, ventricular enlargement, ventricular arrhythmias).

B. Classifications of cardiomyopathy

1. Congestive or dilated cardiomyopathy

—is the **most common form** of cardiomyopathy.

—is characterized by dilatation of both ventricles and by both right- and left-sided heart failure.

—is exemplified by cardiomyopathies of **alcoholism** (alcohol cardiomyopathy) and **thiamine deficiency** (beriberi heart).

2. Restrictive cardiomyopathy

—is caused by infiltrative processes within the myocardium that result in stiffening of the heart muscle, which interferes with pumping action.

—is exemplified by **cardiac amyloidosis,** which may result in both right- and left-sided heart failure.

3. Hypertrophic cardiomyopathy

—is characterized grossly by **hypertrophy of the ventricular wall, especially the ventricular septum** (asymmetric septal hypertrophy).

—is characterized microscopically by **disoriented and tangled myocardial fibers**.

—is often inherited as an **autosomal dominant characteristic**.

—may result in **left ventricular outflow obstruction,** placing the patient in danger of syncope and even sudden death.

VII. Diseases of the Pericardium

A. Noninflammatory conditions

1. Hydropericardium

—is an accumulation of **serous transudate in the pericardial space**.

—may result from any condition causing systemic edema.

—is most frequently caused by congestive heart failure or by edematous conditions due to hypoproteinemia, such as the nephrotic syndrome or chronic liver disease.

2. Hemopericardium

—is an **accumulation of blood in the pericardial sac**.

—is usually caused by traumatic perforation of the heart or aorta, or by myocardial rupture associated with acute myocardial infarction.

B. Acute pericarditis

1. Serous pericarditis

—is associated with **systemic lupus erythematosus, rheumatic fever,** and a variety of **viral infections**.

—is characterized by production of a clear, straw-colored, **protein-rich exudate** containing small numbers of inflammatory cells.

2. Fibrinous or serofibrinous pericarditis

—may be caused by **uremia, myocardial infarction, or acute rheumatic fever**.

—is characterized by a **fibrin-rich exudate**.

3. Purulent or suppurative pericarditis

—is almost always caused by **bacterial infection**.

—is characterized by a grossly cloudy or frankly purulent **inflammatory exudate**.

4. Hemorrhagic pericarditis

—usually results from **tumor invasion of the pericardium**.

—can also result from **tuberculosis or other bacterial infection**.

—is characterized by a **bloody inflammatory exudate**.

C. Chronic (constrictive) pericarditis

—is usually of **tuberculous or pyogenic staphylococcal etiology**.

—is characterized by **obliteration of the pericardial cavity** with resulting interference with cardiac action and venous return, often mimicking the signs and symptoms of right-sided heart failure.

—is marked by **proliferation of fibrous tissue** with occasional small foci of calcification.

VIII. Tumors of the Heart

A. Primary tumors

—are very rare and are most frequently **atrial myxomas**.

B. Metastatic tumors

—are more frequent than primary tumors.

IX. Congestive Heart Failure

—may be failure of the left ventricle, right ventricle, or both.

A. Left-sided heart failure

1. Causes

a. Ischemic heart disease, especially myocardial infarction

b. Hypertension

c. Aortic and mitral valvular disease

d. Myocardial diseases, such as cardiomyopathies and myocarditis

2. Clinical manifestations

    a. Dyspnea and orthopnea caused by pulmonary congestion and edema regularly occurs.

    b. Pleural effusion with hydrothorax often results.

    c. Reduction in renal perfusion, causing activation of the renin-angiotensin-aldosterone system and leading to retention of salt and water, is less frequent.

    d. Cerebral anoxia is less frequent.

B. Right-sided heart failure

    —may be mimicked by the cardiac compression of constrictive pericarditis.

    1. Causes

        a. Left-sided heart failure

        b. Left-sided lesions such as mitral stenosis

        c. Pulmonary hypertension often caused by chronic lung disease (cor pulmonale)

        d. Various types of cardiomyopathy and diffuse myocarditis

        e. Tricuspid or pulmonary valvular disease

    2. Clinical manifestations

        a. Renal hypoxia, leading to greater **fluid retention and peripheral edema** than seen in left-sided failure. Edema occurs first in dependent areas and often manifests early as so-called pitting edema of the ankles. Other manifestations of fluid retention include pleural effusion and sometimes ascites.

        b. Enlarged and congested liver and spleen. Congestion of the centrilobular veins of the liver surrounded by relatively pale, sometimes fatty, peripheral regions leads to a "nutmeg" pattern.

        c. Distention of the neck veins

X. Hypertrophy of the Heart

A. Hypertrophy of the left ventricle

    —is most commonly caused by **hypertension and aortic or mitral valvular disease**.

B. Hypertrophy of the right ventricle

    1. Causes

        a. Left ventricular failure

        b. Chronic lung disease

        c. Mitral valve disease

        d. Congenital heart disease with left-to-right shunt

    2. Cor pulmonale

        —is heart disease secondary to disorders of the lungs, such as emphysema, or pulmonary vessels.

        —is characterized by pulmonary arterial hypertension, the common characteristic among the primary entities that lead to cor pulmonale.

Review Test

Directions: Each of the numbered items or incomplete statements in this section is followed by answers or by completions of the statement. Select the **one** lettered answer or completion that is **best** in each case.

1. Prinzmetal's angina is characterized by

(A) chest pain on exertion.
(B) chest pain at rest.
(C) narrowing of coronary ostia by syphilitic aortitis.
(D) coronary embolism.

2. A myocardial infarct that exhibits early granulation tissue has most likely occurred

(A) less than 1 hour previously.
(B) within 24 hours.
(C) within 1 week.
(D) within 1 month.
(E) within 3 months.

3. Following acute myocardial infarction, rupture of the left ventricle is most likely to occur within

(A) 6–8 hours.
(B) 16–24 hours.
(C) 4–10 days.
(D) 2–3 weeks.
(E) 2–3 months.

4. The most common cause of death immediately following the onset of acute myocardial infarction is

(A) arrhythmia.
(B) left ventricular rupture.
(C) congestive heart failure.
(D) shock.
(E) pulmonary edema.

5. Manifestations of acute rheumatic fever include all of the following conditions EXCEPT

(A) mitral stenosis.
(B) pancarditis.
(C) subcutaneous nodules.
(D) erythema marginatum.
(E) chorea.

6. Characteristic lesions or complications of rheumatic heart disease include all of the following conditions EXCEPT

(A) mitral stenosis.
(B) mitral insufficiency.
(C) aortic stenosis.
(D) pulmonary stenosis.
(E) infective endocarditis.

7. The myocardial lesions shown in the illustration below can be observed in patients with which one of the following conditions?

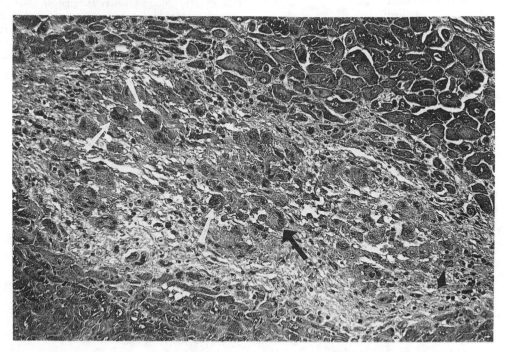

(Reprinted with permission from Golden A, Powell D, and Jennings C: *Pathology: Understanding Human Disease,* 2nd ed. Baltimore, Williams & Wilkins, 1985, p 171.)

(A) Chorea
(B) Unstable angina
(C) Systemic embolization
(D) Wasting diseases
(E) Systemic lupus erythematosus

8. Most deaths that occur during acute rheumatic fever are caused by

(A) pericarditis.
(B) endocarditis.
(C) streptococcal sepsis.
(D) myocarditis.

9. Nonbacterial thrombotic endocarditis is most frequently associated with which of the following conditions?

(A) Terminal neoplastic disease
(B) Systemic lupus erythematosus
(C) Old rheumatic endocarditis
(D) Subdiaphragmatic abscess
(E) Congenital heart disease

10. Which of the two valves listed below is least commonly associated with rheumatic heart disease?

(A) Aortic and pulmonary
(B) Mitral and tricuspid
(C) Aortic and mitral
(D) Pulmonary and tricuspid
(E) Aortic and tricuspid

11. Which of the following conditions characteristically results in aortic valvular insufficiency?

(A) Carcinoid syndrome
(B) Marantic endocarditis
(C) Bicuspid aortic valve
(D) Syphilitic heart disease
(E) Libman-Sacks endocarditis

12. Mitral stenosis most often results from

(A) rheumatic endocarditis.
(B) bacterial endocarditis.
(C) congenital heart disease.
(D) Marfan's syndrome.
(E) syphilitic heart disease.

13. Cyanosis in congenital heart disease is caused by

(A) a left-to-right shunt.
(B) pulmonary valvular insufficiency.
(C) aortic stenosis.
(D) a right-to-left shunt.

14. All of the following conditions are associated with a left-to-right shunt EXCEPT

(A) patent ductus arteriosus.
(B) atrial septal defect.
(C) ventricular septal defect.
(D) tetralogy of Fallot.

15. Tetralogy of Fallot most often includes all of the following features EXCEPT

(A) early left-to-right shunting.
(B) overriding aorta.
(C) pulmonary infundibular or valvular stenosis.
(D) right ventricular hypertrophy.
(E) ventricular septal defect.

16. Which one of the following conditions is associated with paradoxical embolism?

(A) Rheumatic heart disease
(B) Pulmonary stenosis
(C) Pulmonary hypertension
(D) Atrial septal defects
(E) Infective endocarditis

17. Notching of the undersurface of the ribs is characteristic of

(A) atrial septal defect.
(B) ventricular septal defect.
(C) tetralogy of Fallot.
(D) coarctation of aorta.
(E) patent ductus arteriosus.

18. A 42-year-old man is seen because of a long history of slowly developing congestive heart failure. His blood pressure is normal. Coronary artery angiography reveals no vascular disease. No heart murmurs are heard. The white blood cell count, differential, and erythrocyte sedimentation rate are normal. The most likely diagnosis is

(A) cardiomyopathy.
(B) constrictive pericarditis.
(C) carcinoid heart disease.
(D) myocardial infarction.
(E) coarctation of the aorta.

19. Which of the following diseases is classified as a restrictive cardiomyopathy?

(A) Alcoholic heart disease
(B) Hypertensive heart disease
(C) Ischemic heart disease
(D) Amyloid heart disease
(E) Asymmetric septal hypertrophy

20. Which of the following is the most common primary tumor of the heart?

(A) Leiomyoma
(B) Rhabdomyoma
(C) Myxoma
(D) Fibroma
(E) Lipoma

21. Right ventricular failure is commonly characterized by all of the following changes EXCEPT

(A) distended neck veins.
(B) hepatomegaly.
(C) ankle edema.
(D) sodium and water retention.
(E) pulmonary edema.

22. Right ventricular hypertrophy is caused by all of the following conditions EXCEPT

(A) chronic lung disease.
(B) mitral valve disease.
(C) tetralogy of Fallot.
(D) hypertension.
(E) pulmonary arterial hypertension.

23. The most frequent cause of cor pulmonale with right-sided heart failure is

(A) constrictive pericarditis.
(B) disease of the lungs or pulmonary vessels.
(C) left-sided heart failure.
(D) pulmonary infundibular or valvular stenosis.
(E) systemic hypertension.

Answers and Explanations

1–B. Prinzmetal's angina is a variant of angina thought to result from coronary artery spasm and is often seen in patients with anatomically normal coronary vessels. Discomfort is similar to that of classic angina but characteristically occurs at rest rather than upon exertion.

2–C. By the end of the first week following myocardial infarction, early granulation tissue is seen at the periphery of the necrotic area, followed shortly by the appearance of newly formed collagen. Granulation tissue is gradually replaced by scar tissue within several weeks.

3–C. Rupture of the left ventricle, a catastrophic complication of acute myocardial infarction, usually occurs when the necrotic area has the least tensile strength, which is at about 4–10 days following infarction when repair is just beginning. The anterior wall of the heart is the most frequent site of rupture, usually leading to fatal cardiac tamponade. Internal rupture of the interventricular septum or of a papillary muscle may also occur.

4–A. Arrhythmias are the most important early complication of acute myocardial infarction, accounting for almost 50% of deaths shortly after myocardial infarction.

5–A. Severe valvular disease, often manifest as mitral stenosis, is a feature of rheumatic heart disease, the chronic stage of rheumatic disease, in which damaged, fibrotic valves may become stenotic, insufficient, or both. Pancarditis, subcutaneous nodules, erythema marginatum, and chorea are all manifestations of acute rheumatic fever.

6–D. The pulmonary valve is only rarely involved in rheumatic heart disease, and pulmonary stenosis is usually congenital in origin. Fibrous scarring secondary to endocardial involvement in rheumatic fever leads to rheumatic heart disease (chronic valvular disease occurring as a sequela of rheumatic fever). The valve most commonly affected is the mitral valve. The damaged fibrotic valves can become the site of bacterial infection, as in subacute bacterial endocarditis.

7–A. The figure illustrates an Aschoff body, the characteristic lesion of rheumatic fever. This myocardial lesion is most often oval in shape and characterized by swollen fragmented collagen and fibrinoid material and by characteristic large mesenchymal cells (Anitschkow myocytes) and multinucleated cells (Aschoff cells). Chorea is a major manifestation of rheumatic fever.

8–D. The most common cause of death that occurs during acute rheumatic fever is cardiac failure secondary to myocarditis.

9–A. Nonbacterial thrombotic endocarditis, or marantic endocarditis, has been associated with a variety of wasting diseases and is observed most frequently in patients with cancer.

10–D. Valvular deformities caused by rheumatic fever tend to occur in the mitral valve or mitral and aortic valves, most likely because of the hemodynamic factors associated with the left side of the heart. Tricuspid valve involvement is seen in 10%–15% of cases and is almost always associated with mitral and aortic lesions. The pulmonary valve is rarely involved.

11–D. In syphilitic aortitis, the elastica of the aorta is replaced by fibrous tissue, resulting in dilatation of the ascending aorta and separation of the aortic commissures, with resultant aortic insufficiency.

12–A. Mitral stenosis is most often a late sequela of rheumatic fever. Bacterial endocarditis is a complication, not a cause, of mitral stenosis. Congenital heart disease is sometimes complicated by mitral stenosis, which is often of rheumatic origin. Marfan's syndrome is sometimes associated with mitral valve prolapse. Syphilitic heart disease is characterized by widening of the aortic commissures, resulting in aortic insufficiency.

13–D. Cyanosis, which occurs when the arterial concentration of reduced hemoglobin exceeds 5 mg/ml, is seen with a right-to-left shunt in which venous blood gains direct access to the arterial circulation.

14–D. In tetralogy of Fallot, the increased right ventricular pressure caused by pulmonary stenosis results, along with the overriding aorta, in right-to-left shunting. In contrast, patent ductus arteriosus and atrial and ventricular septal defects are associated with left-to-right blood flow because of the pressure gradient from left to right. Reversal of shunting may occur as time passes.

15–A. Most cases of tetralogy of Fallot are cyanotic at birth because of right-to-left shunting. This is not invariable, however, since the direction of blood flow is dependent on the severity of pulmonary infundibular or valvular stenosis.

16–D. The term paradoxical embolism denotes the passage of an embolus of venous origin into the arterial circulation through a right-to-left shunt (e.g., patent foramen ovale, atrial septal defect). The likelihood of right-to-left passage of the embolus is often enhanced by pulmonary hypertension secondary to pulmonary thromboembolism.

17–D. Coarctation of the aorta is characterized by aortic narrowing, most often near the ductus arteriosus. This condition results in hypertension proximal to the obstruction and hypotension distal to it. Eventually, collateral circulation develops, involving the subclavian, internal mammary, and intercostal arteries as well as others. Notching of the undersurface of the ribs is the result of atrophy caused by pressure on the adjacent ribs from the dilated, pulsating intercostal arteries.

18–A. Cardiomyopathies are noninflammatory myocardial disorders not associated with coronary artery obstruction, hypertension, valvular disease, congenital heart disease, or infectious disease. They are most often characterized by otherwise unexplained ventricular dysfunction, such as cardiac failure, ventricular enlargement, or ventricular arrhythmias.

19–D. Restrictive, or obliterative-restrictive, cardiomyopathy is characterized by restricted ventricular filling, most often associated with amyloidosis. Congestive, or dilated, cardiomyopathy is characterized by biventricular dilation associated with alcoholism, thiamine deficiency (beriberi), and cobalt toxicity. Hypertrophic cardiomyopathy is characterized by marked increase in ventricular wall thickness with small ventricular cavities, often with outflow tract obstruction, as in asymmetric septal hypertrophy.

20–C. Myxoma of the heart, while rare, is the most common primary cardiac tumor. Because of the jelly-like appearance and myxoid histology similar to that of some organized thrombi, the neoplastic nature of this lesion was debated for many years. However, authorities now generally believe that the myxoma is indeed a true neoplasm.

21–E. Pulmonary edema characteristically results from severe left ventricular failure. Right ventricular failure results in increased right atrial pressure, leading to distention of neck veins and passive congestion and enlargement of the liver. Renin-mediated release of aldosterone results in sodium and water retention, hypervolemia, and peripheral edema.

22–D. Systemic arterial hypertension results in hypertrophy of the left ventricle. Right ventricular hypertrophy most often results from pulmonary hypertension, as in chronic lung disease; from increased left atrial pressure, as in mitral valve disease; or from congenital cardiac defects, as in the tetralogy of Fallot with its overriding aorta and pulmonary infundibular stenosis.

23–B. The term *cor pulmonale* refers to right ventricular hypertrophy caused by pulmonary hypertension secondary to disorders of the lungs or pulmonary vessels. Other causes of right ventricular hypertrophy and failure, such as valvular disease, congenital defects, and left-sided heart failure, are precluded by this definition. Constrictive pericarditis can clinically mimic right-sided heart failure but is entirely unrelated to cor pulmonale.

11

Anemia

I. General Concepts—Anemia

A. Definitions

–anemia is a decrease in whole body red cell mass, a definition that precludes relative decreases in red blood cell count, hemoglobin, or hematocrit, which occur when the plasma volume is increased.

–anemia of pregnancy is not anemia but is rather a manifestation of increased plasma volume.

–a practical working definition of anemia is a decrease in red blood cell count, hemoglobin, or hematocrit, commonly measured red cell parameters.

B. Causes of anemia (Table 11.1)

–anemia may be caused by two major mechanisms:

1. Decreased red cell production resulting from:

    a. Hemopoietic cell damage from infection, drugs, radiation, and other similar agents

    b. Deficiency of factors necessary for heme synthesis (iron) or DNA synthesis (vitamin B_{12} or folate)

2. Increased red cell loss due to:

    a. External blood loss

    b. Red cell destruction (hemolytic anemia)

II. Acute Post-hemorrhagic Anemia

–within the first few hours of acute blood loss, prior to hemodilution (compensatory increase in plasma volume), there may be no decrease in the hemoglobin, hematocrit, and red cell count because of a parallel loss of both red cells and plasma. There is often a marked reactive increase in platelet count.

–significant clinical findings are related to **hypovolemia**.

Table 11.1. Examples of Anemia Resulting from Decreased Red Cell Production

Type	Mechanisms	Diagnostic Features	Major Etiologic Factors
Iron deficiency anemia	Impaired heme synthesis	Hypochromia and microcytosis; decreased serum iron and increased total iron binding capacity; decreased serum ferritin	Dietary deficiency in infants and preadolescents; excess menstrual bleeding; chronic blood loss from gastrointestinal tract
Pernicious anemia	Chronic gastritis leading to lack of gastric intrinsic factor and failure of vitamin B_{12} absorption; vitamin B_{12} deficiency causes delayed DNA replication	Pancytopenia, oval macrocytes, and hypersegmented neutrophils; megaloblastic hyperplasia; achlorhydria; anti-intrinsic factor antibodies; absent position and vibration sensations; impaired vitamin B_{12} absorption corrected by intrinsic factor (abnormal Schilling test)	
Folate deficiency	Delayed DNA replication	Pancytopenia, oval macrocytes, and hypersegmented neutrophils; megaloblastic hyperplasia	Dietary deficiency; malabsorption syndromes
Aplastic anemia	Markedly diminished hematopoiesis	Pancytopenia, reticulocytopenia, marked hypocellularity of bone marrow	Toxic drugs and chemicals; often idiopathic
Anemia of chronic disease	Diverse mechanisms	Anemia most often normochromic and normocytic or macrocytic; may be hypochromic and microcytic with decreased serum iron and decreased serum iron binding capacity	Various chronic diseases, especially rheumatoid arthritis, renal disease, and chronic infection
Myelophthisic anemia	Bone marrow replacement, usually by malignant tumor	Severe anemia; small numbers of nucleated red cells and immature granulocytes in peripheral blood; tumor cells in bone marrow	

III. Iron Deficiency Anemia (see Table 11.1)

A. Causes

1. Increased iron requirement

—may occur during **pregnancy;** iron demands of the fetus can deplete maternal iron stores.

—may also occur in **infants and preadolescents** who may outgrow borderline iron stores.

2. Dietary deficiency

—is rare except in infants; because human milk is low in iron, newborn storage iron will be depleted within the first 6 months unless it is replaced by dietary supplementation. Premature infants are at special risk.

—may rarely occur in elderly persons.

3. Chronic blood loss

—is the major cause of iron deficiency anemia in adults.

—is most often caused by **menorrhagia** or **bleeding gastrointestinal lesions**.

B. Clinical manifestations—iron deficiency anemia

—may include **pallor, fatigue,** or **dyspnea on exertion**.

—sometimes includes angina pectoris in persons with coronary artery narrowing caused by atherosclerotic disease.

—when extreme, may be associated with glossitis, gastritis, koilonychia (spooning of the nails), or Plummer-Vinson syndrome, in which iron deficiency is associated with a partially obstructing upper esophageal web.

C. Laboratory findings

1. Decreased hemoglobin, hematocrit, and red cell count

2. Hypochromic microcytic erythrocytes on peripheral smear

3. Decreased serum iron and increased total iron binding capacity (TIBC)

4. Decreased body iron stores, measured by bone marrow examination for stainable hemosiderin or by decreased serum ferritin

IV. Megaloblastic Anemias

A. General characteristics—megaloblastic anemias

—are defined by large, abnormal-appearing **erythroid precursor cells** (megaloblasts) in the bone marrow.

—are caused by **deficiency of vitamin B_{12} or folate**.

—are characterized by decreased DNA synthesis, with a consequent delay in DNA replication and nuclear division, and by relatively unimpeded cytoplasmic maturation.

—manifest morphologically as nuclear–cytoplasmic asynchrony of large erythroid precursor cells with an open, loose-appearing chromatin pattern.

—result in anemia caused by impaired red cell production; to a lesser degree, red cell destruction occurs within the bone marrow prior to release of mature erythrocytes into the peripheral blood (ineffective erythropoiesis).

B. **Laboratory abnormalities**

1. **Peripheral blood and bone marrow** findings are identical in all forms of megaloblastic anemias.

   a. **Peripheral blood**
      (1) **Pancytopenia** (decreased red cells, white cells, and platelets)
      (2) **Oval macrocytosis**
      (3) **Hypersegmented neutrophils** (more than five lobes)

   b. **Bone marrow: megaloblastic hyperplasia**

2. **Vitamin B_{12} and folate levels** further define the specific type of megaloblastic anemia.

C. **Types of megaloblastic anemia**

1. **Vitamin B_{12} deficiency**

   a. **Pernicious anemia (PA)**
      (1) **General features—pernicious anemia**
         −is the most common form of vitamin B_{12} deficiency megaloblastic anemia.
         −is considered to be an **autoimmune disorder;** other autoimmune diseases (especially thyroid diseases) occur with unusual frequency in persons with pernicious anemia.
         −is caused by **chronic (fundal [type A]) gastritis,** which is associated with failure of production of intrinsic factor, essential for vitamin B_{12} absorption. The chronic gastritis is also associated with:
         (a) **Achlorhydria** (absent gastric-free hydrochloric acid)
         (b) **Anti-intrinsic factor and antiparietal cell antibodies**
         (c) **Increased incidence of gastric carcinoma**
      (2) **Clinical findings**
         (a) **Insidious onset** with extreme reduction of red blood cell count
         (b) Characteristic **lemon yellow skin color**
         (c) **Stomatitis and glossitis**
         (d) **Subacute combined degeneration of the cord** (combined systems disease, posterolateral degeneration), an associated neurologic disorder that manifests clinically by ataxic gait, hyperreflexia, and impaired position and vibration sensation. (Neurologic abnormalities are associated with vitamin B_{12} deficiency but not with folate deficiency.)
      (3) **Laboratory findings**
         (a) **Pancytopenia, hypersegmented neutrophils, and megaloblastic hyperplasia** of the bone marrow (findings characteristic of all megaloblastic anemias)
         (b) **Anti-intrinsic factor antibodies,** which are rarely found in other conditions; antiparietal cell antibodies may be seen in other conditions but are most frequent in pernicious anemia.
         (c) **Abnormal Schilling test,** characterized by impaired absorption of vitamin B_{12} correctable by intrinsic factor

   b. **Other forms of vitamin B_{12} deficiency megaloblastic anemia**
      −a pernicious anemia-like illness can be caused by a number of other mechanisms that result in vitamin B_{12} deficiency.

    (1) **Total gastric resection;** intrinsic factor is produced in the gastric fundus.

    (2) **Disorders of the distal ileum;** intrinsic factor–vitamin B_{12} complex is absorbed in the distal ileum.

    (3) **Strict vegetarian diet;** vitamin B_{12} is found only in foods of animal origin.

    (4) **Intestinal malabsorption syndromes**

    (5) **Blind-loop syndrome;** bacterial overgrowth in a surgically induced intestinal blind loop results in depletion of vitamin B_{12}.

    (6) **Broad-spectrum antibiotic therapy;** can result in intestinal bacterial overgrowth with vitamin B_{12} depletion.

    (7) *Diphyllobothrium latum* **infestation;** the giant fish tapeworm of man, acquired by ingestion of freshwater fish, inhabits the intestine and causes vitamin B_{12} depletion.

2. Folate deficiency

    –folate deficiency megaloblastic anemia can be caused by a number of diverse mechanisms.

    a. Severe dietary deprivation (most often occurs in chronic alcoholics or fad dieters)

    b. Pregnancy (combination of additional demands of the fetus and borderline maternal diet)

    c. Intestinal malabsorption caused by:

        (1) **Sprue**

        (2) *Giardia lamblia* **infection**

        (3) **Dilantin (phenytoin),** or **oral contraceptive therapy**

        (4) **Folic acid antagonist chemotherapy** for cancer

        (5) **Relative folate deficiency** (increased demand because of compensatory accelerated erythropoiesis in hemolytic anemia)

V. Anemia of Chronic Disease

–is a common form of anemia, second in incidence to iron deficiency anemia.

–can be **secondary to a wide variety of primary disorders,** including rheumatoid arthritis, renal disease, or chronic infection.

–is often **normochromic and normocytic**.

–when associated with renal disease, may be moderately macrocytic.

–when associated with **chronic inflammatory states** (e.g., rheumatoid arthritis), may be accompanied by decreased serum iron and hypochromia and microcytosis, mimicking iron deficiency anemia; however, in contrast to iron deficiency anemia, TIBC is characteristically decreased.

VI. Aplastic Anemia

–is severe anemia resulting from the loss of erythroid precursor cells.

–is most often **secondary to toxic exposure;** it also may occur without evident cause.

–is characterized by markedly **hypocellular bone marrow** with loss of erythrocytic and granulocytic precursor cells and megakaryocytes and by **peripheral pancytopenia**.

–can be induced by the following **etiologic agents:**

A. Radiation exposure

B. **Chemicals,** such as **benzene** and related organic compounds

C. **Therapeutic drugs,** such as **chloramphenicol,** sulfonamides, gold salts, various anti-inflammatory and anti-malarial drugs, and **alkylating agents** used in the treatment of neoplastic diseases

   1. In some persons who have been given chloramphenicol, there is a predictable, dose-related, usually reversible marrow response.

   2. In other persons, there is an idiosyncratic, severe, frequently irreversible effect.

D. **Viral infection,** such as **human parvovirus** or **hepatitis C virus**

VII. Myelophthisic Anemia

—is a form of bone marrow failure caused by replacement of the marrow, most often by a malignant neoplasm.

—is less commonly due to bone marrow destruction from non-neoplastic causes such as marrow fibrosis.

VIII. Hemolytic Anemias (Table 11.2)

—are defined as anemias due to shortening of red cell life span (increased red cell destruction).

A. **General features**

   1. **Increased red cell destruction** with liberation of hemoglobin or its degradation products manifest by:

      a. **Increased unconjugated (indirect reacting) bilirubin,** resulting in **acholuric jaundice,** which is jaundice not accompanied by bilirubinuria. Hyperbilirubinemia may lead to **pigment-containing gallstones** as a late complication.

      b. **Hemoglobinemia and hemoglobinuria,** which, along with methemalbuminemia and hemosiderinuria, occur if red cell destruction is very rapid and within the circulation (intravascular hemolysis).

      c. **Disappearance of serum haptoglobin,** a group of hemoglobin-binding protein, which combines with liberated hemoglobin and is no longer demonstrable. Elevation of serum hemoglobin does not occur until serum haptoglobin is no longer detectable.

      d. **Hemosiderosis,** systemic iron deposition

   2. **Increased erythropoiesis,** compensating in part for the shortened red cell survival and manifest by:

      a. **Normoblastic erythroid hyperplasia** in marrow

      b. **Reticulocytosis** (increased number of circulating newly formed red cells identified by residual stainable RNA)

      c. **Polychromatophilia** (increased number of red cells that stain with a bluish cast, roughly equivalent to increased reticulocyte count)

B. **Terminology**

   1. **Intracorpuscular hemolytic anemia**

      —is marked by defects, most often **genetically determined,** in the red cell itself.

Table 11.2. Examples of Anemias Resulting from Increased Red Cell Destruction

Type	Mechanisms	Diagnostic Features	Comments
Warm antibody autoimmune hemolytic anemia (primary and secondary forms)	IgG autoantibodies combine with red cell surface antigens; Fc combining site of IgG antibody further reacts with Fc receptor of phagocytic cells	Anemia, spherocytosis, and reticulocytosis; unconjugated hyperbilirubinemia and acholuric jaundice; positive direct Coombs' test	Often secondary to lymphocytic neoplasms, Hodgkin's disease, or autoimmune disease; sometimes associated with α-methyldopa or penicillin therapy
Hemolytic disease of the newborn (erythroblastosis fetalis)	Maternal alloimmunization to fetal red cell antigens, classically of Rh system	Rising titer of maternal anti-Rh antibodies during latter part of pregnancy; cord blood at delivery contains immature red cell precursors; direct Coombs' test positive on cord blood; progressive postnatal increase in unconjugated bilirubin	Prevented by administration of anti-Rh antibody (anti-D IgG) to mother at time of delivery of first and subsequent children, removing Rh-positive red cells from maternal circulation; treated by exchange transfusion to remove unconjugated bilirubin from serum of newborn infant to prevent kernicterus
Hereditary spherocytosis	Red cell membrane protein abnormality	Autosomal dominant inheritance; anemia, spherocytosis, and reticulocytosis; increased mean corpuscular hemoglobin concentration; unconjugated hyperbilirubinemia and acholuric jaundice; splenomegaly; increased erythrocyte osmotic fragility to hypotonic saline	Quantitative deficiency of spectrin due to diverse mechanisms
Glucose-6-phosphate dehydrogenase (G6PD) deficiency	Failure of erythrocyte hexose monophosphate shunt under oxidative stress	Self-limited hemolytic anemia; reduced activity of erythrocyte G6PD	X-linked inheritance
Sickle cell anemia	β-globin hemoglobinopathy (mutation in coding sequence of β-globin gene, GAG [glu] → GTG [val])	Anemia and reticulocytosis; sickle-shaped erythrocytes demonstrable on peripheral blood smear; homozygosity for hemoglobin S demonstrable by electrophoresis	Characterized by severe anemia, recurrent painful and aplastic crises, and nonhealing leg ulcers; recurrent splenic infarcts with progressive fibrosis result in autosplenectomy
β-Thalassemia major (Cooley's anemia, Mediterranean anemia)	Diverse mutations in β-globin gene causing decreased synthesis of β-globin chains; aggregation of excess α-chains causes hemolytic anemia and ineffective erythropoiesis.	Severe anemia; thalassemic red cell morphology; increased hemoglobin F	Occurs frequently in Mediterranean populations
α-Thalassemias	Deletion of one or more of the four α-globin genes (α-globin gene is reduplicated in tandem on each chromosome 16)	Differ according to number of deletions	No clinical abnormalities with one gene deletion; mild to moderate thalassemic state with two or three deletions; intrauterine death with four deletions; hemoglobin Barts (γ$_4$) in fetal life; hemoglobin H (β$_4$) in adult life

2. Extracorpuscular hemolytic anemia

–is marked by defects, most often **acquired,** of the extra-erythrocytic environment, such as circulating antibodies or an enlarged spleen.

C. Immune hemolytic anemias

1. Warm antibody autoimmune hemolytic anemia

–is the **most common form** of immune hemolytic anemia.

–is mediated by **IgG autoantibodies** optimally active at 37° C that react with red cell surface antigens.

–is often secondary to underlying disease states such as systemic lupus erythematosus, Hodgkin's disease, or non-Hodgkin's lymphomas.

–is clinically characterized by the following:

a. General features of hemolytic anemia

b. Spherocytosis due to progressive loss of membrane protein by serial passage of antibody-coated red cells through the spleen

c. Positive direct Coombs' test reflecting the binding of IgG autoantibody to the red cell surface

2. Cold agglutinin disease

–is mediated by **IgM antibodies** optimally active at temperatures below 30° C (cold antibodies, cold agglutinins).

a. Acute cold agglutinin disease

–is often mediated by antibodies with specificity for the **I blood group antigen**.

–is often a complication of infectious mononucleosis or *Mycoplasma pneumoniae* infection. Diagnosis of mycoplasma pneumonia is facilitated by the demonstration of cold agglutinins.

b. Chronic cold agglutinin disease

–is often associated with **lymphoid neoplasms**.

–is often mediated by **anti-i antibodies**.

–is characterized clinically by agglutination and hemolysis in tissue sites exposed to the cold.

–may be associated with Raynaud's phenomenon. These cases are marked by chronic hemolytic anemia exacerbated by cold weather, punctuated by episodes of jaundice, sometimes with hemoglobinemia and hemoglobinuria.

3. Hemolytic disease of the newborn (erythroblastosis fetalis)

–results from **maternal alloimmunization** to fetal red cell antigens, classically the D antigen of the **Rh blood group system**. In the most frequently occurring form of Rh-mediated hemolytic disease of the newborn, the mother is typed as d and the fetus as D.

–can also result from **ABO incompatibility**. In most instances of ABO incompatibility, the mother is blood group O and the child is blood group A or group B.

–occurs when maternal antibodies cross the placenta and react with fetal red cells, resulting in **fetal hemolytic anemia**.

–can result in stillbirth or in **hydrops fetalis,** fetal heart failure with massive generalized edema.

—can result in **kernicterus,** staining of the basal ganglia and other central nervous system (CNS) structures by unconjugated bilirubin. Kernicterus with resultant neurologic damage is the most significant long-term consequence of hemolytic disease of the newborn.

—has been markedly reduced in incidence by preventive measures. Routine administration of anti-D IgG antiserum to D-negative mothers at the time of delivery (or termination of pregnancy) of a D-positive child results in the antibody-mediated removal of fetal red cells from the maternal circulation, preventing maternal alloimmunization.

D. Paroxysmal nocturnal hemoglobinuria

—is an uncommon acquired **intracorpuscular defect**.

—arises from a somatic mutation resulting in an abnormal clone of bone marrow stem cells.

—is characterized by increased sensitivity to complement-induced red cell lysis.

—is often marked by the passage of hemoglobin-containing urine on awakening.

E. Hemolytic anemias caused by membrane protein abnormalities

1. Hereditary spherocytosis

—is an autosomal dominant hemolytic anemia characterized by sphere-shaped erythrocytes (spherocytes) that are selectively trapped or sequestered in the spleen.

—is the most common intracorpuscular inherited hemolytic anemia observed in whites.

—is caused by a variety of molecular defects in the genes coding for spectrin, ankyrin, protein 4.1, and other erythrocyte cytoskeletal proteins.

2. Hereditary elliptocytosis (ovalocytosis)

—is an autosomal dominant disorder characterized by elongated, oval red cells.

—does not always cause anemia.

—may be marked by hemolytic anemia and splenomegaly.

F. Enzyme deficiency hemolytic anemias

1. Glucose-6-phosphate dehydrogenase (G6PD) deficiency

—is the most common form of enzyme deficiency hemolytic anemia.

—is an **X-linked** disorder occurring in approximately 10% of blacks and also in persons of Mediterranean origin.

—is manifest by acute self-limited hemolytic anemia caused by oxidative stress induced by a wide variety of therapeutic drugs or, in some persons of Mediterranean origin, by fava beans.

2. Pyruvate kinase deficiency

—is the second most common enzyme deficiency hemolytic anemia.

—is an autosomal recessive disorder characterized by congenital non-spherocytic hemolytic anemia; in contrast to G6PD deficiency, the anemia is chronic and nonepisodic.

G. Hemoglobinopathies

—are hemolytic anemias caused by **genetically determined** abnormalities of hemoglobin structure.

—in the United States, are most importantly represented by disorders involving hemoglobin S; to a lesser extent, hemoglobin C; and in some urban centers, hemoglobin E.

1. Hemoglobin S disorders

a. General considerations

(1) Approximately 7% of American blacks carry the hemoglobin S gene. In some parts of Africa, more than one-third of the population is affected; possibly the hemoglobin S gene confers resistance to malarial infection.

(2) Similar resistance may be conferred by erythrocyte G6PD deficiency or by the absence of Duffy blood group antigens. Both G6PD deficiency and the Duffy Fy(a- b-) phenotype occur with high incidence in black populations.

(3) Hemoglobin S arises from a point mutation in codon 6 of the globin gene and results in a substitution of valine for glutamic acid.

(4) Hemoglobin S polymerizes at low oxygen tension, forming tactoids that distort the shape of red cells to elongated, sickle shapes; repeated sickling episodes stiffen red cell membranes, making affected cells more subject to hemolysis; rigid, sickled cells are more apt to obstruct the microvasculature, causing hemolysis.

(5) All hemoglobin S disorders are characterized by a positive sickle cell preparation (in vitro sickling of red cells on exposure to reducing agents). The sickle cell preparation is positive whenever hemoglobin S is present (e.g., sickle cell anemia, sickle cell trait, sickle C disease, sickle cell thalassemia).

b. Sickle cell anemia

—the homozygous form of hemoglobin S leads to sickle cell anemia (sickle cell disease), which is characterized by:

(1) **Severe lifelong hemolytic anemia**

(2) **Chronic leg ulcers**

(3) Vaso-occlusive **painful crises** (severe pain in the limbs, back, chest, and abdomen), often precipitated by infection or dehydration

(4) **Repeated infarctions in the lungs and spleen;** the spleen is characteristically congested and enlarged in childhood but becomes progressively smaller through repeated infarcts and fibrosis (**autosplenectomy**).

(5) **Aplastic crises** (distinguished from painful crises), characterized by a precipitous fall in hemoglobin concentration, usually provoked by viral infection such as human parvovirus

c. Sickle cell trait

—hemoglobin S in the heterozygous form leads to sickle cell trait, which is generally without clinical consequence.

2. Hemoglobin C disorders

—are primarily observed in blacks.

—when homozygous, are characterized by a mild hemolytic anemia accompanied by prominent splenomegaly, target cells, and, on occasion, intraerythrocytic crystals.

—when heterozygous, result in disease only with coinheritance of other abnormal hemoglobins, most often hemoglobin S.

3. Hemoglobin E disorders

—are prevalent in Southeast Asia.

—have increased significantly in incidence in the United States in recent years and are now more common than hemoglobin S disorders in some urban areas.

—have clinical and laboratory manifestations similar to hemoglobin C disorders.

H. Thalassemias

—are a heterogeneous group of **genetic disorders** characterized by deficient production of either of the two globin chains of hemoglobin.

—are widespread throughout the world, occurring with high frequency in Africa, India, Southeast Asia, and the Mediterranean area.

1. β-Thalassemias

—are the most common forms of thalassemia found in Mediterranean areas and in the United States.

—are caused by defects in the promoter sequence, in introns, or in coding regions of the β globin gene.

a. β-Thalassemia major

—is also known as **Mediterranean anemia** or **Cooley's anemia**.

—results from double heterozygosity or homozygosity for thalassemic variants of the β-globin gene.

—is characterized clinically by:

(1) Marked anemia resulting from:

    (a) Modest decrease in hemoglobin synthesis

    (b) Marked shortening of red cell life span due to aggregation of insoluble excess α-chains

    (c) Ineffective erythropoiesis

    (d) Relative folate deficiency

(2) Marked splenomegaly

(3) Distortion of skull, facial bones, and long bones because of erythroid marrow expansion

(4) Thalassemic red cell morphology (marked microcytosis, hypochromia, extensive changes in size and shape)

(5) Increased hemoglobin F ($\alpha_2\gamma_2$) throughout life

(6) Generalized hemosiderosis due to chronic hemolysis, ineffective erythropoiesis, and repeated transfusions

b. β-Thalassemia minor

—results from heterozygous inheritance of thalassemic variants of the β-globin gene.

—manifests clinically as minimal hypochromic microcytic anemia and an increase in hemoglobin A_2 ($\alpha_2 \delta_2$), a normally occurring minor hemoglobin fraction.

c. Sickle cell thalassemia

—results from coinheritance of hemoglobin S gene and a thalassemic variant of the β-globin gene (double heterozygosity).

—is clinically similar to, but often less severe than, sickle cell anemia.

2. α-Thalassemias

—are the most common forms of thalassemia in Southeast Asia.

—are caused by deletions of one or more of the four globin genes (see Table 11.2).

—in normal persons, there is duplication of the globin gene, with a pair of identical α-globin genes on each member of the chromosome 16 pair.

Review Test

Directions: Each of the numbered items or incomplete statements in this section is followed by answers or by completions of the statement. Select the **one** lettered answer or completion that is **best** in each case.

1. The peripheral blood smear of an anemic one-year-old child is shown in the illustration below. The most likely diagnosis is

(A) hereditary spherocytosis.
(B) thalassemia major.
(C) anemia of chronic disease.
(D) iron deficiency anemia.
(E) aplastic anemia.

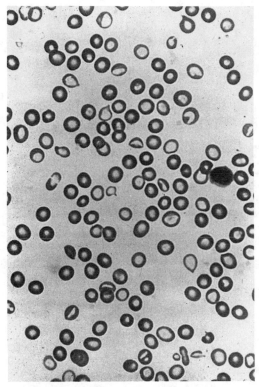

(Courtesy of Dr. Jae O. Ro, Veterans Affairs Medical Center and University of Health Sciences, The Chicago Medical School)

Questions 2 and 3

2. The peripheral blood smear of a severely anemic patient reveals oval macrocytes, hypersegmented neutrophils, and decreased platelets. The most likely cause of the anemia is

(A) a red cell membrane protein defect.
(B) vitamin B_{12} or folate deficiency.
(C) an amino acid substitution in the β-globin chain.
(D) marrow hypoplasia.
(E) iron deficiency.

3. The patient is found to be a severely malnourished alcoholic. The most likely cause of his disorder is

(A) folate deficiency.
(B) pernicious anemia.
(C) fish tapeworm infestation.
(D) aberrant intestinal bacterial flora.
(E) Crohn's disease.

4. A primiparous D-negative (Rh-negative) mother has just delivered a D-positive child. Administration of which of the following substances would be indicated?

(A) D-positive red cells to mother
(B) D-positive red cells to child
(C) Anti-D IgG to mother
(D) Anti-D IgG to child

5. Which one of the following manifestations of hemolytic disease of the newborn has the greatest potential for lifelong disability?

(A) Kernicterus
(B) Renal failure
(C) Cardiogenic shock
(D) Cardiac failure

6. All of the following pairings of red cell Rh types and ABO groups of mother and child may lead to hemolytic disease of the newborn EXCEPT

(A) mother cde, A; child cDe, O.
(B) mother CDe, AB; child cdE, O.
(C) mother cde, O; child CDe, A.
(D) mother cDE, O; child Cde, A.
(E) mother Cde, B; child cDe, B.

Questions 7 and 8

7. A 23-year-old black male with a history of severe lifelong anemia requiring many transfusions has nonhealing leg ulcers and recurrent bouts of abdominal and chest pain. These signs and symptoms are most likely associated with which one of the following laboratory abnormalities?

(A) Sickle cells on peripheral blood smear
(B) Increased erythrocyte osmotic fragility
(C) Schistocytes
(D) Teardrop-shaped cells
(E) Decreased erythropoietin

8. The spleen in this patient would be expected to be

(A) enlarged.
(B) shrunken.
(C) normal sized.

9. Ineffective erythropoiesis is characteristic of which one of the following conditions?

(A) Hereditary spherocytosis
(B) Erythroblastosis fetalis
(C) β-Thalassemia major
(D) Anemia of chronic disease
(E) Sickle cell anemia

10. A 23-year-old man of northern European lineage presents with anemia. His father and paternal aunt had had a similar illness treated successfully by splenectomy. His peripheral blood smear was similar to that shown in the following illustration. All of the following additional abnormalities are expected EXCEPT

(A) acholuric jaundice.
(B) positive direct Coombs' test.
(C) reticulocytosis.
(D) polychromatophilic erythrocytes on peripheral blood smear.
(E) increased osmotic fragility.

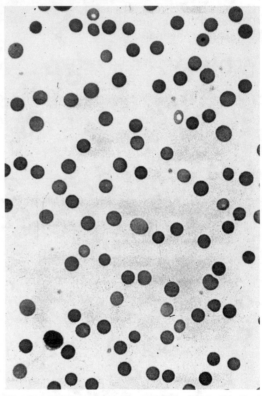

(Courtesy of Dr. Jae O. Ro, Veterans Affairs Medical Center and University of Health Sciences, The Chicago Medical School)

Answers and Explanations

1–D. The illustration shows hypochromia and microcytosis. Iron deficiency is the most frequent cause of hypochromic microcytic anemia. In infants and preadolescents, iron deficiency is most often nutritional in origin. In young women, the cause is most often related to menstrual blood loss compounded by deficient dietary intake. In men, the usual cause is occult gastrointestinal blood loss.

2–B. Megaloblastic anemia due to deficiency of vitamin B_{12} or folate is characterized by oval macrocytes, hypersegmented neutrophils, and decreased platelets.

3–A. Megaloblastic anemia associated with severe malnutrition is most often due to folate deficiency.

4–C. Administration of anti-D antiserum to a D-negative mother at the time of delivery of a D-positive child prevents maternal alloimmunization by removing fetal red cells from the maternal circulation.

5–A. Kernicterus, staining of a variety of CNS structures by unconjugated bilirubin, often results in permanent neurologic damage.

6–B. Hemolytic disease of the newborn does not occur when the mother is D (Rh-positive) and the child is d (Rh-negative) or when the mother is AB and the child is O. Rh-system incompatibility is seen when the mother is d (Rh-negative) and the child is D (Rh-positive). ABO system incompatibility is seen when the mother is O and the child is A, B, or AB.

7–A. Sickle cell anemia is the most common hereditary anemia of blacks. Leg ulcers and recurring painful crises are characteristic. In sickle cell anemia, in contrast to sickle cell trait, sickle cells are frequently seen on the peripheral blood smear.

8–B. Repeated episodes of splenic infarction followed by fibrotic healing lead to a fibrotic, shrunken spleen (autosplenectomy) in adult patients with sickle cell anemia. The spleen is enlarged and congested in children with sickle cell anemia.

9–C. Ineffective erythropoiesis, red cell destruction in marrow prior to red cell release, is a major characteristic of β-thalassemia major and is caused by aggregation of excess α-chains.

10–B. Spherocytes are present on the peripheral blood smear and, along with the history, strongly suggest a diagnosis of hereditary spherocytosis (HS). Since similar cells are also observed in warm antibody autoimmune hemolytic anemia, these two conditions must be distinguished by means of the direct Coombs' test, which is negative in HS and positive in warm antibody autoimmune hemolytic anemia.

12

Neoplastic and Proliferative Disorders of the Hematopoietic and Lymphoid Systems

I. Leukemia

A. General considerations

—leukemia is a general term for a group of malignancies of either lymphoid or hematopoietic cell origin. The number of circulating leukocytes is often markedly increased.

—the bone marrow is diffusely infiltrated with leukemic cells, often with encroachment on normal hematopoietic cell development. Consequent failure of normal leukocyte, red cell, and platelet production can result in anemia, infection, or hemorrhage.

—infiltration of leukemic cells in the liver, spleen, lymph nodes, and other organs is common.

B. Acute leukemias

—are characterized by a predominance of **blasts** and closely related cells in the bone marrow and peripheral blood.

—occur most often in **children** and are the most common malignancies of the pediatric age group.

—exhibit a second incidence peak after age 60.

—are frequently associated with cytogenic abnormalities. For example, the 9;22 translocation results in a morphologically unique chromosome, the **Philadelphia chromosome (Ph^1)**. This abnormality, better known for its association with chronic myeloid leukemia, is associated with a poorer prognosis when it occurs in acute leukemias.

—without therapeutic intervention, follow a short and precipitous course, marked by anemia, infection, and hemorrhage, and death occurs within 6 to 12 months.

1. Acute lymphoblastic leukemia (ALL)

—is characterized by a predominance of **lymphoblasts**.

—occurs most often in **children** and is the form of acute leukemia that is most **responsive to therapy**.

—is further classified into a number of subgroups based on differences in morphology, antigenic cell-surface markers, or rearrangement of the immunoglobulin heavy-chain or T-cell receptor genes.

2. Acute myeloblastic leukemia (AML)

—is also referred to as acute granulocytic leukemia or acute nonlymphoblastic leukemia.

—is characterized by a predominance of **myeloblasts** and early promyelocytes.

—occurs most frequently in **adults**.

—responds more poorly to current therapy than does ALL.

—is further classified into a number of subgroups based on morphology and cytochemical characteristics.

C. Chronic leukemias

—are characterized by proliferations of lymphoid or hematopoietic cells that are more mature than those of the acute leukemias.

—have a longer, less devastating clinical course than the acute leukemias.

1. Chronic lymphocytic leukemia (CLL)

a. General considerations

(1) CLL is characterized by a proliferation of **neoplastic lymphoid cells** (almost always B cells) with widespread infiltration of the bone marrow, peripheral blood, lymph nodes, spleen, liver, and other organs.

(2) Leukemic cells are incapable of differentiating into antibody-producing plasma cells.

(3) CLL most often occurs in persons over the age of 60 and more frequently in men.

b. Characteristics

(1) The leukemic cells closely resemble normal mature peripheral blood lymphocytes.

(2) The cells are susceptible to mechanical disruption, often appearing on the peripheral blood smear as **smudge cells**.

(3) The peripheral white cell count varies from 50,000/µl to 200,000/µl, with a preponderance of leukemic cells.

(4) Leukemic cells diffusely infiltrate the bone marrow.

c. Complications

(1) **Warm antibody autoimmune hemolytic anemia**

(2) Hypogammaglobulinemia and increased susceptibility to bacterial infection, often occurring early in the course of this disorder

d. Clinical features

(1) The clinical course is usually described as indolent, often with few symptoms and minor disability for protracted periods.

(2) Generalized **lymphadenopathy** and moderate **hepatosplenomegaly** are frequent features.

(3) Mean survival is 3 to 7 years; treatment relieves symptoms but has little effect on overall survival.

2. Chronic myeloid leukemia (CML)

—is also referred to as chronic myelocytic leukemia or chronic granulocytic leukemia (CGL).

—is a neoplastic clonal proliferation of **myeloid stem cells,** the precursor cells of erythrocytes, granulocytes, and platelets.

—is one of the myeloproliferative syndromes.

a. Molecular changes

(1) CML is characterized by a reciprocal chromosomal translocation between chromosomes 9 and 22, resulting in the **Philadelphia chromosome**.

(2) The *c-abl* proto-oncogene on chromosome 9 is transposed to an area on chromosome 22, adjacent to a putative oncogene, forming a hybrid, or fusion, gene, *bcr-abl*.

(3) *Bcr-abl* codes for a protein (p210) with tyrosine kinase activity, which may play a critical role in the etiopathogenesis of CML.

b. Characteristics

(1) **Marked leukocytosis,** with white cell counts varying from 50,000/μl to 200,000/μl

(2) Leukemic cells in the peripheral blood and bone marrow, mainly middle-to-late myeloid (granulocytic) precursor cells, including myelocytes, metamyelocytes, bands, and segmented forms

(3) Small numbers of blasts and promyelocytes

(4) The Philadelphia chromosome, found in granulocytic and erythroid precursor cells and in megakaryocytes

(5) Marked reduction in leukocyte alkaline phosphatase activity in the leukemic leukocyte

c. Clinical features

(1) Prominent splenomegaly and modestly enlarged liver and lymph nodes

(2) Peak incidence in middle-age group (ages 35–50)

(3) Terminates, in most instances, in an accelerated phase (blastic crisis) signaled by increasing numbers of blast cells and promyelocytes

II. Myeloproliferative Syndromes

—are neoplastic clonal proliferations of myeloid stem cells.

—represent a group of closely related disorders, which include chronic myeloid leukemia, polycythemia vera, agnogenic myeloid metaplasia, and essential thrombocythemia.

A. Common characteristics

1. Peak incidence in middle-aged and elderly persons

2. Proliferation of one or more of the myeloid series cells

3. Increase in peripheral blood basophils

4. Increase in serum uric acid

5. Prominent splenomegaly

B. Polycythemia vera

1. Clinical characteristics

a. Marked erythrocytosis

b. Moderate increase in circulating granulocytes and platelets

    c. Splenomegaly

    d. Decreased erythropoietin

2. Other features

    a. Sludging of high hematocrit blood often leads to **thrombotic or hemorrhagic phenomena**.

    b. Polycythemia vera often progresses to a late phase in which anemia supervenes. This phase is often marked by bone marrow fibrosis and extramedullary hematopoiesis and a rising white cell count, and it can mimic CML.

    c. Acute leukemia may supervene in approximately 3% of patients, most of whom have received antimitotic drugs or radiation therapy.

3. Diagnosis–polycythemia vera

    –is marked by **decreased erythropoietin,** which distinguishes it from other forms of polycythemia, all of which are associated with increased erythropoietin.

    –must be distinguished from **secondary polycythemia,** which is associated with the following:

    a. Chronic hypoxia, associated with pulmonary disease, congenital heart disease, residence at high altitudes, and heavy smoking

    b. Inappropriate production of erythropoietin, associated with **adult polycystic disease** and **tumors,** such as renal cell carcinoma, hepatocellular carcinoma, and cerebellar hemangioma

    c. Endocrine abnormalities, prominently including **pheochromocytoma** and adrenal adenoma with **Cushing's syndrome**

C. Myeloid metaplasia with myelofibrosis (agnogenic myeloid metaplasia)

    –is characterized by **extensive extramedullary hematopoiesis** involving the liver and spleen and sometimes the lymph nodes.

    –is further characterized by proliferation of non-neoplastic fibrous tissue within the bone marrow cavity (**myelofibrosis**).

1. Postulated pathogenetic factors

    a. Megakaryocytic proliferation may be the primary abnormality, and the elaboration of platelet-derived growth factor and of transforming growth factor-β (TGF-β) by platelets and megakaryocytes may be the cause of the fibroblastic proliferation.

    b. Megakaryocytes are spared in the marrow fibrotic process and increase in number, resulting in prominent bone marrow megakaryocytosis and peripheral blood thrombocytosis.

2. Clinical features

    a. Peripheral blood smear

        (1) Teardrop-shaped erythrocytes

        (2) Granulocytic precursor cells and nucleated red cell precursors in variable numbers

    b. Anemia and massive **splenomegaly**

D. Essential thrombocythemia

–is characterized by marked **thrombocytosis** in the peripheral blood and **megakaryocytosis** in the bone marrow. Platelet counts in excess of 1,000,000/µl are common (normal value is 150,000–350,000/µl).

–is also characterized by **bleeding and thrombosis**.

III. Non-neoplastic Lymphoid Proliferations

A. General considerations

–these reactions include acute and chronic nonspecific lymphadenitis occurring in response to a number of infectious agents or immune stimuli.

B. Infectious mononucleosis

–is a benign, self-limited disorder caused by **Epstein-Barr virus** (EBV), which has an affinity for B lymphocytes.

–occurs frequently in **young adults**.

–is characterized by circulating **atypical lymphocytes** (reactive CD8+ lymphocytes).

–is marked by a number of serum antibodies, including **anti-EBV antibodies** and **heterophil antibodies** (heterophil agglutinins) directed at sheep erythrocytes.

–is clinically characterized by prominent sore throat, fever, generalized lymphadenopathy, and often by hepatosplenomegaly. The spleen is especially susceptible to traumatic rupture.

IV. Plasma Cell Disorders

–are neoplastic proliferations of well-differentiated immunoglobulin-producing cells.

–include multiple myeloma, Waldenström's macroglobulinemia, primary amyloidosis, benign monoclonal gammopathy, and heavy-chain (Franklin's) disease.

A. Multiple myeloma

–is a **malignant plasma cell tumor** that typically involves bone and is associated with prominent serum and urinary protein abnormalities.

1. Bone lesions and protein abnormalities

a. The neoplastic cell is an end-stage derivative of B lymphocytes clearly identifiable as a plasma cell.

b. The tumor cells produce **lytic lesions in bone,** especially in the skull and axial skeleton. Bone lesions:

–appear lucent on radiographic examination, with characteristic sharp borders and are referred to as **punched-out lesions**.

–may be manifest radiographically as diffuse demineralization of bone (**osteopenia**).

–are caused by an osteoclast-activating factor secreted by the neoplastic plasma cells.

–are often associated with severe bone pain and spontaneous fractures.

c. Multiple myeloma arises from proliferation of a single clone of malignant antibody-producing cells.

      (1) The tumor cells produce massive quantities of identical immunoglobulin molecules demonstrable electrophoretically as a narrow serum band or, after densitometric scanning, as a sharp spike referred to as an **M protein**.

      (2) The M protein in multiple myeloma is most often IgG or IgA immunoglobulin of either kappa or lambda light-chain-specificity.

      (3) The marked serum immunoglobulin increase is often initially detected by laboratory screening as increased total protein with an increase in serum globulin (**hyperglobulinemia**).

      (4) The urine often contains significant quantities of free immunoglobulin light chains, either kappa or lambda, which are referred to as **Bence Jones protein**.

      (5) As a consequence of hyperglobulinemia, the red cells tend to congregate together in a manner reminiscent of a stack of poker chips (**rouleaux formation**). There is also a marked increase in the erythrocyte sedimentation rate.

2. Other clinical characteristics—multiple myeloma

a. Anemia due to neoplastic encroachment on myeloid precursor cells; possible leukopenia and thrombocytopenia

b. Increased susceptibility to infection from possible proliferation of the M protein and impaired production of normal immunoglobulins

c. Hypercalcemia secondary to bone destruction

d. Renal insufficiency with azotemia due to myeloma kidney (myeloma nephrosis). The renal lesion is characterized by prominent tubular casts of Bence Jones protein, numerous multinucleated macrophage-derived giant cells, metastatic calcification, and sometimes by interstitial infiltration of malignant plasma cells.

e. Amyloidosis of the primary amyloidosis type

B. Waldenström's macroglobulinemia

    –is a proliferation of **IgM-producing lymphoid cells** of an intermediate stage between B lymphocytes and plasma cells referred to as **plasmacytoid lymphocytes**.

1. Defining characteristics

a. Serum IgM immunoglobulin of either kappa or lambda specificity occurring as an M protein

b. Plasmacytoid lymphocytes infiltrating the blood, bone marrow, lymph nodes, and spleen

c. Bence Jones proteinuria in about 10% of cases

d. Absence of bone lesions

2. Clinical features

a. Most frequently seen in **males over age 50**

b. Slowly progressive course, often marked by generalized lymphadenopathy and mild anemia

3. Complications

   a. Hyperviscosity syndrome, resulting from marked increase in serum IgM

     –includes **retinal vascular dilation,** sometimes with hemorrhage, confusion, and other CNS changes.

     –sometimes requires **emergency plasmapheresis** to prevent blindness.

   b. Abnormal bleeding, which may be due to vascular and platelet dysfunction secondary to the serum protein abnormality

C. Benign monoclonal gammopathy (monoclonal gammopathy of undetermined significance)

–occurs in 5%–10% of otherwise healthy **older persons**.

–is characterized by a monoclonal **M protein** spike of less than 3 g/100 ml, absence of Bence Jones proteinuria, and less than 5% plasma cells in the bone marrow.

–is most often without clinical consequence.

V. Hodgkin's Disease and the Non-Hodgkin's Lymphomas

A. Hodgkin's disease

–is a **malignant** neoplasm with features (e.g., fever, inflammatory cell infiltrates) resembling an inflammatory disorder.

–characteristically affects **young adults** (predominantly **young men**); an exception is nodular sclerosis, which frequently affects young women.

–is often associated with pruritus and fever, diaphoresis, and leukocytosis reminiscent of an acute infection.

–with modern staging and aggressive therapy, clinical cure is often achieved.

–is characterized in all forms by the presence of Reed-Sternberg cells.

1. Reed-Sternberg cells

–may be the actual malignant cells of Hodgkin's disease.

–are **binucleated, or multinucleated, giant cells** with eosinophilic inclusion-like nucleoli.

–differing numbers are found in varying forms of Hodgkin's disease, and the severity of the disease is directly proportional to the number of Reed-Sternberg cells found in the lesions.

–conversely, the greater the number of reactive lymphocytes in the lesions, the better the prognosis.

2. Classification of Hodgkin's disease

–the **Rye classification** identifies four disease variants.

   a. Lymphocytic predominance

     –is the **least frequently occurring** form of Hodgkin's disease.

     –is characterized by large numbers of lymphocytes and histiocytes and a paucity of Reed-Sternberg cells.

     –is associated with a relatively **good prognosis**.

   b. Mixed cellularity

     –is the **most frequently occurring** variant of Hodgkin's disease.

     –is characterized by a polymorphic infiltrate of eosinophils, plasma cells, histiocytes, and Reed-Sternberg cells, and by areas of necrosis and fibrosis.

c. Lymphocytic depletion

–is marked by few lymphocytes, numerous Reed-Sternberg cells, and extensive necrosis and fibrosis.

–has the **poorest prognosis** among the Hodgkin's disease variants.

d. Nodular sclerosis

–occurs more frequently in **women,** unlike other forms of Hodgkin's disease.

–is characterized by nodular division of affected lymph nodes by **fibrous bands** and by the presence of **lacunar cells,** Reed-Sternberg cell variants.

–often arises in the upper mediastinum or lower cervical or supraclavicular nodes.

–is associated with a relatively **good prognosis**.

3. Clinical staging—Ann Arbor classification

–is based on the degree of dissemination, involvement of extralymphatic sites, and presence or absence of systemic symptoms such as fever (Table 12.1).

–is an essential part of the **diagnostic evaluation** of patients with Hodgkin's disease.

–although grading of histopathologic variants (Rye classification) roughly correlates with clinical behavior, **prognosis is better predicted by staging** (Ann Arbor classification).

B. Non-Hodgkin's lymphomas

–are **malignant neoplasms** arising from lymphoid cells or other cells native to lymphoid tissue.

–originate most frequently within **lymph nodes** or in other lymphoid areas. **Tumor involvement** of periaortic lymph nodes is frequent.

1. Classification systems (Table 12.2)

a. The Working Formulation

–is the current standard classification system based on earlier systems partially in use today.

Table 12.1. Ann Arbor Classification of Hodgkin's Disease and Non-Hodgkin's Lymphomas

Stage*	Site of Involvement
I	Involvement of a single lymph node region (I) or involvement of a single extralymphatic organ or site (I_E)
II	Involvement of two or more lymph node regions on the same side of the diaphragm alone (II) or with involvement of limited contiguous extralymphatic organ or tissue (II_E)
III	Involvement of lymph node regions on both sides of the diaphragm (III), which may include the spleen (III_S), limited contiguous extralymphatic organ or site (III_E), or both (III_{ES})
IV	Multiple or disseminated foci of involvement of one or more extralymphatic organs with or without lymphatic involvement

*Stages are further designated on the basis of absence (A) or presence (B) of systemic symptoms.
(Modified from Carbone PT et al.: Report of the Committee on Hodgkin's Disease Staging. *Cancer Res* 31:1860–1861, 1971.)

Table 12.2. Comparison of Classification Systems for Selected Non-Hodgkin's Lymphomas

Working Formulation	Rappaport	Lukes-Collins
Low grade		
Small lymphocytic lymphoma	Diffuse well-differentiated lymphocytic lymphoma (WDLL)	Small lymphocyte lymphoma
Small lymphocytic plasmacytoid lymphoma	Diffuse WDLL with plasmacytoid features	Plasmacytoid lymphocyte lymphoma
Follicular predominantly small cleaved cell lymphoma	Nodular poorly differentiated lymphocytic lymphoma (PDLL)	Follicular center cell lymphoma
Intermediate grade		
Diffuse large cell cleaved or noncleaved lymphoma	Diffuse histiocytic lymphoma	B-cell or T-cell diffuse large cell cleaved or noncleaved lymphoma
High grade		
Lymphoblastic lymphoma	Lymphoblastic lymphoma	T-cell convoluted lymphocyte lymphoma
Small noncleaved cell (Burkitt's) lymphoma	Diffuse undifferentiated lymphoma (Burkitt's type)	Small cell transformed (noncleaved) lymphoma

—emphasizes **clinical behavior,** subdividing the non-Hodgkin's lymphomas into low, intermediate, and high grades based on clinical severity.

b. The Rappaport classification

—divides lymphomas into **nodular** (follicular) and **diffuse** varieties.
—emphasizes that nodular forms are associated with a better prognosis.

c. The Lukes-Collins classification

—emphasizes **cytologic characteristics** of cells and presumed **site of origin** in lymph nodes.
—notes distinctive morphologic characteristics of follicular center cells.
—emphasizes better prognosis of small cell lymphomas as compared to large cell lymphomas.

2. Small lymphocytic lymphoma

—is a **low grade B-cell lymphoma** that follows an indolent course and occurs most often in **older persons**.
—is characterized by diffuse **effacement of lymph node architecture** by small mature-appearing lymphocytes.
—is frequently characterized by **widespread nodal involvement** and involvement of the liver, spleen, and bone marrow.
—is **closely related to CLL.**
—in a plasmacytoid variant, is closely related to Waldenström's macroglobulinemia.

3. Follicular predominantly small cleaved cell lymphoma

—is a **low grade B-cell lymphoma,** frequently following an indolent course in **older persons**.

–is the **most common form** of non-Hodgkin's disease.

–is characterized by proliferation of **angulated grooved cells** that closely resemble the cells of the lymphoid follicular center, commonly in a follicular (**nodular**) pattern.

–is marked by a characteristic **cytogenetic change,** t(14;18), and by expression of *bcl-2,* an oncogene; *bcl-*2 codes for an inner mitochondrial protein that apparently interferes with apoptotic cell death.

4. Large cell lymphomas

–are a group of intermediate and high grade lymphomas that share a number of clinical features.

–most commonly occur in **older persons;** however, the age range is wide and many of these lymphomas occur in **children**.

–most often originate from **B cells**.

–usually present as a large, often extranodal mass followed by widespread aggressive dissemination. Leukemic involvement is rare.

5. Lymphoblastic lymphoma

–is a **high grade T-cell lymphoma** characterized by convoluted appearing nuclei.

–occurs most often in **children**.

–most often arises from **thymic lymphocytes**.

–rapidly disseminates and **progresses to T-ALL** (a subgroup of acute lymphoblastic leukemia of T-cell origin).

–often presents with a **combination of T-ALL and a mediastinal mass**.

6. Small noncleaved cell (Burkitt's) lymphoma

–is a **high grade B-cell lymphoma**. The African form frequently involves the maxilla or mandible; the American form usually involves abdominal organs.

–is closely linked to **EBV infection** (especially in the African variety).

–is characterized histologically by a **"starry-sky"** appearance. As a result of rapid cell turnover, the lesions contain abundant cellular debris that is taken up by non-neoplastic macrophages, resulting in this appearance.

–is closely **related to B-ALL** (a subgroup of acute lymphoblastic leukemia of B-cell origin).

–is associated with a characteristic **cytogenic change,** t(8;14).

a. In this translocation, the *c-myc* proto-oncogene located on chromosome 8 is transposed to a site adjacent to the immunoglobulin heavy-chain locus on chromosome 14.

b. Increased expression of the *c-myc* gene, presumably caused by the proximity of regulatory sequences of the immunoglobulin heavy chain gene, is characteristic.

7. Cutaneous T-cell lymphomas

a. Mycosis fungoides

–presents as an erythematous, eczematoid, or psoriasiform process, progressing to raised plaques and then to a tumor stage.

—is marked histologically by dermal infiltrates of atypical CD4 + T cells with **cerebriform nuclei**. Small pockets of tumor cells within the epidermis are referred to as **Pautrier's microabscesses**.

—eventually disseminates to lymph nodes and internal organs.

b. Sézary syndrome

—is a leukemic form of cutaneous T-cell lymphoma.

—is characterized by the combination of skin lesions and circulating neoplastic cells with cerebriform nuclei.

Review Test

Directions: Each of the numbered items or incomplete statements in this section is followed by answers or by completions of the statement. Select the **one** lettered answer or completion that is **best** in each case.

1. Which one of the following neoplastic diseases is characterized by a specific chromosome marker?

(A) Chronic lymphocytic leukemia
(B) Chronic myeloid leukemia
(C) Adenocarcinoma of the pancreas
(D) Carcinoma of the stomach
(E) Carcinoma of the colon

2. Which of the following clinical and laboratory findings is characteristic of chronic myeloid leukemia?

(A) Autosplenectomy
(B) Increased leukocyte alkaline phosphatase
(C) Peak incidence at age 65
(D) *Bcr-abl* hybrid gene formation
(E) Initial presentation with predominance of blast cells

3. All of the following characteristics are associated with chronic lymphocytic leukemia EXCEPT

(A) autoimmune hemolytic anemia.
(B) hypogammaglobulinemia.
(C) neoplastic cells of B-cell lineage.
(D) peak incidence over age 60.
(E) frequently cured by aggressive chemotherapy.

4. Polycythemia vera is associated with all of the following findings EXCEPT

(A) erythrocytosis.
(B) leukocytosis.
(C) thrombocytosis.
(D) increased erythropoietin.
(E) splenomegaly.

5. The peripheral blood smear of an asymptomatic 68-year-old white male exhibiting generalized lymphadenopathy and hepatosplenomegaly is shown in the following illustration. What is the most likely diagnosis?

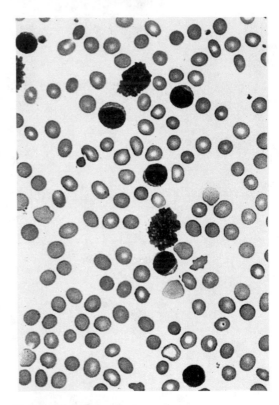

(Courtesy of Dr. Jae O. Ro, Veterans Affairs Medical Center and University of Health Sciences, The Chicago Medical School)

(A) Acute lymphoblastic leukemia
(B) Acute myeloblastic leukemia
(C) Chronic lymphocytic leukemia
(D) Chronic myeloid leukemia

6. X-ray examination of a 65-year-old white male with back pain due to a compression fracture of T12 reveals multiple "punched-out" lytic bone lesions. All of the following additional abnormalities are likely EXCEPT

(A) serum IgM kappa M protein.
(B) urinary free kappa chains.
(C) hypercalcemia.
(D) red cell rouleaux formation.
(E) renal insufficiency.

7. Examination of a lymph node from the neck of a 26-year-old man reveals total effacement of architecture and the histologic picture shown below. Which additional studies are needed to confirm the diagnosis?

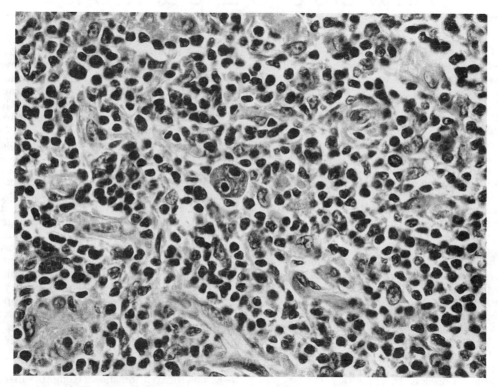

(Reprinted with permission from Golden A, Powell D, and Jennings C: *Pathology: Understanding Human Disease,* 2nd ed. Baltimore, Williams & Wilkins, 1985, p 351.)

(A) Urine for Bence Jones protein
(B) Gene rearrangement studies
(C) Osteoclastic factor assay
(D) Angiotensin converting factor
(E) No additional studies

8. All of the following characteristics apply to Burkitt's lymphoma EXCEPT

(A) Epstein-Barr virus infection.
(B) 8;14 translocation.
(C) transposition of *c-myc* proto-oncogene to site near the immunoglobulin heavy-chain locus.
(D) "starry-sky" appearance.
(E) classification as low grade lymphoma in the Working Formulation.

Answers and Explanations

1–B. Chronic myeloid leukemia (CML) is almost invariably associated with the Philadelphia chromosome, a small residual chromosome 22 resulting from a 9;22 translocation.

2–D. As a result of the 9;22 translocation, the *c-abl* proto-oncogene on chromosome 9 is transposed to the *bcr* region of chromosome 22, forming a hybrid *bcr-abl* gene, which codes for a protein with tyrosine kinase activity. Autosplenectomy is a term for the progressive scarring and shrinking of the spleen in sickle cell disease. In contrast, the spleen is markedly enlarged in CML. The peak incidence of CML is in the middle-age group, and leukocyte alkaline phosphatase is characteristically decreased. Although blast cells and early promyelocytes may predominate during a blastic crisis, there are few of these cells at the time of presentation.

3–E. Although chronic lymphocytic leukemia has an indolent clinical course characterized by long periods without symptoms and frequent instances of long survival, it is not considered curable by present therapeutic regimens.

4–D. The combination of erythrocytosis, leukocytosis, and thrombocytosis along with splenomegaly is highly characteristic of polycythemia vera. Polycythemia vera is a clonal proliferative disorder characterized by a decrease in erythropoietin concentration.

5–C. The illustration shows predominance of mature-appearing lymphocytes and several cells distorted mechanically in preparation of the blood smear (smudge cells), both characteristic of chronic lymphocytic leukemia (CLL). CLL most often affects older persons, many of whom are asymptomatic for many years. Generalized lymphadenopathy and hepatosplenomegaly are frequent findings.

6–A. Widespread "punched-out" lytic bone lesions in a patient in the older age group are highly suggestive of multiple myeloma. IgM paraproteinemia (IgM M protein) is characteristic of Waldenström's macroglobulinemia, in contrast to the IgG or IgA M proteins almost always found in multiple myeloma. Frequent additional laboratory abnormalities of multiple myeloma include hypercalcemia, urinary excretion of Bence Jones protein (free kappa or lambda light chains), and red cell rouleaux formation resulting from hyperglobulinemia. Renal insufficiency from myeloma kidney is not infrequent.

7–E. The illustration shows Hodgkin's disease, mixed cellularity type. A prominent Reed-Sternberg cell can be seen. The diagnosis is based entirely on the biopsy findings, and there are no confirmatory laboratory tests.

8–E. Burkitt's lymphoma is classified in the high grade group in the Working Formulation.

13

Hemorrhagic Disorders

I. Disorders of Primary Hemostasis

—are **defects of initial platelet plug formation**.

—are characterized by bleeding from small vessels and capillaries, resulting in mucocutaneous bleeding. **Petechial hemorrhages** occur in the skin and mucous membranes, with bleeding and oozing from the nose, gums, and gastrointestinal tract.

—are often marked by **prolonged bleeding time**.

—can be caused by lesions of the vasculature, platelet dysfunction, or alterations in the plasma proteins required for adhesion of platelets to vascular subendothelium.

A. Lesions of the vasculature

—usually no laboratory abnormalities are associated with bleeding due to small blood vessel dysfunction, but **prolonged bleeding time** is sometimes noted.

—examples include the following:

1. Simple purpura

—is **easy bruising,** especially of the upper thighs, in otherwise healthy persons.

2. Senile purpura

—is marked by hemorrhagic areas on the back of the hands and forearms of older persons.

—is presumed to arise from age-dependent atrophy of vascular supportive tissues.

3. Scurvy

—is vitamin C deficiency.

—causes **gingival hemorrhages,** bleeding into muscles and subcutaneous tissue, and cutaneous petechiae characteristically occurring about hair follicles.

179

4. Henoch-Schönlein purpura (allergic purpura)

–is a form of leukocytoclastic angiitis, hypersensitivity vasculitis resulting from an immune reaction that damages the vascular endothelium.

–is marked by hemorrhagic urticaria (palpable purpura) accompanied by fever, arthralgias, and gastrointestinal and renal involvement.

5. Hereditary hemorrhagic telangiectasia (Osler-Weber-Rendu syndrome)

–is an autosomal dominant disorder marked by localized malformations of venules and capillaries of the skin and mucous membranes, often complicated by **hemorrhage**.

6. Connective tissue disorders

–include **Ehlers-Danlos syndrome,** an inherited disorder caused by abnormalities of collagen or elastin, and manifested by vascular bleeding, articular hypermobility, dermal hyperelasticity, and tissue fragility.

7. Waldenström's macroglobulinemia

–produces vascular damage from sludging of hyperviscous blood.

–can also cause platelet functional abnormalities.

8. Amyloidosis

–can cause **vessel damage**.

9. Rickettsial and meningococcal diseases

–include Rocky Mountain spotted fever and meningococcemia.

–involve the vascular endothelium, leading to necrosis and rupture of small blood vessels.

B. Platelet disorders

1. Thrombocytopenia (quantitative platelet dysfunction)

–is dominated clinically by **petechial cutaneous bleeding,** intracranial bleeding, and oozing from mucosal surfaces.

–is characterized by **decreased platelet count** and **prolonged bleeding time;** bone marrow aspiration reveals decreased megakaryocytes when caused by decreased platelet production and increased megakaryocytes when caused by increased platelet destruction.

–is a result of decreased production, increased destruction, unreplaced loss, or dilution of platelets, brought about by a wide variety of etiologic factors.

a. Irradiation, exposure to drugs or chemicals

–causes decreased production.

b. Acute leukemia

–causes decreased production because of replacement of bone marrow by blast cells.

c. Splenic sequestration

–results in loss of circulating platelets.

d. Multiple transfusions

–result in dilution.

e. Disseminated intravascular coagulation (DIC)

–results in increased destruction and utilization of platelets.

f. Secondary to other diseases

–include disorders such as **AIDS** and **systemic lupus erythematosus** (SLE).

g. Idiopathic thrombocytopenic purpura (ITP)

–in children, is usually an acute, self-limiting reaction to viral infection or immunization; in adults, is a chronic disorder.

–is characterized by **antiplatelet antibodies** that coat and damage platelets, which are then selectively removed by splenic macrophages.

–is diagnosed based on **thrombocytopenia** with normal or **increased megakaryocytes,** no known exposure to thrombocytopenic agents, and lack of palpable splenomegaly.

h. Thrombotic thrombocytopenic purpura (TTP)

–is characterized by **hyaline microthrombi** in small vessels, **thrombocytopenia,** and **microangiopathic hemolytic anemia**. The microcirculatory lesions produce mechanical damage to red blood cells as they squeeze through the narrowed vessels, resulting in **helmet cells** and **schistocytes**.

–is also marked by transient **neurologic abnormalities, renal insufficiency,** and **fever**.

2. Platelet functional abnormalities (qualitative platelet dysfunction)

–are platelet-mediated bleeding disorders that occur in spite of a **normal platelet count**.

–result in mucocutaneous bleeding, associated with **prolonged bleeding time**.

–are caused by:

a. Defects of platelet adhesion, as in **von Willebrand's disease** or **Bernard-Soulier disease,** an autosomal recessive disorder characterized by unusually large platelets and by lack of platelet-surface glycoprotein Ib (GPIb), needed for platelet adhesion.

b. Defects of platelet aggregation

–can be either acquired or inherited.

–include the following examples:

(1) Aspirin-induced acetylation and inactivation of cyclooxygenase, which causes **failure of synthesis** of the **platelet aggregant thromboxane A$_2$**

(2) Glanzmann's thrombasthenia, inaggregability of platelets due to hereditary deficiency of platelet-surface GPIIb and GPIIIa, required for formation of fibrinogen bridges between adjacent platelets

II. Disorders of Secondary Hemostasis (Table 13.1)

–are caused by **deficiencies of plasma clotting factors**.

–are manifest by **bleeding from larger vessels,** resulting in hemarthroses, large hematomas, large ecchymoses, and extensive bleeding with trauma.

–do not affect the bleeding time or platelet count (thus distinguishing secondary hemostatic disorders from primary hemostatic disorders).

Table 13.1. Laboratory Screening Tests in Selected Hemorrhagic Disorders

Disorder	Screening Tests					Confirmatory Tests or Other Significant Findings
	Bleeding Time	Platelet Count	PT	APTT	Thrombin Time/ Fibrinogen Assay	
Vascular bleeding	Usually prolonged	Normal	Normal	Normal	Normal	....
Thrombocytopenia	Prolonged	Decreased	Normal	Normal	Normal	Megakaryocytes normal or increased when thrombocytopenia is caused by increased platelet destruction, decreased when due to decreased production
Qualitative platelet defects	Prolonged	Normal	Normal	Normal	Normal	Platelet aggregation and other specialized studies
Classic hemophilia	Normal	Normal	Normal	Prolonged	Normal	Factor VIII assay
Christmas disease	Normal	Normal	Normal	Prolonged	Normal	Factor IX assay
Von Willebrand's disease	Prolonged	Normal	Normal	Prolonged	Normal	VWF assay
DIC	Prolonged	Decreased	Prolonged	Prolonged	Prolonged	Fibrin and fibrinogen degradation products

DIC = disseminated intravascular coagulation; APTT = activated partial thromboplastin time; PT = prothrombin time.

—may result in abnormalities in the **prothrombin time (PT),** reflecting deficiencies of factors II, V, VII, and X; **activated partial thromboplastin time (APTT),** reflecting deficiencies of all of the coagulation factors with the exception of factors VII and XIII; and **thrombin time,** reflecting fibrinogen defects. (The whole blood clotting time is an older test that detects the same abnormalities as the APTT.)

A. Classic hemophilia (hemophilia A, factor VIII deficiency)

  —is a common **X-linked disorder** with worldwide distribution that varies in severity, depending on factor VIII activity. Severe cases have less than 1% residual factor VIII activity.

  —is characterized by bleeding into muscles, subcutaneous tissues, and joints.

B. Christmas disease (hemophilia B, factor IX deficiency)

  —occurs in approximately one-fifth to one-tenth the incidence of classic hemophilia.

  —is **indistinguishable from classic hemophilia** in mode of inheritance and clinical features.

C. Vitamin K deficiency

  —in adults, is most often caused by **fat malabsorption** from pancreatic or small-bowel disease.

  —in neonates, is caused by **deficient exogenous vitamin K** in breast milk and by **incomplete intestinal colonization** by vitamin K-synthesizing bacteria.

  —results in **decreased activity of clotting factors II, VII, IX, and X,** and is reflected by **prolonged PT and APTT.**

III. Combined Primary and Secondary Hemostatic Defects

A. Von Willebrand's disease

  —is the most common hereditary bleeding disorder.

  —is an autosomal dominant disorder marked by **deficiency of von Willebrand's factor (vWF),** a large multimeric protein synthesized by endothelial cells and megakaryocytes.

  —is characterized by impaired platelet adhesion, prolonged bleeding time, and a functional deficiency of factor VIII.

1. Function—vWF

  —is a carrier protein for factor VIII, the antihemophilic factor, and the two proteins circulate together as a complex.

  —also mediates adhesion of platelets to subendothelium at sites of vascular injury, reacting with the subendothelium and platelet-surface GPIb.

2. Dual hemostatic defects

  a. Deficiency of vWF leads to a **failure of platelet adhesion,** resulting in deficient platelet plug formation manifest clinically by primary hemostatic bleeding and prolonged bleeding time.

  b. A **functional deficiency of factor VIII** occurs as a consequence of the deficit of vWF, its carrier protein. Deficiency is manifest by secondary hemostatic bleeding and prolonged APTT.

B. **Disseminated intravascular coagulation**
  —is characterized by widespread clotting with resultant **consumption of platelets and coagulation factors,** especially factors II, V, and VIII, and **fibrinogen**.
  —is clinically manifest by **thrombotic phenomena** and **hemorrhage**.
  —is marked by microangiopathic hemolytic anemia, increased fibrin and fibrinogen degradation products, thrombocytopenia, and prolonged bleeding time, PT, APTT, and thrombin time.
  —is caused by **release of tissue thromboplastin** (tissue factor) or **activation of the intrinsic pathway of coagulation,** as well as by secondary **activation of the fibrinolytic system**.
  —is seen most commonly in **obstetric complications,** such as toxemia, amniotic fluid emboli, retained dead fetus, or abruptio placentae; can also result from **cancer,** notably of the lung, pancreas, prostate, or stomach; from tissue damage caused by **infection,** especially gram-negative sepsis; **trauma,** as in chest surgery; or **immunologic mechanisms,** especially immune complex disease or hemolytic transfusion reactions.

C. **Coagulopathy of liver disease**
  —arises because all coagulation factors except vWF are produced in the liver; therefore, as hepatocellular damage progresses, the PT, APTT, and thrombin time are prolonged. In addition, **prolonged bleeding time** due to platelet functional defects or overt thrombocytopenia may occur.
  —may be alleviated in some cases by administration of **vitamin K derivatives,** which promote synthesis of factors II, VII, IX, and X.

D. **Dilutional coagulopathy**
  —may result from **multiple transfusions** of stored blood deficient in platelets and factors II, V, and VIII.
  —is often manifest by **persistent bleeding** from surgical wounds.
  —may result in thrombocytopenia or prolonged PT or APTT.

Review Test

Directions: Each of the numbered items or incomplete statements in this section is followed by answers or by completions of the statement. Select the **one** lettered answer or completion that is **best** in each case.

1. Which one of the following laboratory determinations is abnormally prolonged in idiopathic thrombocytopenic purpura?

(A) Activated partial thromboplastin time (APTT)
(B) Bleeding time
(C) Coagulation time
(D) Prothrombin time (PT)
(E) Thrombin time

2. Which of the following laboratory determinations is abnormally prolonged in classic hemophilia?

(A) APTT
(B) Bleeding time
(C) PT
(D) Thrombin time

3. The association of thrombocytopenia, hemolytic anemia, schistocytes, and helmet cells with changing neurologic signs, fever, and renal insufficiency suggests

(A) idiopathic thrombocytopenic purpura (ITP).
(B) thrombotic thrombocytopenic purpura (TTP).
(C) von Willebrand's disease.
(D) Bernard-Soulier disease.
(E) Glanzmann's thrombasthenia.

4. A 25-year-old man has a lifelong hemorrhagic diathesis. The PT and bleeding time are normal, but the APTT is prolonged. The most likely cause of the bleeding disorder is

(A) factor VIII deficiency.
(B) factor IX deficiency.
(C) factor VII deficiency.
(D) a platelet functional disorder.
(E) von Willebrand's disease.

5. Which of the following defects is associated with hemophilia?

(A) Deficiency of hemoglobin S
(B) Deficiency of hemoglobin A
(C) A defective gene in the X chromosome
(D) A defective gene in the Y chromosome
(E) Absence of the X chromosome

6. Well-known causes of disseminated intravascular coagulation (DIC) include all of the following conditions EXCEPT

(A) retained dead fetus.
(B) prostatic carcinoma.
(C) hemolytic transfusion reaction.
(D) gram-negative sepsis.
(E) heparin administration.

7. Von Willebrand's disease is associated with which one of the following laboratory findings?

(A) Prolonged APTT
(B) Decreased platelet count
(C) Prolonged PT
(D) Prolonged thrombin time

8. All of the following conditions are associated with a prolonged bleeding time EXCEPT

(A) von Willebrand's disease.
(B) deficiency of factor IX.
(C) long-term treatment with aspirin.
(D) idiopathic thrombocytopenic purpura.
(E) Bernard-Soulier disease.

Answers and Explanations

1–B. Thrombocytopenia, regardless of the cause, results in a prolonged bleeding time.

2–A. Classic hemophilia (factor VIII deficiency) is an abnormality of the intrinsic pathway of coagulation proximal to the final common pathway, which begins at factor X → Xa activation. This defect leads to a prolonged APTT. The other laboratory tests listed remain normal since the bleeding time is a measure of platelet plug formation, the PT a measure of the extrinsic pathway of coagulation, and the thrombin time an assay of the conversion of fibrinogen to fibrin.

3–B. TTP is characterized by thrombocytopenia, hemolytic anemia with fragmented circulating red blood cells (helmet cells and schistocytes), changing neurologic abnormalities, renal insufficiency, and fever. The diagnosis is based on histopathologic demonstration of hyaline microthrombi in small vessels.

4–A. The bleeding disorder is probably caused by factor VIII deficiency. The patient has a disorder of the intrinsic pathway of coagulation (prolonged APTT). The abnormality is localized proximal to factor X → Xa activation since the PT is normal. Significant platelet-related problems such as von Willebrand's disease are ruled out by the normal bleeding time. The two most comon intrinsic pathway factor deficiencies are factor VIII and factor IX. Of these, factor VIII deficiency occurs 5 to 10 times more frequently than factor IX deficiency, and therefore is the most likely cause of the bleeding disorder.

5–C. Both classic hemophilia (hemophilia A) and factor IX deficiency (hemophilia B) are X-linked disorders.

6–E. Heparin is an antithrombotic drug that interferes with coagulation by activation of antithrombin III, which in turn neutralizes activated serine proteases, including thrombin and factors IXa, Xa, XIa, and XIIa. Heparin administration is sometimes used to inhibit the progression of DIC. DIC is a generalized activation of thrombosis due to release of thromboplastic substances. DIC may be caused by obstetric complications, such as amniotic fluid emboli, retained dead fetus, and abruptio placentae; tumors of the lung, pancreas, prostate, and stomach; gram-negative endotoxemia; tissue damage, most notably from chest surgery; and immune-mediated injuries such as hemolytic transfusion reactions.

7–A. The APTT will be prolonged. Von Willebrand's disease is due to deficiency of von Willebrand's factor (vWF), which functions as a carrier protein for the antihemophilic procoagulant, factor VIII. Functional deficiency of factor VIII secondary to lack of the carrier protein results in a prolonged APTT. The PT and thrombin time are unaffected by vWF deficiency. Although platelet adhesion is impaired, the platelet count remains normal.

8–B. Factor IX deficiency does not interfere with platelet plug formation and thus does not affect the bleeding time. Deficiency of vWF in von Willebrand's disease results in impaired platelet adhesion. Administration of aspirin, a cyclooxygenase inhibitor, results in impaired production of thromboxane A_2, an important platelet aggregant. Idiopathic thrombocytopenic purpura is an immune-mediated quantitative deficiency of platelets. Bernard-Soulier disease is a hereditary platelet adhesion disorder. All of the platelet-mediated disorders are manifest by impaired platelet plug formation and prolonged bleeding time.

14

Respiratory System

I. Disorders of the Upper Respiratory Tract

A. Acute rhinitis

1. **Common cold**
   - is the most common of all illnesses and is caused by viruses, especially the **adenoviruses**.
   - is manifest by ("runny nose") coryza, sneezing, nasal congestion, and mild sore throat.

2. **Allergic rhinitis**
   - is mediated by IgE **type I immune reaction** involving submucosal mast cells.
   - is characterized by increased **eosinophils** in peripheral blood and nasal discharge.

3. **Bacterial infection**
   - may be superimposed on acute viral or allergic rhinitis by injury to mucosal cilia, which may also occur from other environmental factors.
   - is caused most commonly by streptococci, staphylococci, or *Haemophilus influenzae*.
   - can lead to fibrous scarring, decreased vascularity, and atrophy of the epithelium and mucous glands.

B. Sinusitis

- is **inflammation of the paranasal sinuses** often caused by extension of nasal cavity or dental infection.
- results in obstructed drainage outlets from the sinuses, leading to accumulation of mucoid secretions or exudate.

C. Laryngitis

- is **acute inflammation of the larynx** produced by viruses or bacteria, irritants, or overuse of the voice.
- is characterized by inflammation and edema of the vocal cords, with resultant hoarseness.

D. Acute epiglottitis

—is **inflammation of the epiglottis,** and is life-threatening in young children.
—is usually caused by *H. influenzae*.

E. Acute laryngotracheobronchitis

—is acute **inflammation of the larynx, trachea, and epiglottis** that is potentially life-threatening in infants.
—is most often caused by **viral infection**.
—is characterized by a harsh cough and inspiratory stridor, which are referred to as **croup**.

II. Tumors of the Upper Respiratory Tract

A. Malignant tumors of the nose and nasal sinuses

1. Nasopharyngeal carcinoma

—is most common in Southeast Asia and East Africa.
—is caused by the **Epstein-Barr virus**.

2. Squamous cell carcinoma

—is the most frequently occurring malignant nasal tumor.

3. Adenocarcinoma

—accounts for 5% of malignant tumors of the nose and throat.

4. Plasmacytoma

—is a plasma cell neoplasm that, in its extraosseous form, produces tumors in the upper respiratory tract.

B. Tumors of the larynx

1. Singers' nodule

—is a small, **benign laryngeal polyp,** usually induced by chronic irritation, such as excessive use of the voice, and is associated most commonly with **heavy cigarette smoking**.
—is usually localized to the **true vocal cords**.

2. Laryngeal papilloma

—is a **benign neoplasm** usually located on the true vocal cords.
—in adults, usually occurs singly and sometimes undergoes malignant change.
—in children, multiple lesions, caused by human papillomavirus, appear.

3. Squamous cell carcinoma

—is the **most common malignant tumor of the larynx,** and is usually seen in men over age 40; it is often associated with the combination of cigarette smoking and alcoholism.

a. Glottic carcinoma

—arises from the true vocal cords.
—is the most common laryngeal carcinoma and has the best prognosis.

b. Supraglottic and subglottic carcinomas

—are less common and typically have poorer prognosis.

III. Chronic Obstructive Pulmonary Disease (COPD)

–is a group of disorders characterized by **airflow obstruction** (Table 14.1).

–is often contrasted with restrictive pulmonary disease, a group of disorders characterized by reduced lung capacity due either to chest wall or skeletal dysfunction or to interstitial or infiltrative parenchymal disease. Examples of restrictive pulmonary disease include the adult and neonatal respiratory distress syndromes as well as pneumoconioses and interstitial lung diseases.

A. Bronchial asthma

1. Types include **extrinsic** and **intrinsic asthma,** as well as non–immune-mediated variants such as **exercise- or cold-induced asthma**.

   a. Extrinsic asthma

   –is mediated by a **type I hypersensitivity response** involving IgE bound to mast cells.

   –begins in **childhood,** usually in patients with a family history of allergy.

   b. Intrinsic asthma

   –usually begins in **adult life** and is not associated with a history of allergy.

   –may be complicated by **chronic bronchitis**.

2. **Characteristics—bronchial asthma**

   –is marked by **dyspnea** and **wheezing expiration** caused by episodic narrowing of the airways.

   –is related to increased sensitivity of air passages to stimuli.

3. **Complications**

   –include **superimposed infection, chronic bronchitis,** and **pulmonary emphysema**.

   –may lead to **status asthmaticus,** a prolonged bout of bronchial asthma that can last for days and responds poorly to therapy; can result in death.

Table 14.1. Pathologic Findings in Chronic Obstructive Pulmonary Disease

Disorder	Pathologic Findings
Bronchial asthma	Bronchial smooth muscle hypertrophy Hyperplasia of bronchial submucosal glands and goblet cells Airways plugged by viscid mucus containing Curschmann's spirals, eosinophils, and Charcot-Leyden crystals
Chronic bronchitis	Hyperplasia of bronchial submucosal glands, leading to increased Reid index, ratio of the thickness of the gland layer to that of the bronchial wall
Pulmonary emphysema	Abnormal dilatation of air spaces with destruction of alveolar walls Reduced lung elasticity
Bronchiectasis	Abnormally dilated bronchi filled with mucus and neutrophils Inflammation and necrosis of bronchial walls and alveolar fibrosis

B. Chronic bronchitis

−is clinically defined as productive cough occurring during at least 3 consecutive months over at least 2 consecutive years.

−is clearly linked to **cigarette smoking,** and is also associated with air pollution, infection, and genetic factors.

−is typically characterized by **hypersecretion of mucus**.

−may lead to **cor pulmonale**.

C. Emphysema

−is **dilatation of air spaces** with destruction of alveolar walls.

−is strongly associated with cigarette smoking.

1. Types of emphysema

a. Centrilobular emphysema

−is dilatation of the respiratory bronchioles.

−is most often localized to the upper part of the pulmonary lobes.

b. Panacinar emphysema

−is dilatation of the entire acinus, including the alveoli, alveolar ducts, respiratory bronchioles, and terminal bronchioles.

−is most often distributed uniformly throughout the lung.

−is associated with loss of elasticity and sometimes with genetically determined **deficiency of α_1-antitrypsin** (α_1-protease inhibitor).

c. Paraseptal emphysema

−is dilatation involving mainly the distal part of the acinus, including the alveoli and, to a lesser extent, the alveolar ducts.

−tends to localize subjacent to the pleura and interlobar septa.

−is associated occasionally with large subpleural bullae, or blebs, which may rupture, resulting in pneumothorax.

d. Irregular emphysema

−is irregular involvement of the acinus with scarring within the walls of enlarged air spaces.

−is usually a complication of various inflammatory processes.

2. Complications—emphysema

−is often complicated by, or coexistent with, **chronic bronchitis**.

−may be complicated by **interstitial emphysema,** in which air escapes into the interstitial tissues of the chest from a tear in the airways.

3. Postulated causes—emphysema

−may result from action of proteolytic enzymes such as elastase on the alveolar wall. Elastase can induce destruction of elastin unless neutralized by the antiproteinase–antielastase activities of α_1-antitrypsin.

a. Cigarette smoking

−attracts neutrophils and macrophages, sources of elastase.

−inactivates α_1-antitrypsin.

b. Hereditary α_1-antitrypsin deficiency

−accounts for a small subgroup of cases of **panacinar emphysema**.

−is caused by variants in the *pi* (proteinase inhibitor) gene, localized to chromosome 14.

(1) The **piZ allele** codes for a structural alteration in the protein that interferes with its hepatic secretion. Hepatic cytoplasmic droplets accumulate, with resultant liver damage.

(2) The **homozygous state (piZZ)** is associated with markedly decreased activity in α_1-antitrypsin, panacinar emphysema, and often in hepatic cirrhosis.

D. Bronchiectasis

–is **permanent abnormal bronchial dilatation** caused by chronic infection with inflammation and necrosis of the bronchial wall.

–is predisposed by **bronchial obstruction,** most often by tumor.

–is also predisposed by **chronic sinusitis** accompanied by postnasal drip.

–is characterized by production of **copious purulent sputum,** hemoptysis, and recurrent pulmonary infection that may lead to **lung abscess**.

IV. Pneumoconioses

–are environmental diseases caused by **inhalation of inorganic dust particles**.

–are exemplified by the following conditions.

A. Anthracosis

–is caused by inhalation of **carbon dust;** it is endemic in urban areas and causes no harm.

–is marked by **carbon-carrying macrophages,** resulting in irregular black patches visible on gross inspection.

B. Coal workers' pneumoconiosis

–is caused by inhalation of **coal dust,** which contains both carbon and silica.

1. Simple coal workers' pneumoconiosis

–is marked by **coal macules** around the bronchioles, formed by ingestion of coal dust particles by macrophages.

–in most instances is inconsequential and produces no disability.

2. Progressive massive fibrosis

–is marked by fibrotic nodules filled with necrotic black fluid.

–can result in **bronchiectasis, pulmonary hypertension,** or death from respiratory failure or right-sided heart failure.

C. Silicosis

–is a chronic occupational lung disease caused by **exposure to free silica dust;** it is seen in miners, glass manufacturers, and stone cutters.

–is initiated by ingestion of silica dust by alveolar macrophages; damage to macrophages initiates an inflammatory response mediated by lysosomal enzymes and a variety of chemical mediators.

–is marked by **silicotic nodules** that enlarge, eventually obstructing airways and blood vessels.

–is associated with increased susceptibility to tuberculosis; the frequent concurrence is referred to as **silicotuberculosis**.

D. Asbestosis

–is caused by **inhalation of asbestos fibers**.

—is initiated by uptake of asbestos fibers by alveolar macrophages. A fibroblastic response occurs, probably from release of fibroblast-stimulating growth factors by macrophages, and leads to **diffuse interstitial fibrosis,** principally in the lower lobes.

—is characterized by **ferruginous bodies,** yellow-brown, rod-shaped bodies with clubbed ends that stain positively with Prussian blue; these arise from iron and protein coating on fibers. Dense **hyalinized fibrocalcific plaques of the parietal pleura** are also present.

—results in marked predisposition to **bronchogenic carcinoma** and to **malignant mesothelioma** of the pleura or peritoneum. Cigarette smoking further increases the risk of bronchogenic carcinoma.

V. Interstitial Lung Disease

—is a heterogenous group of disorders affecting the alveolar wall.

—is characterized by **diffuse interstitial fibrosis** of the alveolar wall, producing a characteristic honeycomb appearance.

—involves similar pathogenetic mechanisms in spite of multiple etiologies.

—includes hypersensitivity pneumonitis (extrinsic allergic alveolitis), Goodpasture's syndrome, and idiopathic pulmonary hemosiderosis (Table 14.2), as well as the following:

A. Eosinophilic granuloma

—is a localized proliferation of histiocytic cells closely related to the Langerhans' cells of the skin. These cells have characteristic cytoplasmic inclusions (**Birbeck granules**) resembling tennis rackets.

—is also characterized by prominent monocytes–macrophages, lymphocytes, and eosinophils.

—is found in the lung or in bony sites such as the ribs.

—is often grouped with Hand-Schüller-Christian disease and Letterer-Siwe syndrome as a variant of **histiocytosis X** syndrome.

B. Idiopathic pulmonary fibrosis (Hamman-Rich syndrome)

—is characterized by **chronic inflammation and fibrosis of the alveolar wall**.

Table 14.2. Interstitial Lung Diseases

Disorder	Description
Hypersensitivity pneumonitis (extrinsic allergic alveolitis)	Interstitial pneumonia caused by inhalation of various antigenic substances
Goodpasture's syndrome	Hemorrhagic pneumonitis and glomerulonephritis caused by antibodies directed against glomerular basement membranes
Idiopathic pulmonary hemosiderosis	Resembles pulmonary component of Goodpasture's syndrome without renal component
Eosinophilic granuloma	Proliferation of histiocytic cells related to Langerhans' cells of the skin
Idiopathic pulmonary fibrosis (Hamman-Rich syndrome)	Immune complex disease with progressive fibrosis of the alveolar wall
Sarcoidosis	Granulomatous disorder of unknown etiology

—begins with alveolitis, progresses to fibrosis, and ends in a distorted fibrotic lung filled with cystic spaces (honeycomb lung).

—often results in death within 5 years.

C. Sarcoidosis (Boeck's sarcoid)

—is of unknown etiology.

—is characterized by **noncaseating granulomas,** often involving **multiple organ systems;** can involve almost any organ system.

—occurs most frequently in **blacks**.

—usually becomes clinically apparent during the **teenage or young adult years**.

1. Common pathologic changes

   a. Interstitial lung disease

   b. Enlarged hilar lymph nodes

   c. Anterior uveitis

   d. Erythema nodosum of the skin

   e. Polyarthritis

2. Immunologic phenomena

   a. Reduced sensitivity and often anergy to skin test antigens (characteristically negative tuberculin test)

   b. Polyclonal hyperglobulinemia

3. Clinical abnormalities

   —on routine chest x-ray, most often presents with

   a. Bilateral hilar lymphadenopathy

   b. Interstitial lung disease

4. Laboratory findings

   a. Hypercalcemia and hypercalciuria

   b. Hypergammaglobulinemia

   c. Increased activity of serum angiotensin-converting enzyme

5. Definitive diagnosis requires biopsy demonstrating noncaseating granulomas.

VI. Pulmonary Vascular Disease

A. Pulmonary embolism

—is found in more than half of all autopsies.

—most often originates from **venous thrombosis** in the lower extremities or pelvis.

—can rarely be due to nonthrombotic particulate material such as fat, amniotic fluid, clumps of tumor cells or bone marrow, or foreign matter such as bullet fragments.

—occurs in clinical settings marked by **venous stasis,** including primary venous disease, congestive heart failure, prolonged bed rest or immobilization, and prolonged sitting while traveling.

—is also predisposed by cancer, multiple fractures, and the use of oral contraceptives.

—results in **hemorrhagic, or red, infarcts,** usually in patients with compromised circulation, but can occur without infarction because of the dual blood supply to the lungs.

—can be of variable clinical consequence, ranging from asymptomatic disease to sudden death.

B. Pulmonary hypertension

1. Primary pulmonary hypertension

—is a disorder of **unknown etiology** and poor prognosis that arises in the absence of heart or lung disease.

2. Secondary pulmonary hypertension

—is more common than the primary form.

—is most often caused by **COPD;** can also be caused by **increased pulmonary blood flow,** as in congenital right-to-left shunt; **increased resistance within the pulmonary circulation,** from embolism or vasoconstriction secondary to hypoxia; or **increased blood viscosity** from polycythemia.

—often leads to **right ventricular hypertrophy**.

C. Pulmonary edema

—is **intra-alveolar accumulation of fluid**.

—may be caused by:

1. Increased hydrostatic pressure, as a result of left ventricular failure or mitral stenosis

2. Increased alveolar capillary permeability, as in inflammatory alveolar reactions, resulting from inhalation of irritant gases, pneumonia, shock, sepsis, pancreatitis, uremia, or drug overdose

VII. Pulmonary Infection

A. Pneumonia

1. General characteristics—pneumonia

—is an inflammatory process of infectious origin affecting the pulmonary parenchyma.

—is characterized by **chills and fever,** productive cough, blood-tinged or **rusty sputum,** pleuritic pain, hypoxia with shortness of breath, and sometimes cyanosis.

2. Morphologic types of pneumonia

—occurs in three morphologic and clinical patterns, **lobar pneumonia, bronchopneumonia,** and **interstitial pneumonia** (Table 14.3).

3. Etiologic types of pneumonia

—is most commonly caused by bacteria or viruses. See Table 14.4 for a discussion of the most common bacterial pneumonias. Other important forms include the following:

a. Hospital-acquired gram-negative pneumonias

—are often fatal and occur in hospitalized patients, usually those with serious, debilitating diseases.

Table 14.3. Morphologic Variants of Pneumonia

Variant	Causative Organism	Characteristics
Lobar pneumonia	Most frequently *Streptococcus pneumoniae* (pneumococcus)	Predominantly intra-alveolar exudate resulting in consolidation May involve entire lobe
Bronchopneumonia	Many organisms, including *Staphylococcus aureus, Haemophilus influenzae, Klebsiella pneumoniae,* and *Streptococcus pyogenes*	Acute inflammatory infiltrates extending from bronchioles into adjacent alveoli Patchy distribution involving one or more lobes
Interstitial pneumonia	Most frequently viruses or *Mycoplasma pneumoniae*	Diffuse, patchy inflammation localized to interstitial areas of alveolar walls Distribution involving one or more lobes

—are caused by many **gram-negative organisms,** including *Klebsiella, Pseudomonas aeruginosa,* and *Escherichia coli.* Endotoxins produced by these organisms play an important role in the infection.

b. *Mycoplasma* pneumonia (primary atypical pneumonia)

—is the most common nonbacterial form of pneumonia; it usually occurs in children and young adults, and it may occur in epidemics.

—has a more insidious onset than bacterial pneumonias and usually follows a mild, self-limiting course.

—is characterized by an inflammatory reaction confined to the interstitium, with no exudate in alveolar spaces, and by **intra-alveolar hyaline membranes**.

—is diagnosed by **sputum cultures,** requiring several weeks of incubation, and by complement-fixing antibodies and **nonspecific cold agglutinins** reactive to red blood cells.

c. *Pneumocystis carinii* pneumonia

—is the most common **opportunistic infection in AIDS** patients; also occurs in other forms of immunodeficiency.

—is caused by *P. carinii,* usually classified as a protozoan.

—is diagnosed by morphologic demonstration of organism in biopsy or bronchial washing specimens.

d. Q fever

—is the most common **rickettsial pneumonia;** it is caused by *Coxiella burnetii.*

—may infect persons working with infected cattle or sheep, who inhale dust particles containing the organism, or those who drink **unpasteurized milk** from infected animals.

e. Ornithosis

—is caused by an organism of the genus *Chlamydia,* which is transmitted by inhalation of dried excreta of infected birds.

Table 14.4 Important Features of Selected Bacterial Pneumonias

Organism	Characteristics	Complications
Streptococcus pneumoniae	Most common in elderly or debilitated patients, especially those with cardiopulmonary disease, and malnourished persons	May lead to empyema (pus in the pleural cavity)
Staphylococcus aureus	Often a complication of influenza or viral pneumonias or a result of blood-borne infection in intravenous drug users; seen principally in debilitated hospitalized patients, the elderly, and those with chronic lung disease	Abscess formation frequent; may lead to empyema or to other infectious complications, including bacterial endocarditis and brain and kidney abscesses
Streptococcus pyogenes	Often a complication of influenza or measles	Lung abscess
Klebsiella pneumoniae	Most frequent in debilitated hospitalized patients and diabetic or alcoholic patients; high mortality in elderly patients	Considerable alveolar wall damage, leading to necrosis, sometimes with abscess formation
Haemophilus influenzae	Usually seen in infants and children, but may occur in debilitated adults, most often those with chronic obstructive pulmonary disease	Meningitis in infants and children
Legionella pneumophila	Infection from inhalation of aerosol from contaminated stored water, most often in air-conditioning systems	

   f. Viral pneumonias
   —are the most common pneumonias of childhood.
   —are caused most commonly by **influenza and parainfluenza viruses,** adenoviruses, and respiratory syncytial virus; may also arise after childhood exanthems; the measles virus produces **giant cell pneumonia,** marked by numerous giant cells and often complicated by tracheobronchitis.

B. Lung abscess
   —is a **localized area of suppuration** within the parenchyma, usually resulting from bronchial obstruction (often by cancer), or from aspiration of gastric contents; may also be a complication of bacterial pneumonia.
   —is especially seen in patients predisposed to aspiration by **loss of consciousness** from alcohol or drug overdose, neurologic disorders or general anesthesia.
   —is frequently caused by *Staphylococcus, Pseudomonas, Klebsiella,* or *Proteus,* often in combination with anaerobic organisms.

C. Tuberculosis

1. General characteristics

—tuberculosis occurs worldwide, with greatest frequency in disadvantaged groups.

—in the pulmonary form, it is spread by inhalation of droplets containing the organism *Mycobacterium tuberculosis.*

—in the nonpulmonary form, it is most often caused by the ingestion of infected milk.

2. Types of tuberculosis

a. Primary tuberculosis

—**is initial infection, characterized by the primary, or Ghon, complex,** the combination of a peripheral subpleural parenchymal lesion and involved hilar lymph nodes. Granulomatous inflammation is characteristic of these lesions. The granuloma of tuberculosis is referred to as a tubercle and is characterized by central caseous necrosis and often by Langhans giant cells. The calcified lesions are often visible by x-ray.

—is most often asymptomatic.

—usually does not progress to clinically evident disease.

b. Secondary tuberculosis

—usually results from activation of a prior Ghon complex, with blood-borne spread to a new pulmonary site.

—rarely occurs without preceding primary tuberculosis.

—is characterized clinically by progressive disability, fever, hemoptysis, pleural effusion (often bloody), and generalized wasting.

(1) Pathologic changes

(a) Localized lesions, usually in the apical or posterior segments of the upper lobes

(b) Tubercle formation. The lesions frequently coalesce and rupture into the bronchi. The caseous contents may liquefy and be expelled, resulting in **cavitary lesions**.

(c) Scarring and calcification

(2) Spread of disease

(a) Secondary tuberculosis may be complicated by lymphatic and hematogenous spread, resulting in **miliary tuberculosis,** seeding of distal organs with innumerable small millet seed-like lesions.

(b) Hematogenous spread may also result in larger granulomatous lesions, which may involve almost any organs.

(c) Prominent examples of **extrapulmonary tuberculosis** include tuberculous meningitis, Pott's disease, paravertebral abscess, or psoas abscess.

3. Immune mechanisms in pathogenesis of tuberculosis

a. The organisms are ingested by macrophages, which process the bacterial antigens for presentation to T cells.

b. The T cells proliferate and secrete lymphokines, attracting lymphocytes and macrophages.

    c. The macrophages are morphologically altered to form epithelioid cells and Langhans multinucleated giant cells.

    d. Delayed hypersensitivity results in a **positive tuberculin skin test**. The test is positive in both primary and secondary infection, represents hypersensitivity and relative immunity, and ordinarily remains positive throughout life.

D. *Mycobacterium avium-intracellulare* **infection**

—is an infection with nontuberculous mycobacteria.

—is most often seen in patients with AIDS and other immunodeficiency diseases.

—is often manifest by nonpulmonary involvement.

E. Infections caused by fungi and fungus-like bacteria (Table 14.5)

—usually result from inhalation of the organism or from inoculation through the skin.

—in most instances, are manifest as inflammatory reactions similar to tuberculosis.

VIII. Miscellaneous Disorders of the Lungs

A. Atelectasis

    1. Acquired atelectasis

    —is **alveolar collapse** caused by bronchial obstruction or external compression of lung parenchyma by tumors or by pleural accumulation of fluid.

    2. Atelectasis neonatorum

    —is failure of alveolar spaces to expand adequately at birth; it occurs in two forms.

        a. Primary atelectasis

        —is failure of initial aeration of the lungs at birth; the alveoli remain collapsed and respiration is never fully established.

        —is associated with **prematurity** and **intrauterine fetal anoxia**.

        b. Secondary atelectasis

        —is collapse of previously aerated bronchi.

B. Adult respiratory distress syndrome (ARDS)

—is produced by **diffuse alveolar damage** with resultant increase in alveolar capillary permeability, causing leakage of protein-rich fluid into alveoli.

—is marked by the formation of an **intra-alveolar hyaline membrane** composed of fibrin and cellular debris.

—results in severe impairment of respiratory gas exchange with consequent severe hypoxia.

—is caused by a wide variety of mechanisms and toxic agents, including shock, sepsis, trauma, uremia, aspiration of gastric contents, acute pancreatitis, inhalation of chemical irritants such as chlorine, oxygen toxicity, or overdose with street drugs such as heroin or therapeutic drugs such as bleomycin.

—is initiated by damage to alveolar capillary endothelium and alveolar epithelium and is influenced by the following pathogenetic factors:

    1. Neutrophils release substances toxic to the alveolar wall.

Table 14.5. Characteristics of Pulmonary Infections Caused by Fungi and Fungus-like Bacteria

Disorder	Organism	Characteristics
Actinomycosis	*Actinomyces,* gram-positive anaerobic filamentous bacteria no longer classified as fungus	Abscess and sinus tract formation Exudate containing characteristic sulfur granules, yellow clumps of the organism
Nocardiosis	*Nocardia,* gram-positive aerobic, filamentous, weakly acid-fast bacteria closely related to *Actinomyces*	Typically opportunistic infection May disseminate to the brain and meninges
Candidiasis	*Candida albicans*	In immunocompromised patients, invasive form produces blood-borne dissemination Pulmonary, renal, and hepatic abscesses and vegetative endocarditis
Cryptococcosis	*Cryptococcus neoformans*	Infection usually begins in the lungs but can also produce cryptococcal meningitis Organism's characteristic encapsulated appearance visualized in India ink preparations
Aspergillosis	*Aspergillus*	Invasive form has predilection for growth into vessels, with consequent widespread hematogenous dissemination
Histoplasmosis	*Histoplasma capsulatum*	Pulmonary manifestations similar to tuberculosis; occurs in primary and secondary forms Results in multiple pulmonary lesions with late calcification Disseminated form, marked by multisystem involvement with infiltrates of macrophages filled with fungal yeast forms
Coccidioidomycosis	*Coccidioides immitis*	Occurs in primary and disseminated forms Fungal spherules containing endospores found within granulomas

    2. Activation of the coagulation cascade is suggested by the presence of microemboli.

    3. Oxygen toxicity is mediated by formation of oxygen-derived free radicals.

C. Neonatal respiratory distress syndrome (hyaline membrane disease)
    —is the most common cause of respiratory failure in the newborn, and is the most common cause of death in premature infants.
    —is marked by dyspnea, cyanosis, and tachypnea shortly after birth.
    —results from a deficiency of surfactant, most often as a result of immaturity.

1. Pathogenesis

a. Role of surfactant

(1) Surfactant reduces surface tension within the lung, facilitating expansion during inspiration and preventing atelectasis during expiration.

(2) Surfactant consists primarily of dipalmitoyl lecithin and is secreted by type II pneumocytes.

(3) **Fetal pulmonary maturity** can be assessed by measuring the ratio of surfactant lecithin to sphingomyelin in the amniotic fluid; lecithin concentration increases from about the 33rd week of pregnancy while the sphingomyelin concentration remains stable. A lecithin-sphingomyelin ratio of 2:1 or greater indicates pulmonary maturity.

b. Predisposing factors

(1) **Prematurity**

(2) **Maternal diabetes mellitus**

(3) Birth by **caesarean section**

2. Pathologic findings

a. Lungs are heavier than usual with areas of atelectasis alternating with occasional dilated alveoli or alveolar ducts.

b. Small pulmonary vessels are engorged, with leakage of blood products into the alveoli and formation of intra-alveolar hyaline membranes consisting of fibrin and cellular debris.

3. Complications and associated conditions

a. **Bronchopulmonary dysplasia,** which appears to be precipitated by treatment with high-concentration oxygen and mechanical ventilation

b. **Patent ductus arteriosus,** caused by failure of closure of the ductus caused by immaturity and hypoxia

c. **Intraventricular brain hemorrhage**

d. **Necrotizing enterocolitis,** a fulminant inflammation of the small and large intestines

D. Pulmonary alveolar proteinosis

—is uncommon and is characterized by accumulation of amorphous, PAS-positive material in the alveolar air spaces. Sometimes this material appears to be surfactant.

IX. Cancers of the Lung

A. General characteristics

—most lung tumors are malignant; those that arise from **metastases** from primary tumors elsewhere occur more frequently than those that originate in the lung (Table 14.6).

B. Bronchogenic carcinoma

—is the leading cause of death from cancer in both men and women.

—is increasing in incidence, especially in women, in parallel with cigarette smoking.

Table 14.6. Tumors of the Lung

Type	Location	Characteristics
Bronchogenic carcinoma: Squamous cell carcinoma	Central	Appears as a hilar mass, and frequently results in cavitation; clearly linked to smoking; incidence greatly increased in smokers
Adenocarcinoma Bronchial-derived	Peripheral	Develops on site of prior pulmonary inflammation or injury (scar carcinoma); less clearly linked to smoking
Bronchioloalveolar	Peripheral	Apparently unrelated to smoking; tumor cells line alveolar walls
Small cell (oat cell) carcinoma	Central	Undifferentiated tumor; most aggressive bronchogenic carcinoma; usually already metastatic at diagnosis; often associated with ectopic hormone production; incidence greatly increased in smokers
Large cell carcinoma	Peripheral	Undifferentiated tumor; may show features of squamous cell or adenocarcinoma on electron microscopy
Other carcinomas of the lung: Carcinoid	Major bronchi	Low malignancy, spreading by direct extension into adjacent tissues; may result in carcinoid syndrome
Carcinoma metastatic to lung	. . .	Higher incidence than primary lung cancer

—is directly proportional in incidence to the number of cigarettes smoked daily and to the number of years of smoking.

—is preceded in cigarette smokers by a variety of histologic changes, including squamous metaplasia of respiratory epithelium, often with atypical changes ranging from dysplasia to carcinoma in situ.

1. Other etiopathogenic factors

a. Air pollution

b. Radiation; incidence increased in radium and uranium workers

c. Asbestos; increased incidence with asbestos and greater increase with combination of asbestos and cigarette smoking

d. Industrial exposure to nickel and chromates

2. Clinical features

—has a 5-year survival rate of less than 10%.

—is manifest clinically by cough, hemoptysis, and bronchial obstruction, often with atelectasis and pneumonitis.

—often spreads by local extension into the pleura, pericardium, or ribs.

—may also be manifest by the following **clinical features**

a. **Superior vena cava syndrome;** obstruction of the superior vena cava, resulting in facial swelling and cyanosis along with dilation of the veins of the head and neck

b. **Pancoast's tumor** (superior sulcus tumor); involvement of the apex of the lung, often with **Horner's syndrome** (ptosis, miosis, and anhidrosis); due to involvement of the cervical sympathetic plexus

c. **Hoarseness** from recurrent laryngeal nerve paralysis

d. **Pleural effusion,** often bloody; bloody pleural effusion suggests malignancy, tuberculosis, or trauma.

e. **Paraneoplastic endocrine syndromes,** the most frequent of which is ACTH-like activity with small cell carcinoma; also of note are antidiuretic hormone-like activity with small cell carcinoma of the lung and parathyroid-like activity with squamous cell carcinoma.

3. **Classification**
   −bronchogenic carcinoma is subclassified, into squamous cell carcinoma, adenocarcinoma, small cell carcinoma, and large cell carcinoma; it appears all share a common endodermal origin in spite of morphologic differences.

Review Test

Directions: Each of the numbered items or incomplete statements in this section is followed by answers or by completions of the statement. Select the **one** lettered answer or completion that is **best** in each case.

1. All of the following disorders are correctly paired with related characteristics EXCEPT

(A) atelectasis—bronchial obstruction.
(B) adult respiratory distress syndrome—hyaline membranes.
(C) cystic fibrosis—α_1-antitrypsin deficiency.
(D) acute epiglottitis—*Haemophilus influenzae*.
(E) asbestosis—ferruginous bodies.

2. Which of the following neoplasms is closely associated with the Epstein-Barr virus?

(A) Extramedullary plasmacytoma
(B) Laryngeal papilloma
(C) Nasopharyngeal carcinoma
(D) Bronchioloalveolar carcinoma
(E) Carcinoid tumor of the lung

3. Adult respiratory distress syndrome is caused by all of the following conditions EXCEPT

(A) shock.
(B) sepsis.
(C) inhalation of toxic irritants.
(D) bronchial obstruction by foreign body.
(E) head injury.

4. All of the following conditions are associated with the neonatal respiratory distress syndrome EXCEPT

(A) prematurity.
(B) maternal diabetes mellitus.
(C) birth by caesarean section.
(D) increased alveolar surfactant.

5. A biopsy with findings similar to those shown in the figure below was obtained from the hilar lymph nodes of a 23-year-old man who presented with radiographic evidence of bilateral hilar lymphadenopathy and interstitial lung disease. This condition is associated with all of the following findings EXCEPT

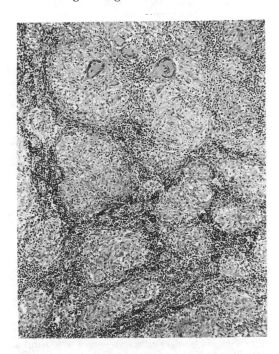

(Reprinted with permission from Golden A, Powell D, and Jennings C: *Pathology: Understanding Human Disease,* 2nd ed. Baltimore, Williams & Wilkins, 1985, p 42.)

(A) anergy to tuberculin.
(B) involvement of almost any organ system.
(C) increased incidence in blacks.
(D) hypercalcemia.
(E) hypogammaglobulinemia.

6. All of the following disorders are correctly paired with related characteristics EXCEPT

(A) sarcoidosis—noncaseating granulomas.
(B) idiopathic pulmonary hemosiderosis—antiglomerular basement membrane antibodies.
(C) idiopathic pulmonary fibrosis—immune complex disease.
(D) eosinophilic granuloma—Birbeck granules.
(E) Goodpasture's syndrome—renal lesions.

7. A patchy distribution of lesions throughout the lungs is characteristic of pneumonia caused by all of the following agents EXCEPT

(A) *Staphylococcus aureus.*
(B) viruses.
(C) *Mycoplasma pneumoniae.*
(D) *Streptococcus pneumoniae.*
(E) *Haemophilus influenzae.*

8. All of the following types of pneumonia are correctly paired with related findings EXCEPT

(A) *Streptococcus pyogenes* pneumonia—lobar involvement.
(B) staphylococcal pneumonia—abscess formation.
(C) *Mycoplasma* pneumonia—cold agglutinins.
(D) *Haemophilus* pneumonia—infants and children.
(E) *Klebsiella* pneumonia—high mortality in elderly.

9. All of the following causative microorganisms or disease entities are correctly paired with a frequent association or effect EXCEPT

(A) bronchiectasis—abundant sputum.
(B) bronchogenic carcinoma—lung abscess.
(C) *Mycoplasma pneumoniae*—cold agglutinins.
(D) *Staphylococcus aureus*—lobar pneumonia.
(E) *Streptococcus pneumoniae*—exudate in pleural space.

10. All of the following disorders are correctly paired with related characteristics EXCEPT

(A) Legionnaires' disease—air-conditioning systems.
(B) Q fever—livestock workers.
(C) ornithosis—rickettsial disease.
(D) measles—giant cells.

11. Which of the following changes does not occur in primary tuberculosis?

(A) Calcification
(B) Caseating granulomas
(C) Cavitation
(D) Langhans giant cells
(E) Positive tuberculin test

12. All of the following terms related to tuberculosis are correctly paired EXCEPT

(A) Ghon complex—primary infection.
(B) apical segments of upper lobes—secondary infection.
(C) hematogenous spread—miliary pattern.
(D) Langhans cells—Birbeck granules.
(E) nonpulmonary tuberculosis—unpasteurized milk.

13. All of the following terms are correctly paired EXCEPT

(A) actinomycosis—sulfur granules.
(B) cryptococcosis—India ink preparations.
(C) histoplasmosis—overwhelming pneumonia.
(D) coccidioidomycosis—spherules with endospores.
(E) nocardiosis—opportunistic infection.

14. All of the following phenomena related to lung cancer are correctly matched with the appropriate association EXCEPT

(A) bronchial squamous metaplasia—cigarette smoking.
(B) facial swelling and cyanosis—recurrent laryngeal nerve paralysis.
(C) Pancoast's tumor—superior sulcus.
(D) ptosis, miosis, and anhidrosis—Horner's syndrome.
(E) paraneoplastic syndrome—small cell carcinoma.

15. All of the following forms of lung cancer are correctly paired with the appropriate characteristic EXCEPT

(A) squamous cell carcinoma—central location.
(B) small cell carcinoma—almost never resectable.
(C) large cell carcinoma—lung tumor most clearly related to cigarette smoking.
(D) adenocarcinoma—peripheral location.
(E) bronchioloalveolar carcinoma—tumor cells lining alveolar walls.

16. All of the following statements concerning respiratory tract neoplasms are correct EXCEPT

(A) the most common site of extramedullary plasmacytoma is the upper respiratory tract.
(B) a singers' nodule is a small, benign laryngeal polyp induced by chronic irritation.
(C) papillomas of the larynx tend to be single in adults and multiple in children.
(D) squamous cell carcinoma is the most common malignant tumor of the larynx.
(E) most laryngeal carcinomas have a subglottic location.

Directions: Each group of items in this section consists of lettered options followed by a set of numbered items. For each item, select the **one** lettered option that is most closely associated with it. Each lettered option may be selected once, more than once, or not at all.

Questions 17–20

Match each of the following disorders with the most appropriate associated finding.

(A) Bronchial asthma
(B) Chronic bronchitis
(C) Emphysema
(D) Bronchiectasis

17. α_1-Antitrypsin deficiency

18. Charcot-Leyden crystals

19. Bronchial submucosal gland hyperplasia

20. Copious purulent sputum

Questions 21–24

Match each of the following disorders with the most appropriate pulmonary finding or complication.

(A) Progressive massive fibrosis
(B) Silicosis
(C) Asbestosis
(D) Anthracosis

21. Tuberculosis

22. Mesothelioma

23. Carbon-laden macrophages

24. Black fibrotic nodules

Answers and Explanations

1–C. Cystic fibrosis is associated with a mutation in the cystic fibrosis transmembrane conductance regulator (CFTR) gene; it is not associated with α_1-antitrypsin deficiency.

2–C. Nasopharyngeal carcinoma, a lesion that is most common in Southeast Asia and East Africa, is caused by EBV.

3–D. Although bronchial obstruction by a foreign body might result in atelectatic collapse of the pulmonary parenchyma distal to the obstruction, the diffuse alveolar damage and increased capillary permeability characteristic of ARDS would be an unlikely complication of this occurrence. A variety of conditions can cause this syndrome, including shock, sepsis, inhalation of toxic irritants, and head injury.

4–D. The neonatal respiratory distress syndrome is due to a deficiency of pulmonary surfactant. Surfactant reduces surface tension within the lung, facilitating expansion by inspiration, and thus preventing atelectasis during expiration. Important predisposing factors include prematurity, diabetes mellitus, and caesarean section.

5–E. The illustration shows noncaseating granulomas and Langhans giant cells, which, in the clinical setting described, are diagnostic of sarcoidosis. A frequent abnormal laboratory finding is polyclonal hypergammaglobulinemia along with hypercalcemia. Anergy to tuberculin is often demonstrable. Patients most often present with lung findings and hilar lymphadenopathy, but any organ system can be involved. The disorder is much more common in blacks.

6–B. Idiopathic pulmonary hemosiderosis is characterized by hemorrhagic lung involvement similar to Goodpasture's syndrome, but notable differences include the absence of antiglomerular basement membrane antibodies or renal involvement.

7–D. Patchy distribution of lesions throughout the lungs is characteristic of bronchopneumonia, which is caused by a number of organisms, most notably *S. aureus* and *H. influenzae*. A similar distribution is observed in the interstitial pneumonias caused by viruses and mycoplasma. In contrast, involvement of a single lobe, often in its entirety (lobar pneumonia), is characteristic of infection with *S. pneumoniae*.

8–A. The most frequent etiologic agent of lobar pneumonia is *S. pneumoniae,* not *S. pyogenes.* Staphylococcal pneumonia is often complicated by pulmonary or extrapulmonary abscess formation as well as by empyema, bronchopleural fistula, or bacterial endocarditis. Diagnosis of *Mycoplasma* pneumonia, the most common nonbacterial pneumonia, is facilitated by laboratory demonstration of nonspecific cold agglutinins directed against red blood cells as well as by complement-fixing antibodies and microbiologic culture techniques. *Haemophilus* pneumonia is most often observed in infants and young children. *Klebsiella* pneumonia has a high mortality rate in the elderly.

9–D. Lobar pneumonia is typically caused by *S. pneumoniae.* In contrast, pulmonary infection with *S. aureus* is most often associated with bronchopneumonia, often with formation of multiple small abscesses.

10–C. Ornithosis, caused by an organism of the genus *Chlamydia,* is not a rickettsial disease. Legionnaires' disease, *Legionella pneumophila* infection, has often been traced to contamination of air-conditioning systems. Q fever, the most common rickettsial pneumonia, often affects livestock workers who handle cattle or sheep. Pneumonia from the measles virus can take the form of giant cell pneumonia.

11–C. Cavitation occurs only in secondary tuberculosis. Both primary and secondary tuberculosis are characterized by caseating granulomas, often with Langhans giant cells, that heal by scarring and calcification. The skin test for tuberculin sensitivity is positive in both forms.

12–D. Birbeck granules are associated with the Langerhans'-like cells of histiocytosis X. Langhans cells are multinucleated giant cells that have a horseshoe-like arrangement of their multiple nuclei.

13–C. Histoplasmosis exhibits pulmonary manifestations similar to those of tuberculosis, and overwhelming pneumonia does not occur. The most frequent form is the asymptomatic primary pulmonary disease, marked by a positive skin test and residual calcifications. Secondary pulmonary histoplasmosis can result in cavitary disease, and disseminated histoplasmosis involves the lymphoreticular system.

14–B. Facial swelling and cyanosis, often with dilatation of the veins of the head and neck, is characteristically caused by partial obstruction of the superior vena cava and is referred to as the superior vena cava syndrome. These findings are most often a manifestation of lung cancer. Another quite unrelated complication of lung cancer is hoarseness caused by involvement of the recurrent laryngeal nerve.

15–C. Large cell carcinomas are poorly differentiated carcinomas, some of which prove to be squamous cell carcinoma or adenocarcinoma on electron microscopy. Since the relationship of cigarette smoking to adenocarcinoma is not as clear as with squamous cell or small cell carcinoma, large cell carcinomas display a somewhat less clear relationship to cigarette smoking than other forms of bronchogenic carcinoma.

16–E. The most common location of laryngeal carcinoma is on the true vocal cords (glottis). Tumors in this region have the best prognosis since the glottis has almost no lymphatic drainage. The second most common location is supraglottic, and tumors in this location have a poorer prognosis. The least common location is the subglottic region, and tumors in this region have the poorest prognosis.

17–C. Homozygous inheritance of the mutant Z allele of the pi (proteinase inhibitor) gene results in marked α_1-antitrypsin deficiency. Absence of this antiproteinase results in panacinar emphysema and liver damage.

18–A. Charcot-Leyden crystals, thought to be derived from eosinophil membrane proteins, are found in the sputum in bronchial asthma.

19–B. The characteristic pathologic change in chronic bronchitis is hyperplasia of bronchial submucosal glands and bronchial smooth muscle hypertrophy, which can be quantified by the Reid index, a ratio of glandular layer thickness to bronchial wall thickness.

20–D. The cardinal clinical sign of bronchiectasis is the production of large amounts of purulent sputum, often more than one cup a day.

21–B. Pulmonary tuberculosis is a major complication of silicosis. The cause of this association is unknown but may be due to altered macrophage activity.

22–C. Asbestos exposure is associated with malignant mesothelioma of the pleura and peritoneum. Exposure to asbestos is also a risk factor for bronchogenic carcinoma as well as for carcinoma of the oropharynx, esophagus, and colon. The risk of bronchogenic carcinoma is markedly increased in cigarette smokers with exposure to asbestos.

23–D. Anthracosis, a common finding in the lungs of city dwellers, is characterized by subpleural collections of carbon-laden macrophages. The carbon deposits ordinarily do not result in a significant tissue reaction and are of no clinical consequence.

24–A. Progressive massive fibrosis, a generalized pulmonary fibrotic change, sometimes complicates simple coal workers' pneumoconiosis. Progressive massive fibrosis is characterized by fibrotic nodules filled with necrotic black India ink-like liquid. The lesions may lead to bronchiectasis and pulmonary hypertension.

15

Gastrointestinal Tract

I. Diseases of the Mouth and Jaw

A. Inflammatory disorders

1. Herpes labialis (fever blisters, cold sores)
- is a common vesicular lesion caused by herpes simplex virus (HSV), most often by HSV type 1 (HSV-1).
- tends to recur, with activation by febrile illness, trauma, sunshine, or menstruation.

2. Aphthous stomatitis
- is characterized by painful, recurrent, erosive oral ulcerations.

3. Oral candidiasis (thrush, moniliasis)
- is a local white, membranous lesion caused by *Candida albicans*.
- occurs most commonly in debilitated infants and children, immunocompromised patients, and diabetics.

4. Acute necrotizing ulcerative gingivitis (trench mouth, Vincent's infection, fusospirochetosis)
- is a severe gingival inflammation occurring in patients with decreased resistance to infection.
- is due to concurrent infection with the symbiotic bacteria *Fusobacterium fusiforme* and *Borrelia vincentii*.

B. Tumors and tumor-like conditions

1. Benign tumors of the oral mucosa

a. Papilloma
- is the most common benign epithelial tumor of the oral mucosa.
- can occur anywhere in the mouth; the most common sites are the tongue, lips, gingivae, or buccal mucosa.

b. Fibroma
- is most often a non-neoplastic hyperplastic lesion resulting from chronic irritation.

209

c. Hemangioma

—occurs most commonly on the tongue, lip, or buccal mucosa.

d. Epulis

—refers to any benign (usually non-neoplastic) growth of the gingivae.

—is most often a reparative growth rather than a true neoplasm.

2. Leukoplakia

—is a clinical term describing irregular white mucosal patches.

—results from hyperkeratosis, usually secondary to chronic irritation.

—is usually benign but may represent dysplasia or carcinoma in situ.

3. Odontogenic tumors

a. Odontoma

—is the most common odontogenic tumor.

—is a **hamartoma** derived from odontogenic epithelium and odonto-blastic tissue.

b. Ameloblastoma (adamantinoma)

—is an **epithelial tumor arising from precursor cells of the enamel organ**.

—occurs most frequently in the mandible.

—usually appears before age 35.

—although benign, can lead to slow expansion of the jaw because of ir-regular local extension.

4. Oral cancer

—is most frequently squamous cell carcinoma.

—involves the tongue in more than 50% of cases.

—may be associated with irritants such as pipe smoking, chewing tobacco or betel nuts, and alcohol consumption.

II. Diseases of the Salivary Glands

A. Sialadenitis

—is **inflammation of the salivary glands**.

—may be caused by infection, immune-mediated mechanisms, or occlusion of the salivary ducts by stones (sialolithiasis).

B. Acute parotitis

—occurs in mumps.

—may also be caused by other infectious agents.

C. Sjögren's syndrome

—is most likely of autoimmune origin.

—is characterized by **keratoconjunctivitis sicca** (dry eyes), **xerostomia** (dry mouth), and an associated **connective tissue disease,** most often rheumatoid arthritis.

—is associated with an increased incidence of malignant lymphoma.

D. Mucocele

—is a cyst-like pool of mucus, lined by granulation tissue, near a minor sal-ivary gland.

—results from mucus leakage caused by rupture of obstructed or traumatized ducts.

E. Ranula

–is a **large mucocele, of salivary gland origin,** characteristically localized to the floor of the mouth.

F. Tumors of the salivary gland (Table 15.1)

–the majority of salivary gland tumors occur in the parotid gland.

1. Pleomorphic adenoma (mixed tumor)

–is the most frequently occurring salivary gland tumor.

–occurs with greatest frequency in women between the ages of 20 and 40.

–is a benign tumor but frequently recurs; it rarely becomes malignant.

–has been termed "mixed tumor" because of the presence of myxoid and cartilage-like elements as well as epithelial cells.

–varies histologically but most often demonstrates irregular masses or anastomosing strands of stellate or fusiform epithelial cells, some forming ducts or tubules, all of which are embedded in a myxoid stroma that may display fibrous, cartilage-like, or hyalinized areas.

–is **most often localized to the parotid gland** (about 90%).

–usually presents as a firm, nontender swelling.

–often is difficult to remove completely because of its proximity to the facial nerve.

Table 15.1. Salivary Gland Tumors

Type	Typical Location	Histology	Characteristics
Pleomorphic adenoma (mixed tumor)	Parotid gland; can occur in submandibular or minor salivary glands	Variable mix of epithelial and mesenchyme-like elements	Most common salivary gland tumor; benign; tends to recur after resection; malignant transformation occurs but is rare
Papillary cystadenoma lymphomatosum (Warthin's tumor, adenolymphoma)	Parotid gland	Cystic spaces lined by double-layered eosinophilic epithelium, all embedded in lymphoid stroma	Benign
Mucoepidermoid tumor	Parotid gland	Comprised of mucus-producing and epidermoid components and cells intermediate between the two	Behavior varies from benign to highly malignant; tumors with greater number of epidermoid cells and nonparotid tumors tend to be more aggressive
Adenoid cystic carcinoma	Minor salivary glands	Variable; most characteristic appearance consists of cribriform pattern with masses of small, dark-staining cells arrayed around cystic spaces	Tends to infiltrate perineural spaces and cause pain; slow-growing malignancy with late metastasis
Oncocytoma	Parotid gland	Large, granular-appearing, eosinophilic-staining epithelial cells	Benign; peak occurrence in elderly

2. Other salivary gland tumors

a. Papillary cystadenoma lymphomatosum (Warthin's tumor)

b. Mucoepidermoid tumor

c. Adenoid cystic carcinoma

d. Oncocytoma

III. Diseases of the Esophagus

A. Tracheoesophageal fistula

—is a congenital disorder.

—is suggested in a newborn by copious salivation associated with choking, coughing, and cyanosis on attempts at food intake.

—presents in three distinct variants:

1. In the **most common variant** (90%), the lower portion of the esophagus communicates with the trachea near the tracheal bifurcation. The upper esophagus ends in a blind pouch. Maternal polyhydramnios (increased amniotic fluid) is a frequently associated abnormality.

2. The **second most common variant** is characterized by a fistulous connection between the upper esophagus and the trachea; the lower esophageal segment is not connected to the upper esophagus.

3. In a **third variant,** there is a fistulous connection between the trachea and a completely patent esophagus.

B. Esophageal diverticula

—are pouches lined by one or more layers of the esophageal wall.

—are most commonly false (**pulsion**) diverticula resulting from herniation of the mucosa through defects in the muscular layer.

—are less commonly true (**traction**) diverticula consisting of mucosal, muscular, and serosal layers. Traction diverticula result from periesophageal inflammation and scarring.

—occur in three characteristic **locations**:

1. Immediately above the upper esophageal sphincter (**Zenker's diverticulum**)

2. Near the midpoint of the esophagus

3. Immediately above the lower esophageal sphincter (**epiphrenic diverticulum**)

C. Achalasia

—is persistent contraction of the lower esophageal sphincter and absence of esophageal peristalsis leading to dilation of the esophagus.

—is caused by a loss of ganglion cells in the myenteric plexus, which leads to the progressive dilation of the esophagus.

—is characterized clinically by difficulty in swallowing.

D. Esophageal varices

—are **dilated submucosal esophageal veins** secondary to portal hypertension.

—can result in upper gastrointestinal hemorrhage; the other important causes of upper gastrointestinal hemorrhage are bleeding peptic ulcer and the Mallory-Weiss syndrome, bleeding from esophagogastric laceration as a result of severe retching.

E. Inflammatory and related disorders of the esophagus

1. Gastroesophageal reflux

–may be caused by hiatal hernia, incompetent lower esophageal sphincter, pregnancy, or scleroderma.
–can cause esophagitis, stricture, ulceration, or columnar metaplasia of esophageal squamous epithelium (Barrett's esophagus).
–often manifests by substernal pain (heartburn).

2. Barrett's esophagus

–is **columnar metaplasia of esophageal squamous epithelium**.
–is a complication of long-standing gastroesophageal reflux.
–is associated with an **increased incidence of esophageal adenocarcinoma**.

3. Esophageal stricture

–most often results from prolonged esophageal gastric acid reflux.
–may also be caused by suicidal or accidental ingestion of corrosive agents.
–is marked by progressive dysphagia.

4. Candida esophagitis (moniliasis)

–often is associated with antibiotic therapy, diabetes mellitus, malignant disease, or immunodeficiency caused by AIDS or immunosuppressive drugs.
–is manifest clinically by white adherent mucosal patches and painful, difficult swallowing.

5. Herpetic esophagitis

–is caused by HSV-1 infection.
–tends to occur in immunosuppressed persons.
–is characterized by painful, difficult swallowing.

F. Esophageal carcinoma

–is an aggressive tumor manifest clinically by dysphagia, weight loss, and anorexia, and occasionally by pain or hematemesis.
–is usually **squamous cell carcinoma**.
–is much less commonly adenocarcinoma, which arises in aberrant gastric mucosa, submucosal glands, or the metaplastic columnar epithelium of Barrett's esophagus.
–may be manifest pathologically by protrusion into the esophageal lumen, by local extension into adjacent structures such as the trachea, bronchi, or aorta, or by diffuse infiltration into the esophageal wall.
–is predisposed by esophagitis.
–occurs with greatly increased incidence among smokers and alcoholics.

IV. Diseases of the Stomach

A. Congenital pyloric stenosis

–is caused by hypertrophy of the circular muscular layer of the pylorus, often resulting in a **palpable mass**.

—results in obstruction of the gastric outlet, causing episodes of **projectile vomiting** beginning in the first two weeks of life.

—is much more common in boys.

—is corrected by surgical incision of the hypertrophied muscle.

B. Gastritis

1. Acute (erosive) gastritis

a. Causes

(1) Nonsteroidal anti-inflammatory drugs

(2) Cigarette smoking

(3) Heavy alcohol intake

(4) Burn injury; **Curling's ulcer,** an acute gastric ulcer in association with severe burns

(5) Brain injury; **Cushing's ulcer,** an acute gastric ulcer in association with brain injury

b. Characteristics

(1) Focal damage to the gastric mucosa, with acute inflammation, necrosis, and hemorrhage

(2) May be manifest as acute gastric ulcer

2. Chronic (nonerosive) gastritis

—is characterized by chronic mucosal inflammation and atrophy of the mucosal glands.

a. Fundal (type A) gastritis

—is associated with the presence of antibodies to parietal cells, achlorhydria, pernicious anemia, and autoimmune diseases such as chronic thyroiditis and Addison's disease.

—is also associated with aging, partial gastrectomy, gastric ulcer, and gastric carcinoma.

b. Antral (type B) gastritis

—is not associated with pernicious anemia, antibodies to parietal cells, or reduced gastric acid secretion.

—is often associated with *Helicobacter (Campylobacter) pylori* infection; this organism is also associated with gastric and duodenal peptic ulcer and with carcinoma of the stomach.

3. Ménétrier's disease (giant hypertrophic gastritis)

—is characterized by extreme enlargement of gastric rugae and sometimes by severe loss of plasma proteins from the altered mucosa.

C. Peptic ulcer of the stomach

—most often occurs at or near the lesser curvature, in the antral and prepyloric regions.

—is not a precursor lesion of carcinoma of the stomach.

—unlike peptic ulcer that occurs elsewhere, is not dependent on increased gastric acid secretion; however, acid and pepsin are believed to play a role since gastric peptic ulcers rarely occur in association with absolute achlorhydria.

Postulated etiopathogenic mechanisms of gastric peptic ulcer production include:

1. Increased permeability of gastric mucosa to hydrogen ion, resulting in back diffusion of hydrogen ion with injury to the gastric mucosa

2. Bile-induced gastritis leading to gastric ulceration

D. Malignant tumors of the stomach

1. Carcinoma of the stomach

–is most common after **age 50,** with an increased incidence in **men**.

–occurs more frequently in persons of **blood group A,** suggesting a genetic predisposition.

–varies markedly in incidence from one geographic area to another, with incidence much higher in Japan, Finland, and Iceland.

a. Etiologic factors—stomach carcinoma

(1) **Nitrosamines** from dietary amines and nitrites used as food preservatives: Incidence of the disease is markedly increased in populations who eat large amounts of smoked fish and meat and pickled vegetables.

(2) Increased incidence is also associated with excessive salt intake and a diet low in fresh fruits and vegetables.

(3) A further etiopathogenic factor is the recently noted association with *H. pylori* infection

(4) Stomach carcinoma is also predisposed by:
  (a) Achlorhydria
  (b) Chronic gastritis with or without pernicious anemia

b. Characteristics—stomach carcinoma

(1) Histologically, stomach carcinoma is almost always **adenocarcinoma**.

(2) Involvement of the distal stomach, along the lesser curvature of the antrum or prepyloric region is most common; rarely involves the fundus.

(3) Aggressive spread to adjacent organs and the peritoneum and by early lymphatic metastasis to regional lymph nodes and the liver.

(4) May involve more distal sites:
  (a) Involvement of a supraclavicular lymph node by metastatic carcinoma of the stomach is referred to as **Virchow's node**.
  (b) Bilateral involvement of the ovaries by metastatic carcinoma of the stomach is referred to as **Krukenberg tumor**. The tumor cells often contain abundant mucin, displacing the nucleus to one side and resulting in so-called **signet-ring cells**.

c. Morphologic variants—stomach carcinoma

(1) **Polypoid (fungating) carcinoma**
  –forms a solid mass projecting into the lumen of the stomach.

(2) **Ulcerated carcinoma**
  –forms an ulcer with an irregular necrotic base and firm, raised margins.

−must be differentiated from peptic ulcer, which usually exhibits a smooth base with nonelevated, punched-out margins.

   (3) **Infiltrating or diffuse carcinoma** (linitis plastica, leather-bottle stomach)

      −is characterized by a thickened, rigid stomach wall, caused by diffuse infiltration of tumor cells with accompanying extensive fibrosis.

2. Lymphoma

−accounts for 4% of malignant gastric tumors.

−has a better prognosis than adenocarcinoma.

V. Diseases of the Small Intestine

A. Peptic ulcer

−occurs most frequently in the first portion of the duodenum, the stomach, or the lower end of the esophagus, all of which are exposed to acid and pepsin.

−except for peptic ulcer of the stomach, is always associated with hypersecretion of gastric acid and pepsin.

−is not a precursor of malignancy.

−occurs with increased frequency in persons of blood group O, suggesting that genetic factors may play a role.

−is frequently complicated by hemorrhage with melena (black stools containing blood). Other important complications include obstruction and perforation.

−is sometimes associated with:

1. Intake of **aspirin** or other nonsteroidal anti-inflammatory drugs. The ulcerogenic effect of these drugs may be mediated by inhibition of prostaglandin synthesis.

2. The incidence of peptic ulcer is twofold greater in **smokers**.

3. Zollinger-Ellison syndrome, increased tendency toward peptic ulcer formation, is caused by gastric acid hypersecretion due to gastrin-secreting islet cell tumor of the pancreas. Recurrent peptic ulcer or peptic ulcer in aberrant sites such as the jejunum is suggestive of the Zollinger-Ellison syndrome.

4. Primary hyperparathyroidism

5. Multiple endocrine neoplasia type I (MEN type I, Wermer's syndrome), an autosomal dominant syndrome characterized by pituitary, thyroid, parathyroid, adrenal cortical, and pancreatic islet cell adenomas or hyperplasias associated with hypergastrinemia and peptic ulcer

B. Crohn's disease (Table 15.2)

−is a **chronic inflammatory condition** of unknown etiology that may affect any part of the gastrointestinal tract but most commonly involves the distal ileocecum, small intestine, or colon.

−tends to affect young people in the second and third decades of life, although no age group is exempt.

−occurs most frequently in people of Jewish descent.

Table 15.2. Comparison of Crohn's Disease and Ulcerative Colitis

Crohn's Disease	Ulcerative Colitis
May involve any portion of gastrointestinal tract, usually ileocecal region, small intestine, or colon	Affects only colon
Chronic inflammatory reaction extends through entire thickness of intestinal wall	Inflammation and ulceration limited to mucosa and submucosa
Lymphocytic infiltrate; noncaseating granulomas; fibrosis; thickening of intestinal wall with narrowing of lumen; fistulous tracts between loops of intestine or between intestine and other sites; mucosal cobblestone appearance; skip lesions	Crypt abscesses, pseudopolyps
Incidence of secondary malignancy much lower than in ulcerative colitis	Markedly increased incidence of colon cancer in long-standing cases

—in about 3% of cases leads to carcinoma involving the small intestine or colon.

1. **Morphology**

   a. Chronic inflammation involving **all layers** of the intestinal wall

   b. **Thickening** of involved segments, with narrowing of lumen

   c. Linear **ulceration** of the mucosa

   d. Submucosal edema with elevation of the surviving mucosa, producing a **cobblestone appearance**

   e. **Skip lesions** (segments of normal intestine between affected regions)

   f. Discrete noncaseating **granulomas** sometimes observed

   g. Submucosal fibrosis

2. **Clinical manifestations**

   a. Abdominal pain and diarrhea

   b. Malabsorption

   c. Fever

   d. Intestinal obstruction resulting from fibrous **stricture**

   e. **Fistulae** between loops of intestine, and between the intestine, bladder, vagina, and skin

C. **Meckel's diverticulum**

   —is the most common congenital anomaly of the small intestine.
   —is a remnant of the embryonic vitelline duct.
   —may contain ectopic gastric, duodenal, colonic, or pancreatic tissue.
   —is usually asymptomatic but complications, including bleeding and peptic ulceration in ectopic gastric mucosa, may occur.
   —on occasion, is associated with:

   1. **Intussusception** (invagination of a proximal segment of bowel into a more distal segment), causing bowel obstruction

2. Volvulus (twisting of a portion of the gastrointestinal tract about itself), often causing bowel obstruction.

D. Malabsorption syndromes (Table 15.3)

1. Celiac disease
  - is caused by **sensitivity to gluten** in cereal products.
  - is diagnosed by biopsy of the small intestinal mucosa, which demonstrates **blunting of small intestinal villi.**
  - is increased in incidence in association with human leukocyte antigens (HLA) antigens HLA-B8 and HLA-DW3. This finding and the presence of antibodies directed against gliadin, a glycoprotein component of gluten, suggests that both **genetic** and **immune-mediated mechanisms** may be involved.
  - in approximately 10%–15% of cases leads to small intestinal malignancy, most often **B-cell lymphoma**.
  - most often becomes **symptomatic in infancy** when cereals are first added to the diet.
  - is manifest clinically by weight loss, weakness, and diarrhea with pale, bulky, frothy, foul-smelling stools.
  - is also characterized by **growth retardation** and general **failure to thrive**.

Table 15.3. Malabsorption Syndromes

Disorder	Morphologic Features	Comments
Celiac disease	Flat mucosal surface with marked villous atrophy; increased lymphocytes and plasma cells in lamina propria	Gluten sensitivity
Tropical sprue	Histologic findings vary from no changes to abnormalities similar to those of celiac disease	Tropical disease of probable infectious origin; often responds to antibiotics
Whipple's disease	Distinctive PAS-positive macrophages in intestinal mucosa Bacteria-like inclusions by electron microscopy	May affect any organ
Disaccharidase deficiency	No characteristic histologic changes	Deficiency of disaccharidases sited in brush border of mucosal cells of small intestine; lactase deficiency, which leads to milk intolerance, is most frequent
Abetalipoproteinemia	No characteristic features in intestine; circulating acanthocytes (red cells with spiny projections) suggest diagnosis	β-lipoprotein deficiency is caused by hereditary deficiency of apoprotein B
Intestinal lymphangiectasia	Generalized dilatation of small intestinal lymphatics	Marked gastrointestinal protein loss with resultant hypoproteinemia and generalized edema

2. Other malabsorption syndromes

—include tropical sprue, Whipple's disease, disaccharidase deficiency, abetalipoproteinemia, and intestinal lymphangiectasia.

E. Tumors of the small intestine

1. General considerations

a. Tumors of the small intestine make up a small percentage of gastrointestinal neoplasms.

b. The most common malignant tumors are **adenocarcinoma,** lymphoma, and carcinoid.

2. Carcinoid

—is classified in the **APUDoma** group of tumors.

—occurs most frequently in the **appendix**.

—is localized to the small intestine in about 30% of cases.

—although characteristically slow growing, is of low grade malignancy; in contrast to other carcinoids, appendiceal carcinoid almost never metastasizes.

—when metastatic to the liver, can be manifest by the **carcinoid syndrome,** which is:

a. Caused by the elaboration of vasoactive peptides and amines, especially serotonin

b. Manifest clinically by:
  (1) Cutaneous **flushing**
  (2) Watery **diarrhea** and abdominal cramps
  (3) Bronchospasm
  (4) Valvular lesions of the right side of the heart

3. Lymphoma

—can arise from the abundant lymphoid tissue of the small intestine.

—may present with **malabsorption** when there is diffuse involvement.

4. Adenocarcinoma

—although rare, is a common primary malignant tumor of the small intestine.

VI. Diseases of the Colon

A. Hirschsprung's disease (congenital megacolon)

—is **dilatation of the colon** due to the absence of ganglion cells of the submucosal and myenteric neural plexuses; dilatation is proximal to the aganglionic segment.

B. Diverticula

—are pulsion (or false) diverticula (pockets of mucosa and submucosa herniated through the muscular layer).

—are most common in older persons.

—most frequently involve the **sigmoid colon**.

—are almost always multiple.

1. Diverticulosis

—is defined by the presence of multiple diverticula without inflammation.

−occurs most commonly in populations that consume low fiber diets.

−is most often asymptomatic or associated with vague discomfort.

2. Diverticulitis

−refers to **inflammation of diverticula**.

−may be complicated by perforation, peritonitis, abscess formation, or bowel stenosis. Bright red rectal bleeding is frequent.

C. Vascular diseases of the colon

1. Ischemic bowel disease

−results in mucosal, mural, or transmural infarction involving the wall of the intestine.

−is almost always caused by **atherosclerotic occlusion** of at least two of the major mesenteric vessels.

−most often affects the **splenic flexure** and the **rectosigmoid junction,** which lie in the relatively poorly vascularized (so-called watershed areas) regions between areas supplied by the superior mesenteric artery and the inferior mesenteric and internal iliac arteries.

2. Hemorrhoids

−are dilated internal and external venous plexuses in the anal canal.

−are predisposed by low fiber diet.

D. Inflammatory disorders of the colon

1. Ulcerative colitis

a. General considerations

(1) Ulcerative colitis is of unknown etiology.

(2) It is often grouped along with Crohn's disease as **inflammatory bowel disease**. The two disorders are compared in Table 15.2.

(3) Crohn's disease and ulcerative colitis share a similar geographical and racial distribution; some patients have a family history of either ulcerative colitis or Crohn's disease.

(4) Both disorders frequently demonstrate **extraintestinal manifestations,** which include:

(a) Arthritis

(b) Iritis and episcleritis

(c) Sclerosing cholangitis, a chronic fibrosing inflammatory process of the biliary system leading to chronic cholestasis and sometimes to portal hypertension

(d) Skin manifestations, including erythema nodosum and pyoderma gangrenosum

b. Characteristics—ulcerative colitis

(1) **Mucosal inflammation and ulceration** limited to the **large intestine;** the rectum is always affected but the entire colon may be involved.

(2) Inflammatory changes almost entirely confined to the mucosa and submucosa; the most characteristic feature is the **crypt abscess,** in which there are infiltrates of neutrophils in the crypts of Lieberkuhn.

    (3) **Red, granular appearance** of the mucosa; ulceration may be minimal or quite extensive, with only islands of surviving mucosa remaining.

    (4) **Pseudopolyps,** mucosal remnants of previous severe ulceration

    (5) Chronic **diarrhea** associated with the passage of **blood** and **mucus;** the **most frequent clinical manifestation is bleeding**.

  c. Complications—ulcerative colitis

    (1) **Toxic megacolon,** a medical emergency in which there is a marked dilation of the colon

    (2) **Perforation** of the colon

    (3) **Carcinoma** of the colon

2. Pseudomembranous colitis

  —is morphologically distinguished by superficial grayish mucosal exudates consisting of necrotic, loosely adherent mucosal debris (**pseudomembrane**).

  —is most frequently caused by overgrowth of enterotoxin-producing *Clostridium difficile*.

  —is clinically characterized by fever, toxicity, and diarrhea, most often occurring in patients on **broad-spectrum antibiotic therapy**.

E. Tumors of the colon

1. Benign polyps (Table 15.4)

a. Terminology

  —polyp is a descriptive term for any elevation of the intestinal surface.

  (1) **Pedunculated polyps** are attached by a narrow stem.

  (2) **Sessile polyps** have a broad based attachment.

Table 15.4. Intestinal Polyps

Type	Comments
Non-neoplastic polyps	
Hyperplastic polyp	No clinical significance
Inflammatory polyps:	
Lymphoid polyp	Most common site rectal mucosa; may be reaction to local irritation
Inflammatory pseudopolyp	Associated with ulcerative colitis and other inflammatory diseases of the colon; consists of granulation tissue and residual and regenerating mucosa
Hamartomatous polyps:	
Juvenile polyp	Occurs most frequently in children
Peutz-Jeghers polyp	Associated with Peutz-Jeghers syndrome
Neoplastic polyps	
Tubular adenoma	Benign but may undergo malignant change; often multiple; hereditary multiple polyposis syndromes associated with greatly increased risk of malignancy
Tubulovillous adenoma	Morphologically resembles tubular adenoma with additional features similar to villous adenoma; greater malignant potential than tubular adenoma
Villous adenoma	Large sessile tumor with velvety surface comprised of finger-like villi; high potential for malignant change

b. Non-neoplastic polyps

(1) Hyperplastic polyps

    —can occur anywhere in the colon.

    —have no clinical significance but may be mistaken for an adenomatous polyp.

(2) Inflammatory polyps

    —include **benign lymphoid polyps** and **inflammatory pseudopolyps** consisting of granulation tissue and remnants of mucosa, caused by chronic inflammatory bowel disease.

(3) Hamartomatous polyps

    (a) Juvenile polyps

        —most often occur in children but are also seen in adults.

    (b) Peutz-Jeghers polyps

2. Adenomatous polyps

—are true **neoplasms** rather than benign proliferations of tissue.

—are usually **asymptomatic** but can result in rectal bleeding.

a. Tubular adenomas

    —are the **most common** type (75%) of adenomatous polyps.

    —are usually **small** and **pedunculated**.

    —can contain **malignant foci;** the likelihood of malignancy is greater in larger polyps.

b. Tubulovillous adenomas

    —account for about 15% of adenomatous polyps.

    —resemble tubular adenomas but the surface is covered by finger-like villi.

    —histologically are similar to tubular adenomas.

    —are intermediate in malignant potential between tubular adenomas and villous adenomas.

c. Villous adenomas

    —account for about 10% of adenomatous polyps.

    —are usually larger than tubular adenomas, usually sessile, and are characterized by large numbers of finger-like villi.

    —**become malignant** in more than **30%** of cases.

3. Multiple polyposis syndromes

—are associated with a **greatly increased risk of malignant transformation**.

a. Familial polyposis

    —is an autosomal dominant condition characterized by the presence of numerous adenomatous polyps. **The risk of malignant transformation approaches 100%.**

b. Gardner's syndrome

    —is an autosomal dominant condition characterized by the presence of numerous adenomatous polyps along with osteomas and soft tissue tumors.

c. Turcot's syndrome
    —is characterized by adenomatous polyps along with tumors of the central nervous system.

4. Peutz-Jeghers syndrome
    —is an **autosomal dominant disorder** characterized by melanin pigmentation of the oral mucosa, lips, hands, and genitalia and by entirely benign hamartomatous polyps at a variety of sites in the gastrointestinal tract, most commonly in the small intestine.
    —is further characterized by an increased incidence of carcinoma arising in a variety of sites such as the stomach, breast, or ovaries.

5. Adenocarcinoma of the colon and rectum
    —is one of the most common neoplasms in the Western world.
    —exhibits a peak age incidence in the sixth to seventh decades.
    —is associated with increased serum concentration of carcinoembryonic antigen (CEA). Since elevated CEA is not specific for colon cancer, this laboratory determination is most useful for following the course of the disease rather than for initial diagnosis.

a. Predisposing factors
    (1) Adenomatous polyps
    (2) Inherited multiple polyposis syndromes
    (3) Long-standing ulcerative colitis
    (4) Genetic factors; up to a fourfold increase in incidence is noted among relatives of patients with colon cancer.
    (5) A **low fiber, high animal fat diet;** the disease is far less common in much of the Third World, where populations consume a high fiber, low animal fat diet.

b. Characteristics
    (1) Adenocarcinoma varies in gross presentation according to the region of the colon involved.
    (2) Carcinoma of the rectosigmoid colon tends to present in an annular manner, producing early obstruction.
    (3) Carcinoma of the right colon usually does not obstruct early and often presents (sometimes quite late) with iron deficiency anemia secondary to chronic blood loss.

VII. Diseases of the Appendix

A. Acute appendicitis
    —occurs most frequently in the second and third decades of life.
    —is thought to be caused by obstruction of the appendiceal lumen, most often by a fecolith, resulting in bacterial proliferation and invasion of the mucosa.
    —is marked grossly by a congested appendix with a swollen distal half covered by purulent exudate; the lumen also contains a purulent exudate and often a fecolith.
    —is characterized histologically by an acute inflammatory infiltrate extending from the mucosa through the full thickness of the appendiceal wall.

—presents with anorexia, nausea, and **abdominal pain,** most commonly localized to the **right lower quadrant**.

—if untreated by **surgical resection,** most often leads to perforation or abscess, or both.

B. Tumors of the appendix

—the most common appendiceal neoplasm is **carcinoid,** which is usually detected as an incidental finding.

Review Test

Directions: Each of the numbered items or incomplete statements in this section is followed by answers or by completions of the statement. Select the **one** lettered answer or completion that is **best** in each case.

1. Which of the following phrases best characterizes ameloblastoma?

(A) Hamartoma derived from odontogenic epithelium and odontoblastic tissue
(B) Originates from osteoclasts
(C) Usually is metastatic at the time of diagnosis
(D) Most often involves mandible
(E) Parotid gland tumor

2. All of the following terms relating to salivary gland disease are correctly matched with the appropriate associations EXCEPT

(A) acute parotitis—mumps.
(B) mucocele—sequela of trauma.
(C) ranula—mucocele.
(D) sialadenitis—occlusion of salivary ducts by stones.
(E) Sjögren's syndrome—immunodeficiency.

3. All of the following conditions are associated with Sjögren's syndrome EXCEPT

(A) mumps parotitis.
(B) keratoconjunctivitis sicca.
(C) malignant lymphoma.
(D) rheumatoid arthritis.
(E) xerostomia.

4. All of the following salivary gland tumors are correctly matched with the appropriate characteristic EXCEPT

(A) pleomorphic adenoma—most common salivary gland tumor.
(B) oncocytoma—eosinophilic-staining cells.
(C) adenolymphoma—Warthin's tumor.
(D) mucoepidermoid tumor—"mixed tumor."
(E) adenoid cystic carcinoma—presents with pain.

5. Which salivary gland is the most frequent site of tumor involvement?

(A) Parotid gland
(B) Submaxillary gland
(C) Sublingual gland
(D) Minor salivary glands

6. Which of the following statements concerning the most common variant of tracheoesophageal fistula is true?

(A) The esophagus is completely patent and is connected to the trachea by a fistula.
(B) Diagnosis is most often delayed until the infant begins to ingest solid food.
(C) Untreated cases are associated with an increased incidence of respiratory infection in middle age.
(D) The condition is often associated with maternal polyhydramnios.

7. All of the following conditions are correctly matched with the appropriate phrase EXCEPT

(A) achalasia—acid gastric reflux.
(B) Mallory-Weiss syndrome—esophageal mucosal tears and hemorrhage due to retching.
(C) esophageal varices—portal hypertension.
(D) Barrett's esophagus—lesion predisposing to malignancy.

8. Predisposing factors that may lead to gastroesophageal reflux include all of the following EXCEPT

(A) hiatal hernia.
(B) pernicious anemia.
(C) pregnancy.
(D) scleroderma.
(E) incompetent esophageal sphincter.

9. The most frequent esophageal malignancy is

(A) adenocarcinoma.
(B) fibrosarcoma.
(C) leiomyosarcoma.
(D) rhabdomyosarcoma.
(E) squamous cell carcinoma.

10. All of the following disorders are correctly matched with the appropriate characteristic or causative agent EXCEPT

(A) congenital pyloric stenosis—palpable mass.
(B) adenocarcinoma of the stomach—*Helicobacter (Campylobacter) pylori.*
(C) acute (erosive) gastritis—alcohol.
(D) fundal (type A) chronic gastritis—lesion predisposing to duodenal ulcer.
(E) Ménétrier's disease—gastric rugal hypertrophy.

11. All of the following phrases concerning peptic ulcer are correctly matched EXCEPT

(A) peptic ulcer of jejunum—pancreatic neoplasm.
(B) Meckel's diverticulum—ectopic gastric mucosa.
(C) gastric peptic ulcer—extreme hypersecretion of hydrochloric acid.
(D) duodenal ulcer—most common peptic ulcer.
(E) blood group O—increased incidence of duodenal ulcer.

12. Which of the following statements concerning the lesion illustrated below is true?

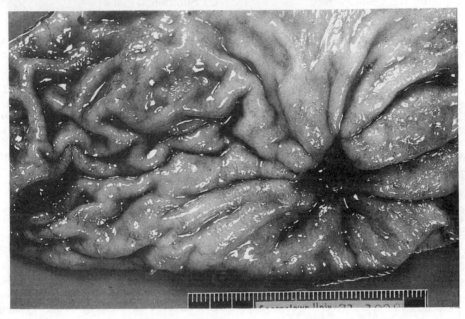

(Reprinted with permission from Golden A, Powell D, and Jennings C: *Pathology: Understanding Human Disease,* 2nd ed. Baltimore, Williams & Wilkins, 1985, p 319.)

(A) Is more frequent in Japan than in the U.S.
(B) Has been decreasing in frequency over the past several decades
(C) Is related to the use of nitrites as food preservatives
(D) Will most likely heal with conservative management
(E) May result in Krukenberg tumor

13. All of the following factors are associated with increased incidence or severity of peptic ulcer EXCEPT

(A) Zollinger-Ellison syndrome.
(B) hypoparathyroidism.
(C) multiple endocrine neoplasia (MEN) type I.
(D) aspirin therapy.
(E) cigarette smoking.

14. Risk factors associated with carcinoma of the stomach include all of the following EXCEPT

(A) use of nitrites as food preservatives.
(B) high intake of animal fat.
(C) blood group A.
(D) chronic gastritis.
(E) pernicious anemia.

15. All of the following diseases are correctly matched with the appropriate feature or complication EXCEPT

(A) Meckel's diverticulum—intussusception.
(B) celiac disease—gluten sensitivity.
(C) Whipple's disease—PAS-positive macrophages.
(D) abetalipoproteinemia—acanthocytes.
(E) intestinal lymphangiectasia—dehydration and hypernatremia.

16. All of the following are characteristics of ulcerative colitis EXCEPT

(A) bleeding most frequent clinical presentation.
(B) crypt abscess formation.
(C) increased risk of adenocarcinoma.
(D) inflammatory changes limited to mucosa and submucosa.
(E) involvement of any portion of gastrointestinal tract.

17. Congenital megacolon is associated with which one of the following characteristics?

(A) Melanin pigmentation of the lips and oral mucosa
(B) Absence of submucosal and myenteric neural plexuses
(C) Cysts in the liver and berry aneurysm of the circle of Willis
(D) Extreme gastric hypersecretion of hydrochloric acid

18. Which of the following characteristics is associated with carcinoma of the colon?

(A) The highest incidence is in Third World countries.
(B) Early obstruction as the first presenting sign suggests right-sided lesion.
(C) Iron-deficiency anemia as the first presenting sign suggests left-sided lesion.
(D) Increased incidence seen with high animal fat, low fiber diet.
(E) High incidence seen with Crohn's disease.

19. All of the following are characteristic features of the lesion depicted in the figure EXCEPT it

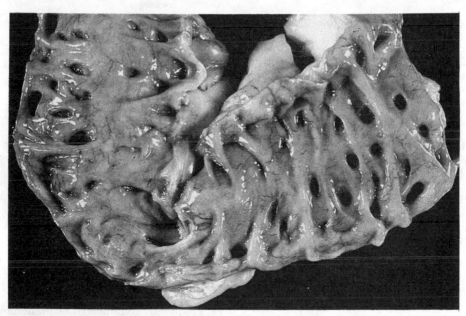

(Reprinted with permission from Golden A, Powell D, and Jennings C: *Pathology: Understanding Human Disease,* 2nd ed. Baltimore, Williams & Wilkins, 1985, p 333.)

(A) most frequently occurs in the sigmoid colon.
(B) is most likely related to low fiber diet.
(C) occurs most often in teenagers.
(D) can be complicated by inflammation, perforation, and peritonitis.

20. The lesion shown below may occur in all of the following syndromes EXCEPT

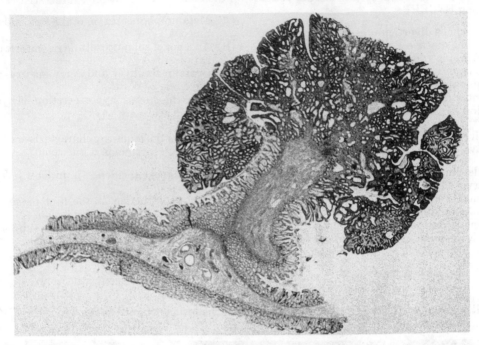

(Reprinted with permission from Golden A, Powell D, and Jennings C: *Pathology: Understanding Human Disease,* 2nd ed. Baltimore, Williams & Wilkins, 1985, p 341.)

(A) Gardner's.
(B) Turcot's.
(C) familial polyposis.
(D) Peutz-Jeghers.

Directions: Each group of items in this section consists of lettered options followed by a set of numbered items. For each item, select the **one** lettered option that is most closely associated with it. Each lettered option may be selected once, more than once, or not at all.

Questions 21–23

Match the causative factor with the appropriate oral infection.

(A) Vincent's infection
(B) Thrush
(C) Aphthous stomatitis
(D) Herpes labialis

21. Activated by febrile illness

22. *Candida albicans*

23. Symbiotic bacteria

Questions 24–26

Match the following characteristics to the appropriate disease

(A) Ulcerative colitis
(B) Crohn's disease
(C) Both ulcerative colitis and Crohn's disease

24. Frequently complicated by malignancy

25. All layers of intestinal wall are involved

26. Extraintestinal manifestations

Answers and Explanations

1–D. Ameloblastoma, a true neoplasm, most commonly originates within the mandible and less often within the maxilla. Origin is from the epithelial tissue involved in the development of teeth. The tumor is benign and does not metastasize; however, local expansion can have serious consequences.

2–E. Sjögren's syndrome is an autoimmune disease. Immunodeficiency is not involved. Sialadenitis is often caused by salivary duct occlusion. Acute parotitis is the most frequent manifestation of mumps infection. A ranula is a large mucocele of salivary gland origin.

3–A. There is no relation of mumps parotitis to Sjögren's syndrome. Sjögren's syndrome is an autoimmune disorder characterized by keratoconjunctivitis sicca and xerostomia, due to lymphocytic infiltration and parenchymal destruction of the parotid and lacrimal glands in association with a connective tissue disorder such as rheumatoid arthritis. Malignant lymphoma is a frequent complication.

4–D. "Mixed tumor" properly refers to pleomorphic adenoma, which often demonstrates myxoid and cartilage-like elements in addition to stellate or fusiform epithelial cells. Oncocytoma is characterized by cells with granular eosinophilic cytoplasm. Adenolymphoma (papillary cystadenoma lymphomatosum) is often called Warthin's tumor. Adenoid cystic carcinoma often presents with pain due to infiltration of perineural spaces.

5–A. Approximately 80% to 90% of salivary gland tumors originate in the parotid gland, and of these, about 70% are pleomorphic adenomas.

6–D. Maternal polyhydramnios is a frequent association that may alert the physician to the diagnosis of tracheoesophageal fistula. In the most common variant, the upper esophagus ends in a blind pouch, and the lower portion has a fistulous connection to the trachea. If not surgically repaired, this condition is incompatible with life, even for a few days.

7–A. Achalasia is characterized by failure of relaxation of the lower esophageal sphincter; acid gastric reflux is not an expected finding. Mallory-Weiss syndrome (hemorrhage from esophagogastric mucosal tears) and bleeding esophageal varices (due to portal hypertension) are important causes of upper gastrointestinal hemorrhage. Barrett's esophagus is a well-recognized precursor of adenocarcinoma.

8–B. Gastroesophageal reflux of hydrochloric acid does not occur in patients with pernicious anemia, which is associated with achlorhydria, total absence of gastric hydrochloric acid. Hiatal hernia, pregnancy, scleroderma, and incompetence of the esophageal sphincter all can lead to gastroesophageal reflux.

9–E. Squamous cell carcinoma is the most frequent form of esophageal malignancy. Adenocarcinoma is much less frequent, and sarcomas are quite rare.

10–D. Fundal (type A) chronic gastritis is associated with reduced secretion of proteolytic enzymes and hydrochloric acid, as well as with antiparietal cell antibodies. It predisposes to pernicious anemia, other autoimmune disorders, and carcinoma of the stomach. Duodenal ulcer is unlikely in the presence of hyposecretion of gastric hydrochloric acid. The hypertrophied pyloric circular muscle layer of congenital (hypertrophic) pyloric stenosis often results in a palpable mass. Adenocarcinoma of the stomach is often associated with *Helicobacter pylori* infection, as are chronic gastritis and peptic ulcer of the stomach and duodenum. Acute (erosive) gastritis is caused by a variety of toxic agents, including alcohol, aspirin and other analgesics, and cigarette smoking. Ménétrier's disease is defined by characteristic enlargement of gastric rugae.

11–C. In contrast to peptic ulcer of the duodenum, gastric acid secretion is often not increased in gastric peptic ulcer. It is rare, however, for gastric peptic ulceration to occur in the total absence of hydrochloric acid.

12–D. The illustration depicts a chronic gastric peptic ulcer with characteristic radiating folds of gastric mucosa starting at the ulcer margins. The lesion has a smooth base and nonelevated, punched-out margins, in contrast to gastric carcinoma, which often has an irregular necrotic base and firm, raised margins. In spite of these characteristic findings, the distinction between gastric peptic ulcer and ulcerated carcinoma must be established by biopsy.

13–B. Hyperparathyroidism (not hypoparathyroidism) may sometimes present with peptic ulcer, a well-known complication. The hypergastrinemia of the Zollinger-Ellison syndrome can be caused by isolated gastrinoma or by a similar tumor or hyperplasia occurring as part of MEN type I. Aspirin and tobacco usage both predispose to peptic ulcer.

14–B. High animal fat intake is associated with a decreased incidence of carcinoma of the stomach. The use of nitrites as food preservatives, blood group A, chronic gastritis, and pernicious anemia are all well-known associations of gastric cancer.

15–E. Intestinal lymphangiectasia is associated with protein-losing enteropathy with resultant hypoalbuminemia and edema, not with dehydration and hypernatremia. Meckel's diverticulum may be the site of a number of complications, including intestinal obstruction due to intussusception or volvulus. On occasion, Meckel's diverticulum is the site of peptic ulcer development within acid-secreting ectopic gastric mucosa. Celiac disease is due to gluten sensitivity. Whipple's disease is characterized by PAS-positive macrophages, often with small bacillary bodies, most frequently found in the mucosal lamina propria of the small intestine. Similar cells may be found in other sites such as the joints, heart, and central nervous system.

16–E. Ulcerative colitis is limited to the large intestine, principally affecting the rectum and left colon and sometimes the entire colon.

17–B. Hirschsprung's disease is characterized by segmental absence of submucosal and myenteric neural plexuses with dilatation of the colon proximal to the aganglionic segment. Mucosal melanin depositions and hamartomatous polyps are associated with Peutz-Jeghers syndrome. Cysts in the liver and berry aneurysm of the circle of Willis are associated with polycystic kidney. Extreme gastric hypersecretion of hydrochloric acid is a feature of the Zollinger-Ellison syndrome.

18–D. Adenocarcinoma of the colon is one of the most common malignancies in the Western world and occurs much less frequently in Third World countries. This difference is thought due to the protective effect of a diet high in fiber and low in animal fat. Early obstruction due to annular lesions is highly suggestive of left-sided lesions. In contrast, right-sided lesions may remain clinically silent for long periods and may often present quite late with iron-deficiency anemia due to blood loss. A minimal increased incidence of cancer is associated with Crohn's disease.

19–C. The illustration demonstrates diverticulosis of the colon. These lesions are most common in older persons and are most frequently found in the sigmoid. Disease incidence is increased in populations that consume low fiber diets. Although most often asymptomatic, diverticula may become the site of acute inflammation (diverticulitis), sometimes with life-threatening complications, such as perforation and peritonitis.

20–D. The illustration shows a tubular adenoma, the most common form of adenomatous polyp. These lesions can be single or multiple, or they can occur as components of a variety of multiple polyposis syndromes. Notable among these syndromes are Gardner's (associated with osteomas and soft tissue tumors), Turcot's (associated with CNS tumors), and familial polyposis. All of the foregoing are associated with an increased incidence of colon malignancy. In contrast, the Peutz-Jeghers polyp is a non-neoplastic hamartomatous lesion and is not associated with colon cancer.

21–D. Herpes labialis is a recurrent vesicular infection of the oral mucosa and adjacent skin, caused by herpes simplex virus type 1. The virus most often resides in the trigeminal ganglion, where it remains latent until activation by stresses such as fever, trauma, sunshine, and menstruation.

22–B. Oral candidiasis (thrush), the most common fungal infection of the mouth, is characterized by white curd-like patches.

23–A. Acute necrotizing ulcerative gingivitis (trench mouth or Vincent's infection) is a severe gingival inflammation most often caused by infection with the two symbiotic bacteria, *Borrelia vincentii* and *Fusobacterium fusiforme*.

24–A. After a decade of disease, approximately one-third of patients with ulcerative colitis develop colon cancer. Although there is some increased risk for malignancy, carcinoma is an unusual complication of Crohn's disease.

25–B. In marked contrast to ulcerative colitis, which is primarily a mucosal disease, Crohn's disease affects all layers of the intestinal wall.

26–C. Extraintestinal manifestations are common in both ulcerative colitis and Crohn's disease. These findings include arthritis, iritis, skin changes such as erythema nodosum and pyoderma gangrenosum, and sclerosing cholangitis.

16

Liver, Gallbladder, and Exocrine Pancreas

I. Diseases of the Liver

A. Jaundice (Table 16.1)

—refers to **yellow discoloration** of skin, sclerae, and tissues caused by hyperbilirubinemia.

—is most often associated with hepatocellular disease, biliary obstruction, or hemolytic anemia.

1. Physiologic jaundice of the newborn

—is commonly noted during the **first week of life** but is not usually clinically important.

—is characterized chemically by **unconjugated hyperbilirubinemia**.

—results from both increased bilirubin production and a relative deficiency of glucuronyl transferase in the immature liver; these phenomena are exaggerated in premature infants.

2. Congenital hyperbilirubinemias

a. Gilbert's syndrome

—is extremely **common,** occurring in almost 5% of the population.

—is a familial disorder characterized by a modest **elevation of serum unconjugated bilirubin;** the liver is otherwise unimpaired, and there are no clinical consequences.

—is caused by a combination of decreased bilirubin uptake by liver cells and reduced activity of glucuronyl transferase.

b. Crigler-Najjar syndrome

—is a severe familial disorder characterized by unconjugated hyperbilirubinemia caused by a deficiency of glucuronyl transferase.

—in one form leads to early death from kernicterus, damage to the basal ganglia and other parts of the central nervous system caused by unconjugated bilirubin.

—in a less severe form, responds to phenobarbital therapy, which decreases the serum concentration of unconjugated bilirubin.

Table 16.1. Differential Diagnosis of Jaundice

Type of Jaundice	Hyper-bilirubinemia	Urine Bilirubin	Urine Urobilinogen	Other Findings
Hepatocellular	Conjugated and unconjugated	Increased	Normal to decreased	Intrahepatic cholestasis may result in retention of conjugated bilirubin; hepatocellular damage may result in impaired conjugation of bilirubin; enzyme activities of ALT and AST increased; increased alkaline phosphatase indicates intrahepatic obstruction
Obstructive	Conjugated	Increased	Decreased	Alkaline phosphatase and cholesterol increased; ALT and AST variable; with complete obstruction, stools pale and clay-colored and urine urobilinogen undetectable.
Hemolytic	Unconjugated	Absent (acholuria)	Increased	Degree of urine urobilinogen increase directly related to increased hemoglobin catabolism

    c. Dubin-Johnson syndrome
        —is an autosomal recessive form of conjugated hyperbilirubinemia characterized by defective bilirubin transport.
        —is characterized by a striking brown-to-black **discoloration of the liver** caused by the deposition of granules of **very dark pigment,** the chemical nature of which is unclear.

    d. Rotor syndrome
        —is similar to the Dubin-Johnson syndrome, but abnormal pigment is not present.

B. Acute viral hepatitis (Table 16.2)
    —may be caused by a variety of viral agents, including Epstein-Barr virus (EBV) or cytomegalovirus, but usually results from hepatic infection by any of the following viruses:

    1. Hepatitis A virus (HAV)
        —is spread by **fecal–oral transmission; parenteral infection does not occur**.
        —has an incubation period of 15–45 days.
        —**does not cause a chronic carrier state;** complete recovery almost always occurs.

    2. Hepatitis B virus (HBV)
        —is composed of a central core containing the viral DNA genome, DNA polymerase, hepatitis B core antigen (HBcAg), and hepatitis B e antigen (HBeAg), and an outer lipoprotein coat containing the hepatitis B surface antigen (HBsAg). The complete virion is known as the Dane particle.

Table 16.2. Viral Hepatitis

Virus	Predominant Modes of Transmission	Clinical Features
Hepatitis A virus	Fecal–oral	No carrier state; does not lead to chronic liver disease
Hepatitis B virus (HBV)	Sexual, fecal–oral, parenteral	Frequently leads to carrier state or chronic liver disease
Hepatitis C virus	Parenteral	Most frequent cause of transfusion-mediated hepatitis; frequently progresses to chronic liver disease
Delta agent (hepatitis D virus)	Sexual, fecal–oral, parenteral	Requires concurrent infection with HBV for multiplication
Hepatitis E virus	Fecal–oral	Occurs in epidemic form in Third World countries; does not lead to chronic liver disease

–is **transmitted via parenteral, sexual, and vertical (mother to neonate) routes**.

–has an incubation period averaging 60–90 days.

–can result in a carrier state or in chronic liver disease. The sequence in which the various antigens or antibodies to these antigens appear in the serum is of clinical significance.

a. **HBsAg**

–appears in serum some weeks before onset of clinical findings, then decreases and generally persists for a total of 3 to 4 months.

–persistence as detectable serum antigen for longer than 6 months denotes the carrier state.

–elicits an antibody response (anti-HBsAg); antibody appears a few weeks after the disappearance of the antigen and indicates recovery as well as immunity to future infection.

b. **Anti-HBcAg**

–appears about 4 weeks after the appearance of HBsAg, is present during the acute illness, and can remain elevated for several years.

–is the only marker of hepatitis infection during the "window period" between the disappearance of HBsAg and the appearance of anti-HBsAg.

c. **HBeAg**

–appears shortly after HBsAg and disappears before HBsAg.

–is closely correlated with viral infectivity.

3. **Hepatitis C virus (HCV)**

–is the most common cause of what was formerly termed non-A, non-B hepatitis.

–is **transmitted parenterally** and is the most frequent cause of **transfusion-mediated hepatitis**.

4. **Hepatitis D virus (HDV, delta agent)**

–is a very small, spherical virus consisting of a single RNA strand and the associated delta protein antigen (HDAg), surrounded by a proteinaceous coat of HBsAg.

      —is **replicatively defective,** requiring **simultaneous infection with HBV** for viral replication.

      —is transmitted via **sexual, fecal—oral, or parenteral routes**.

      —usually causes illness more severe than HBV infection alone.

  5. Hepatitis E virus (HEV)

      —causes an **enterically transmitted** form of viral hepatitis similar to HAV infection that occurs in epidemic form in underdeveloped countries.

      —**does not lead to chronic liver disease.**

C. Chronic hepatitis (Table 16.3)

  —is defined by the persistence of abnormalities for more than 6 months.

  —may result from any of the viral hepatitides except HAV or HEV infection and also from liver damage induced by nonviral agents.

  —appears in three major forms: **chronic persistent hepatitis, chronic active hepatitis,** and **chronic autoimmune (lupoid) hepatitis**.

D. Other inflammatory liver disorders

  1. Neonatal hepatitis

      —is of unknown etiology.

      —is characterized by the presence of multinucleated giant cells.

      —may demonstrate bile pigment and hemosiderin within parenchymal cells.

      —may result in jaundice during the first few weeks of life.

  2. Other viral infections

      —may involve the liver along with other organ systems.

    a. Epstein-Barr virus (EBV)

        —causes **infectious mononucleosis,** which often has a hepatitic component.

    b. Herpes simplex virus type 1 (HSV-1)

        —may involve the liver in infants and immunocompromised persons.

    c. Cytomegalovirus (CMV)

        —may involve the liver in infants and immunocompromised persons.

        —infected liver cells demonstrate characteristic nuclear inclusions surrounded by a halo (owl's eye appearance).

Table 16.3. Chronic Hepatitis

Disease Type	Characteristics
Chronic persistent hepatitis	Inflammation limited to portal triad (triaditis); intact limiting plate, with complete preservation of normal lobular architecture; prognosis almost always excellent
Chronic active hepatitis	Extension of inflammation through limiting plate into hepatic lobule, with destruction of hepatocytes; may progress to cirrhosis
Chronic autoimmune (lupoid) hepatitis	Variant of chronic active hepatitis; anti-smooth muscle, anti-nuclear, anti-mitochondrial, and other autoantibodies demonstrable; LE test often positive; polyclonal hypergammaglobulinemia

  d. Yellow fever
  —characteristically demonstrates a severe hepatitic component characterized by midzonal hepatic necrosis. The dying hepatocytes often condense into eosinophilic contracted forms referred to as **Councilman bodies**. Similar inclusions are observed in all of the viral hepatitides.

3. Leptospirosis
  —is also known as Weil's disease or icterohemorrhagic fever.
  —is caused by *Leptospira* species.
  —is a severe infection characterized by jaundice, renal failure, and hemorrhagic phenomena.

4. *Echinococcus granulosus* infestation
  —is caused by ingestion of tapeworm eggs from the excreta of dogs and sheep.
  —results in **hydatid disease** of the liver, in which large parasitic cysts invade the liver.

5. Schistosomiasis
  —is caused by infestation with *Schistosoma mansoni* or *S. japonicum*. The adult worms lodge in the portal vein and its branches. The eggs are highly antigenic and stimulate granuloma formation, with resultant tissue destruction, scarring, and portal hypertension.

E. Microvesicular fatty liver
  —is a group of serious disorders associated with the presence of small fat vacuoles in parenchymal liver cells, which differ from the large fat-containing vacuoles characteristic of fatty change.

1. Reye's syndrome
  —is an acute disorder of **young children** characterized by encephalopathy, coma, and microvesicular fatty liver.
  —is associated with **aspirin administration** to children with **acute viral infections**.

2. Fatty liver of pregnancy
  —is acute hepatic failure during the third trimester of pregnancy associated with microvesicular fatty liver.
  —has a high mortality rate.

3. Tetracycline toxicity
  —results in an unpredictable hypersensitivity-like reaction with microvesicular fatty change.

F. Alcoholic liver disease
  —refers to the constellation of hepatic changes associated with excessive alcohol consumption.
  —is the most common form of liver disease in the United States.
  —varies from fatty change to alcoholic hepatitis and cirrhosis.
  —may be asymptomatic or may be associated with mild-to-severe hepatic inflammation, cirrhosis, or encephalopathy.

1. Fatty change
  —is the most frequent morphologic abnormality caused by alcohol.
  —is reversible.

2. Alcoholic hepatitis
  —is characterized by fatty change, focal liver cell necrosis, infiltrates of neutrophils, and the presence of intracytoplasmic eosinophilic hyaline inclusions (Mallory bodies, alcoholic hyalin) derived from cytoplasmic intermediate filaments; these inclusions are not entirely specific for alcoholic hepatitis.
  —is often associated with fibrosis that characteristically surrounds central veins and has been referred to as perivenular fibrosis, sclerosing hyaline necrosis, or central hyaline sclerosis. This fibrosis can lead to central vein obstruction and fibrosis surrounding individual liver cells, and can eventuate into cirrhosis.

3. Alcoholic cirrhosis

G. Cirrhosis (Table 16.4)

1. General considerations—cirrhosis
  —is a descriptive term for chronic liver disease characterized by generalized disorganization of hepatic architecture with scarring and nodule formation.
  —liver cell damage, regenerative activity, and generalized fibrosis resulting in a nodular pattern are also characteristic.
  —classification can be morphologic, on the basis of nodule size (micronodular, macronodular, and mixed macromicronodular forms).

Table 16.4. Cirrhosis

Type	Features
Alcoholic (Laennec's, nutritional)	Most frequently occurring form of cirrhosis; associated with alcoholism; micronodular pattern evolving in late stages to typical hobnail liver with large, irregular nodules
Postnecrotic (macronodular, posthepatitic)	Large, irregular nodules containing intact hepatic lobules; diverse etiologies; often end result of viral hepatitis
Biliary Primary	Probable autoimmune origin; anti-mitochondrial antibodies; obstructive jaundice
Secondary	End result of long-standing extrahepatic biliary obstruction
Hemochromatosis Idiopathic (primary)	Familial defect in control of iron absorption; massive accumulation of hemosiderin in hepatic and pancreatic parenchymal cells, myocardium, and other sites; classic triad of cirrhosis, diabetes mellitus, and increased skin pigmentation; cirrhosis micronodular type
Secondary	Caused by chronic iron overload of diverse etiology
Wilson's disease	Accumulation of copper in liver, kidney, brain, and cornea; cirrhosis can be micronodular or macronodular; decreased serum ceruloplasmin
Inborn errors of metabolism	Cirrhosis associated with galactosemia, glycogen storage diseases, or α_1-1-antitrypsin deficiency

−is associated, in all forms, with an **increased incidence of hepatocellular carcinoma**.

−has numerous etiologic agents, including:

a. Prolonged alcohol intake, drugs, and chemical agents

b. Viral hepatitis, biliary obstruction, and hemochromatosis

c. Wilson's disease and other inborn errors of metabolism

d. Heart failure with long-standing chronic passive congestion of the liver

2. Alcoholic (Laennec's, nutritional) cirrhosis

−is the prototype for all forms of cirrhosis.

a. Clinical manifestations

(1) Findings associated with hepatocellular damage and liver failure include:

(a) Jaundice, most often mixed conjugated and unconjugated

(b) Hypoalbuminemia, caused by decreased albumin synthesis in damaged hepatocytes

(c) Coagulation factor deficiencies, caused by decreased synthesis; all coagulation factors, with the exception of von Willebrand's factor, are synthesized in the liver.

(d) Hyperestrinism, manifest as palmar erythema (liver palms); spider nevi (capillary telangiectases) of the face, upper arms, and chest; loss of body and pubic hair; testicular atrophy; and gynecomastia

(2) Consequences of intrahepatic scarring with increased portal venous pressure include:

(a) Esophageal varices, often leading to upper gastrointestinal hemorrhage

(b) Rectal hemorrhoids

(c) Periumbilical venous collaterals (caput medusae)

(d) Splenomegaly

(3) Changes due to both liver cell damage and portal hypertension include:

(a) Peripheral edema, ascites, or hydrothorax, caused by increased **portal venous pressure,** which leads to

(i) Increased production of hepatic lymph

(ii) Decreased plasma oncotic pressure secondary to hypoalbuminemia

(iii) Retention of sodium and water as a result of decreased hepatic degradation of aldosterone, activation of the renin-angiotensin system, or both

(b) Encephalopathy facilitated by portal systemic shunting, with direct delivery of neurotoxic substances such as ammonia and other enteric degradation products directly into the systemic circulation

(c) Neurologic manifestations varying from slight confusion to deep coma; asterixis (flapping tremor of hands) is a characteristic feature.

b. Morphologic abnormalities

(1) The liver may be enlarged or small and shrunken.

(2) The pattern is most often micronodular.

(3) Hepatic architecture is obscured by fibrous bands surrounding nodules of distorted liver cell plates.

(4) The fibrous bands contain proliferating bile ducts and inflammatory cells, most often lymphocytes and plasma cells.

(5) In late stages, the nodules tend to become larger and irregular; this pattern results in a scarred, shrunken liver termed the hobnail liver.

3. Postnecrotic (macronodular, posthepatitic) cirrhosis

–is characterized by broad fibrous bands dividing the liver into **large, irregular nodules,** often containing intact hepatic lobules.

–**is often a sequela of chronic active hepatitis; HBV and HCV are the most common viral etiologies.**

–can be caused by noninfectious hepatotoxic agents.

–sometimes can result from the progression of micronodular alcoholic cirrhosis.

–is often of uncertain etiology (cryptogenic cirrhosis).

–leads to hepatocellular carcinoma more often than other forms of cirrhosis.

4. Biliary cirrhosis

–occurs as a primary, probably autoimmune, disorder and much more frequently as a secondary form due to biliary obstruction.

a. Primary biliary cirrhosis

–is most likely of **autoimmune origin**. There is an increased incidence of other autoimmune disorders in these patients, and **antimitochondrial antibodies** are characteristic.

–is **most common in middle-aged women**.

–is characterized by **severe obstructive jaundice, itching, and hypercholesterolemia;** hypercholesterolemia leads to cutaneous xanthoma formation.

–is marked by increased parenchymal copper concentration, a finding of unknown significance.

b. Secondary biliary cirrhosis

–is caused by **extrahepatic biliary obstruction,** which leads to dilation and increased pressure within intrahepatic bile ducts and cholangioles, further resulting in ductal injury, ductal and periductal inflammation, and resolution by fibrous tissue formation.

–often is complicated by ascending cholangitis, bacterial inflammation of intrahepatic bile ducts.

–is marked histologically by evidence of bile stasis and by bile lakes, accumulation of bile within hepatic parenchyma.

5. Hemochromatosis

a. Idiopathic hemochromatosis

–is a **familial defect of iron absorption** by the intestinal mucosa.

–can be detected and treated successfully before organ damage occurs.

–in its fully developed, neglected state, is characterized by:

(1) The **triad of cirrhosis, diabetes mellitus, and increased skin pigmentation,** giving rise to the older term **bronze diabetes**

      (2) Skin pigmentation caused by hemosiderin and melanin deposition

      (3) Pigment cirrhosis (micronodular cirrhosis with enormous accumulation of parenchymal hemosiderin demonstrable by Prussian blue staining)

      (4) Marked **increase in serum iron**

      (5) Modest **reduction in total iron binding capacity** (TIBC, transferrin)

   b. Secondary hemochromatosis

     —most often is associated with a combination of ineffective erythropoiesis and multiple transfusions, such as occurs in thalassemia major.

     —also can be secondary to a variety of other causes of iron overload.

6. Wilson's disease (hepatolenticular degeneration)

  —is an **autosomal recessive** disorder of copper metabolism.

  —is characterized by **decreased serum ceruloplasmin** (copper-binding protein); probably not a primary defect but it is secondary to increased copper.

  —results in an abnormal major **accumulation of copper** in parenchymal cells of the liver and kidney and in the brain and cornea.

  —is manifest as **liver disease** that varies from chronic active hepatitis to cirrhosis, either micronodular or macronodular in type.

  —results in extrapyramidal motor signs caused by **involvement of the basal ganglia,** especially the putamen of the lenticular nucleus.

  —is marked by the **Kayser-Fleischer ring** circumscribing the periphery of the cornea, representing deposition of copper-containing pigment in Descemet's membrane.

  —may demonstrate aminoaciduria and glycosuria due to renal tubular damage.

7. Cirrhosis due to inborn errors of metabolism

  —results from several disorders, including:

   a. α_1-antitrypsin deficiency

   b. Galactose-1-phosphate uridyl transferase deficiency (galactosemia)

   c. Glycogen storage diseases

H. Vascular disorders of the liver

1. Portal hypertension

  —is characterized by the development of venous collaterals with varices in the submucosal veins of the esophagus, the hemorrhoidal plexus, and other sites.

  —is often classified by the site of portal venous obstruction:

   a. Prehepatic—caused by portal and splenic vein obstruction, most often by thrombosis

   b. Intrahepatic—caused by intrahepatic vascular obstruction, most often by cirrhosis or metastatic tumor, and more rarely by exotic entities such as schistosomiasis

    c. Posthepatic—caused by venous congestion in the distal hepatic venous circulation, most often as a result of constrictive pericarditis, tricuspid insufficiency, congestive heart failure, or hepatic vein occlusion (Budd-Chiari syndrome)

2. Infarction

    —is unusual, since the liver has a double blood supply (mesenteric and hepatic).

3. Budd-Chiari syndrome

    —is caused by thrombotic occlusion of the major hepatic veins, resulting in abdominal pain, jaundice, hepatomegaly, ascites, and eventual liver failure.

    —is most often associated with polycythemia vera, hepatocellular carcinoma, and other abdominal neoplasms; also may occur as a complication of pregnancy.

4. Congestive heart failure

    a. In long-standing chronic right-sided heart failure, the cut surface of the liver can assume an appearance referred to as the nutmeg liver, with dark red congested centrilobular areas alternating with pale portal areas.

    b. Eventually, centrilobular fibrosis occurs, resulting in cardiac cirrhosis (cardiac sclerosis). Similar changes may follow long-standing constrictive pericarditis or tricuspid insufficiency.

I. Hepatic tumors

  1. Benign tumors

    a. Hemangioma

      —is the most common benign tumor of the liver.

    b. Adenoma

      —incidence is apparently related to use of oral contraceptives.

      —when subcapsular in location, may rupture, resulting in severe intraperitoneal hemorrhage.

  2. Malignant tumors

    a. Metastatic tumors

      —account for the majority of hepatic malignancies.

    b. Hepatocellular carcinoma

      —is the most common primary malignancy of the liver.

      —is a frequent complication of cirrhosis, especially when associated with HBV infection; incidence is highest in areas of the world with a high incidence of HBV infection.

      —has been associated with aflatoxin B contamination of nuts and grains; aflatoxin B is thought to be a possible carcinogen.

      —frequently is marked by increased serum concentration of alpha-fetoprotein (AFP).

      —has a propensity for invasion of vascular channels with hematogenous dissemination.

c. Cholangiocarcinoma (bile duct carcinoma)

—is less common than hepatocellular carcinoma.

—occurs most frequently in the Far East, where it is associated with *Clonorchis sinensis* (liver fluke) infestation.

—originates from intrahepatic biliary epithelium.

—like hepatocellular carcinoma, has a propensity for early invasion of vascular channels.

—unlike hepatocellular carcinoma, is not associated with HBV infection or cirrhosis.

—sometimes occurs as a late complication of thorium dioxide (Thorotrast) administration.

d. Hemangiosarcoma (angiosarcoma)

—is a rare malignant vascular tumor.

—is associated with toxic exposure to polyvinyl chloride, Thorotrast, and arsenic.

II. Diseases of the Gallbladder

A. Cholecystitis

1. Acute cholecystitis

—is acute inflammation of the gallbladder, most often pyogenic.

—is manifest clinically by nausea, vomiting, fever, and leukocytosis associated with right upper quadrant and epigastric pain.

2. Chronic cholecystitis

—demonstrates thickening of the gallbladder wall as a result of extensive fibrosis.

—is **frequently complicated by gallstones**.

B. Cholelithiasis (gallstones)

—has a higher incidence in women.

—is often associated with obesity and multiple pregnancies.

1. Stone types

a. Cholesterol stones

—are often solitary and too large to enter the cystic duct or the common bile duct.

b. Pigment stones

—result from precipitation of excess insoluble unconjugated **bilirubin**.

—are often associated with **hemolytic anemia**.

—can be associated with bacterial infection.

c. Mixed stones

—account for the majority of stones (75%–80%).

—are a mixture of cholesterol and calcium salts.

—can often be visualized radiographically because of their calcium content.

2. Clinical manifestations

a. **Cholelithiasis** is often silent and asymptomatic.

b. **Fatty food intolerance** is characteristic.

3. Complications

   a. Biliary colic results from impaction of gallstone in cystic or common bile duct.

   b. Common bile duct obstruction results in obstructive **jaundice** with conjugated hyperbilirubinemia, hypercholesterolemia, increased alkaline phosphatase, and hyperbilirubinuria.

   c. Ascending cholangitis can result from secondary bacterial infection facilitated by obstructed bile flow.

   d. Cholecystitis, acute or chronic

   e. Acute pancreatitis

   f. Gallstone ileus (intestinal obstruction caused by passage of a large gallstone through the eroded gallbladder wall into the adjacent small bowel)

   g. Mucocele (distended, mucus-filled gallbladder secondary to chronic cystic duct obstruction)

   h. Malignancy

C. Cholesterolosis (strawberry gallbladder)

   —is characterized by yellow cholesterol-containing flecks in the mucosal surface.

   —is not associated with inflammatory changes.

   —has no special association with cholelithiasis.

D. Tumors

1. Tumors of the gallbladder

   a. Benign tumors of the gallbladder are rare.

   b. The most common primary tumor of the gallbladder is adenocarcinoma, which is often associated with gallstones.

2. Carcinoma of the extrahepatic biliary ducts and the ampulla of Vater

   —is less common than carcinoma of the gallbladder.

   —is almost always adenocarcinoma.

   —typically presents with progressive, relentless **obstructive jaundice**.

   —often is characterized clinically by the combination of **jaundice** and a **palpably enlarged gallbladder**. Tumors that obstruct the common bile duct result in an enlarged gallbladder; obstructing stones do not, since the gallbladder is typically too scarred to allow enlargement (**Courvoisier's law**).

III. Diseases of the Exocrine Pancreas

A. Acute pancreatitis

   —is caused by activation of pancreatic enzymes, resulting in autodigestion of the organ, with **hemorrhagic fat necrosis** and deposition of **calcium soaps,** and sometimes formation of **pseudocysts** (parenchymal cysts not lined with ductal epithelium).

   —is predisposed by gallstones and excessive alcohol intake.

—is manifest clinically as **severe abdominal pain** and **prostration** closely mimicking an acute surgical abdomen.

—is associated with **increased serum amylase**.

—is characterized by **hypocalcemia** caused by loss of circulating calcium into precipitated calcium–fatty acid soaps.

B. Chronic relapsing pancreatitis

—is characterized by **progressive parenchymal fibrosis**.

—is almost always associated with **alcoholism**.

—is frequently characterized by **calcification**.

—may be characterized by **pseudocysts**.

—is manifest clinically by extremely variable findings, including **abdominal and back pain,** progressive disability, and **steatorrhea**.

C. Carcinoma of the pancreas

—is a common tumor; incidence is increasing.

—is more common in smokers.

—is almost always adenocarcinoma.

—more often arises in the head of the pancreas, causing obstructive jaundice; somewhat less often it originates in the pancreatic body or tail.

—may be manifest clinically by **abdominal pain radiating through to the back,** by weight loss and anorexia, sometimes by **migratory thrombophlebitis** (Trousseau's sign), and frequently by common bile duct obstruction resulting in **obstructive jaundice** (often accompanied by a distended, palpable gallbladder).

—is often silent prior to widespread dissemination.

—usually results in death within a year.

Review Test

Directions: Each of the numbered items or incomplete statements in this section is followed by answers or by completions of the statement. Select the **one** lettered answer or completion that is **best** in each case.

1. Each of the following disorders is matched with the appropriate characteristic or association EXCEPT

(A) physiologic jaundice of newborn—conjugated hyperbilirubinemia.
(B) Gilbert's syndrome—unconjugated hyperbilirubinemia.
(C) Crigler-Najjar syndrome—kernicterus.
(D) Dubin-Johnson syndrome—dark pigment.
(E) The Rotor syndrome—impaired bilirubin transport.

2. All of the following statements concerning serum antigens and antibodies associated with hepatitis B infection are true EXCEPT

(A) detection of hepatitis B surface antigen (HBsAg) for longer than 6 months defines the carrier state.
(B) anti-HBsAg is associated with fulminant hepatitis.
(C) detectable hepatitis B e antigen (HBeAg) correlates with viral infectivity.
(D) antibody to hepatitis B core antigen (anti-HBcAg) can remain elevated for many years.

3. Each of the following disorders is appropriately matched with the corresponding hepatic change EXCEPT

(A) neonatal hepatitis—giant cells.
(B) cytomegalovirus infection—owl's eye inclusions.
(C) yellow fever—cholestasis.
(D) *Echinococcus* infection—large cysts.
(E) schistosomiasis—portal hypertension.

4. Intracytoplasmic eosinophilic hyaline inclusions within hepatocytes are most suggestive of chronic exposure to which of the following agents?

(A) Carbon tetrachloride
(B) Methyltestosterone
(C) Polyvinyl chloride
(D) Ethyl alcohol
(E) Phosphorus

5. Clinical manifestations of the lesion illustrated below frequently include all of the following EXCEPT

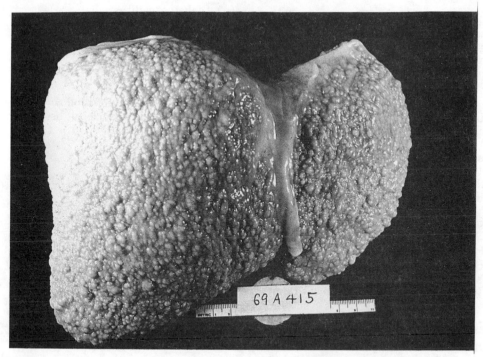

(Reprinted with permission from Golden A, Powell D, and Jennings C: *Pathology: Understanding Human Disease,* 2nd ed. Baltimore, Williams & Wilkins, 1985, p 289.)

(A) hypoalbuminemia.
(B) hypoestrinism.
(C) portal hypertension.
(D) coagulation factor deficiencies.
(E) encephalopathy.

6. Each of the following disorders is correctly matched with the appropriate phrase EXCEPT

(A) postnecrotic cirrhosis—macronodular.
(B) primary biliary cirrhosis—anti-mitochondrial antibodies.
(C) secondary biliary cirrhosis—extrahepatic biliary obstruction.
(D) hemochromatosis—bronze diabetes.
(E) Wilson's disease—increase in ceruloplasmin.

7. The most frequent hepatic malignancy is

(A) hepatocellular carcinoma.
(B) cholangiocarcinoma.
(C) hemangiosarcoma.
(D) adenocarcinoma.
(E) metastatic tumor.

8. Which of the following factors is associated with cholangiocarcinoma of the liver?

(A) Alpha-fetoprotein increase
(B) *Clonorchis sinensis* infestation
(C) Cirrhosis
(D) Hepatitis B virus infection
(E) Intraperitoneal bleeding

9. Complications or well-established associations of gallstones include all of the following EXCEPT

(A) biliary obstruction.
(B) cholesterolosis.
(C) pancreatitis.
(D) intestinal obstruction.
(E) malignancy.

10. All of the following etiologic characteristics or manifestations are suggestive of acute pancreatitis EXCEPT

(A) fat necrosis.
(B) tetracycline toxicity.
(C) gallstones.
(D) alcoholism.
(E) hypocalcemia.

11. Migratory thrombophlebitis is associated with which one of the following diseases?

(A) Diabetes mellitus
(B) Cystic fibrosis
(C) Acute pancreatitis
(D) Chronic relapsing pancreatitis
(E) Pancreatic carcinoma

Directions: Each group of items in this section consists of lettered options followed by a set of numbered items. For each item, select the **one** lettered option that is most closely associated with it. Each lettered option may be selected once, more than once, or not at all.

Questions 12–15

Match the etiologic or clinical feature with the appropriate form of hepatitis.

(A) Hepatitis A virus (HAV)
(B) Hepatitis B virus (HBV)
(C) Hepatitis C virus (HCV)
(D) Hepatitis D virus (HDV)

12. Requires concurrent infection with another virus

13. Not associated with chronic carrier state

14. Dane particle

15. Cause of majority of transfusion-mediated viral hepatitides

Questions 16 and 17

Match the type of hepatitis to the related finding.

(A) Inflammation of portal triads
(B) Piecemeal and bridging necrosis
(C) Hypergammaglobulinemia

16. Chronic active hepatitis

17. Chronic persistent hepatitis

Questions 18 and 19

Match the associated factor with the appropriate hepatic tumor.

(A) Adenoma
(B) Hepatocellular carcinoma
(C) Cholangiocarcinoma
(D) Hemangiosarcoma

18. Polyvinyl chloride

19. HBV infection

Answers and Explanations

1–A. The hyperbilirubinemia of physiologic jaundice of the newborn is primarily due to unconjugated bilirubin. Gilbert's syndrome is characterized by modest elevations of unconjugated bilirubin. The Crigler-Najjar syndrome in its severe variant (sometimes referred to as type I) often results in early death from kernicterus. The Dubin-Johnson syndrome is characterized by striking deposition of dark pigment within hepatocytes and by conjugated hyperbilirubinemia due to defective bilirubin transport across the canalicular membrane. The Rotor syndrome is characterized by a similar defect in bile transport, but pigment deposition does not occur.

2–B. Antibody to hepatitis B surface antigen (anti-HBsAg) appears a few weeks after the disappearance of the corresponding antigen and indicates recovery as well as immunity to future infection.

3–C. Yellow fever characteristically results in midzonal hepatic necrosis, not cholestasis.

4–D. The terms Mallory body and alcoholic hyalin refer to intracytoplasmic hepatic eosinophilic hyaline inclusions derived from intermediate filaments. Mallory bodies are very suggestive of, but not entirely specific for, alcoholic liver disease. Poisoning with carbon tetrachloride results in centrilobular hepatic necrosis; methyltestosterone toxicity results in cholestatic changes; and phosphorus toxicity is manifest by periportal fatty change. Exposure to polyvinyl chloride has been associated with hepatic hemangiosarcoma (angiosarcoma).

5–B. Fine uniform nodularity of the liver, shown by the illustration, is characteristic of micronodular cirrhosis, the gross pattern most typical of alcoholic cirrhosis. Hyperestrinism is characteristic of this disorder. Other characteristics of alcoholic cirrhosis include hypoalbuminemia, portal hypertension, coagulation factor deficiencies, and a predisposition to encephalopathy because of shunting of neurotoxic substances from the portal to the systemic circulation.

6–E. Wilson's disease (hepatolenticular degeneration) is characterized by decreased serum ceruloplasmin. Postnecrotic cirrhosis is the prototype of macronodular change. Primary biliary cirrhosis is associated with antimitochondrial antibodies and is thought to be of autoimmune origin, and secondary biliary cirrhosis is due to extrahepatic biliary obstruction. Hemochromatosis is characterized by bronze diabetes, the triad of cirrhosis, diabetes mellitus, and increased skin pigmentation.

7–E. Although hepatocellular carcinoma is the most common primary hepatic malignancy, metastatic tumors account for the majority of malignant tumors of the liver.

8–B. Cholangiocarcinoma occurs most frequently in the Far East, where it is typically caused by infestation with the liver fluke *Clonorchis sinensis*. Another important association is past exposure to thorium dioxide (Thorotrast). Cirrhosis, hepatitis B virus infection, and elevation of alpha-fetoprotein, all well-known pathogenetic factors or associations of hepatocellular carcinoma, are not linked to cholangiocarcinoma. Intraperitoneal bleeding suggests subcapsular hepatic adenoma.

9–B. Cholesterolosis (strawberry gallbladder), a clinically insignificant aberration characterized by yellow, cholesterol-containing flecks in the mucosal surface of the gallbladder, has no special association with gallstones. Well-known complications of gallstones include biliary obstruction, pancreatitis, and intestinal obstruction (gallstone ileus), often occurring late in life. Carcinoma of the gallbladder is more frequent in the presence of gallstones.

10–B. Intravenous tetracycline therapy has no relation to pancreatic disease. It is, however, a cause of microvesicular liver disease. Factors important in the etiopathogenesis of acute pancreatitis include biliary tract disease and alcoholism. Manifestations or consequences of acute pancreatitis include enzymatic hemorrhagic fat necrosis with calcium soap formation and resultant hypocalcemia.

11–E. Migratory thrombophlebitis is associated with carcinoma of the pancreas and other visceral malignancies.

12–D. Hepatitis D virus (delta agent) is a defective RNA virus requiring simultaneous infection with hepatitis B virus to reproduce or cause infection. The RNA core of the hepatitis D virus requires encapsulation by the HBsAg protein.

13–A. A chronic carrier state is not observed with HAV infection (or with the more recently described hepatitis E virus infection).

14–B. The complete virion of HBV is referred to as the Dane particle. The virus consists of a central core containing double-stranded circular DNA and a virally coded DNA polymerase, both surrounded by an outer lipoprotein coat.

15–C. Hepatitis C virus infection accounts for the majority of transfusion-mediated hepatitides and includes the majority of cases previously grouped as non-A–non-B hepatitis.

16–B. Chronic active hepatitis is a severe form of chronic inflammatory liver disease which often evolves into cirrhosis. The principal morphologic manifestations are piecemeal necrosis and bridging necrosis, as well as fibrotic changes.

17–A. Chronic persistent hepatitis is a mild form of chronic inflammatory liver disease that is almost always clinically inconsequential. The principal morphologic manifestation is inflammation confined to the portal triad (triaditis), with sparing of parenchymal cells.

18–D. Industrial exposure to polyvinyl chloride is associated with increased incidence of hemangiosarcoma of the liver.

19–B. The incidence of hepatocellular carcinoma has been closely linked with the combination of cirrhosis and hepatitis B viral infection. In Africa and Asia, this association is very marked. Hepatitis B viral infection, along with the ingestion of aflatoxin B, a contaminant of nuts and grains, is the presumptive cause of the high incidence of hepatocellular carcinoma in these regions.

17

Kidney and Urinary Tract

I. Congenital Anomalies of the Urinary Tract

A. Kidney

1. Complete or bilateral renal agenesis

—is rare and not compatible with life.

—is absence of both kidneys.

—results in **oligohydramnios,** decreased amniotic fluid, because of failure of renal excretion of fluid swallowed by the fetus.

—results in multiple fetal anomalies (e.g., hypoplastic lung, defects in extremities), all caused by oligohydramnios and collectively known as Potter's syndrome.

2. Unilateral renal agenesis

—is much more common than complete renal agenesis.

—is absence of one kidney.

3. Renal ectopia

—is abnormal location of a kidney, frequently in the pelvis (pelvic kidney).

4. Horseshoe kidney

—may cause urinary tract obstruction because of impingement on the ureters.

B. Ureters

—may be doubled; double ureters may affect the ureters alone or may be part of a duplication of the entire urinary collecting system on one side.

II. Glomerular Diseases (Table 17.1)

A. Nephrotic syndrome

—includes a group of conditions characterized by increased basement membrane permeability, permitting the urinary loss of plasma proteins, particularly low-weight proteins, such as albumin.

1. Clinical manifestations

a. Massive proteinuria

—is generally characterized by more than 4 grams of protein per day.

Table 17.1. Glomerular Diseases

Types	Morphologic Findings
Disorders manifest by nephrotic syndrome	
Minimal change disease (lipoid nephrosis)	No visible basement membrane changes; fused epithelial foot processes; lipid accumulation in renal tubular cells
Focal and segmental glomerulosclerosis	No visible basement membrane changes; segmental sclerosis of scattered juxtamedullary glomeruli
Membranous glomerulonephritis	Basement membrane markedly thickened by intramembranous and epimembranous (subepithelial) immune complex deposits; granular immunofluorescence; "spike and dome" appearance
Diabetic nephropathy	Basement membrane markedly thickened; diffuse or nodular mesangial accumulations of basement membrane-like material
Renal amyloidosis	Amyloid protein identified by special stains (e.g., Congo red), birefringence under polarized light, or electron microscopic criss-cross fibrillary pattern
Lupus nephropathy	Immune complex deposition in subendothelial location may manifest as membranous glomerulonephritis
Disorders manifest by nephritic syndrome	
Poststreptococcal glomerulonephritis	Subepithelial electron-dense "humps"; "lumpy-bumpy" immunofluorescence
Rapidly progressive (crescentic) glomerulonephritis	Crescents
Goodpasture's syndrome	Linear immunofluorescence caused by anti-glomerular basement membrane antibodies
Alport's syndrome	Split basement membrane
Other glomerular disorders	
IgA nephropathy (Berger's disease)	Mesangial IgA deposits
Membranoproliferative glomerulonephritis	Tram-track appearance; deposits of C3, and dense deposits in one variant

b. Hypoalbuminemia

—results from proteinuria and is often marked by a serum concentration of less than 3 grams per 100 ml.

c. Generalized edema

—results from decreased plasma colloid oncotic pressure.

d. Hyperlipidemia and hypercholesterolemia

—are due to increased hepatic lipoprotein synthesis.

2. Minimal change disease (lipoid nephrosis)

—is seen most often in very young children.

—is the prototype of the nephrotic syndrome.

—is characterized by **lipid-laden renal cortices** (lipids are intracytoplasmic in tubular cells, particularly in cells of proximal convoluted tubules).

—demonstrates normal-appearing glomeruli by light microscopy.

—demonstrates normal electron microscopic findings except for the disappearance or **fusing of epithelial foot processes**.

—most often responds well to adrenal steroid therapy.

3. Focal and segmental glomerulosclerosis

—is clinically similar to minimal change disease but occurs in somewhat older patients.

—is characterized by sclerosis within capillary tufts of deep juxtamedullary glomeruli with focal or segmental distribution.

a. Focal distribution

—is involvement of some, but not all, of the glomeruli.

b. Segmental distribution

—is involvement of only a part of the glomerulus.

4. Membranous glomerulonephritis

—is a major primary cause of the nephrotic syndrome.

—is an immune complex disease of unknown etiology.

—has its highest incidence in teenagers and young adults.

—is characterized by markedly **thickened capillary walls** visible by light microscopy and visible by electron microscopy as a 5- to 10-fold thickening of the basement membrane.

—ultrastructurally demonstrates numerous electron-dense **immune complexes in intramembranous and epimembranous locations** within and upon the basement membrane (the term *subepithelial* is often used synonymously with epimembranous).

—demonstrates, with special stains, a **"spike and dome" appearance** resulting from the deposition of new basement membrane between and around the immune deposits; the spikes are basement membrane material, and the domes are immune complex deposits.

—demonstrates granular deposits of immunoglobulin G (IgG) or C3 by immunofluorescence. **Granular immunofluorescence** is a general characteristic of immune complex diseases.

—is a slowly progressive disorder that shows little response to steroid therapy.

—is sometimes associated with hepatitis B, syphilis, or malaria infection; with drugs, such as gold salts or penicillamine; or with malignancy.

—sometimes causes renal vein thrombosis, which was previously thought to be an etiologic factor of the disorder.

—is seen in 10% of patients with systemic lupus erythematosus (SLE).

5. Diabetic nephropathy

—is often manifest clinically by the nephrotic syndrome.

—demonstrates, by electron microscopy, a striking increase in thickness of glomerular basement membrane.

—is characterized by an **increase in mesangial matrix,** resulting in two characteristic morphologic patterns:

a. Diffuse glomerulosclerosis

—is marked by a diffusely distributed increase in mesangial matrix.

b. Nodular glomerulosclerosis

—is marked by nodular accumulations of mesangial matrix material (**Kimmelstiel-Wilson nodules**).

6. Renal amyloidosis

—is another cause of the nephrotic syndrome.

−is characterized by predominantly **subendothelial and mesangial amyloid deposits**.

−can be identified by reactivity of amyloid with special stains (e.g., Congo red, crystal violet, thioflavin T) and by birefringence under polarized light.

−is also demonstrated by a characteristic criss-cross fibrillary pattern of amyloid by electron microscopy.

7. Lupus nephropathy

−is the renal component of systemic lupus erythematosus (**SLE**); the severity of the renal lesion often determines the overall prognosis in patients with SLE.

−is often manifest as the **nephrotic syndrome;** many cases also have major nephritic features.

−is classified by the World Health Organization (WHO) into five distinct renal patterns, termed **WHO types**.

a. Type I

−no observable renal involvement.

b. Type II

−is the **mesangial form** of lupus nephropathy.

−is characterized by focal and segmental glomerular involvement with an increase in the number of mesangial cells and quantitative increase in mesangial matrix.

−results most often in slight proteinuria and minimal hematuria; is usually of little clinical consequence.

c. Type III (focal proliferative form)

−usually involves less than half of the glomeruli.

−can cause extensive damage to individual glomeruli.

d. Type IV (diffuse proliferative form)

−is the prototype of lupus nephropathy and the most severe form of the disease.

−is often associated with a combination of the nephrotic and nephritic syndromes.

−involves almost all of the glomeruli.

−includes glomerular changes, such as marked inflammation with small focal thromboses and mesangial proliferation, all resulting in extensive scarring.

−is characterized by the **wire-loop abnormality,** a light microscopic finding resulting from immune complex deposition and gross thickening of the glomerular basement membrane.

−is also characterized by **endothelial cell proliferation,** which is often prominent by electron microscopy.

−is further characterized by marked **subendothelial immune complex deposition,** which is also a major diagnostic feature.

e. Type V (membranous form)

−is indistinguishable from primary membranous glomerulonephritis.

B. Nephritic syndrome

—is characterized by inflammatory rupture of the glomerular capillaries with resultant bleeding into the urinary space; proteinuria and edema may be present but are usually mild.

1. Clinical findings

a. Oliguria

b. Azotemia

—is increased concentrations of serum urea nitrogen and creatinine.

c. Hypertension

d. Hematuria

—results from leakage of the red cells directly from glomerular capillaries into Bowman's space. Many of the red cells are aggregated into the shape of the renal tubules and embedded in a proteinaceous matrix forming red cell casts that can be observed in the urine; the patient often reports "**smoky brown urine.**"

2. Poststreptococcal glomerulonephritis (acute glomerulonephritis)

—is the prototype of the **nephritic syndrome**.

—most often follows or accompanies infection (tonsillitis, streptococcal impetigo, infected insect bites) with nephritogenic strains of **group A β-hemolytic streptococci**.

—is followed by complete recovery in almost all children and many adults.

—is an **immune complex disease** with the antigen of the antigen–antibody complexes of streptococcal origin.

—is marked by several laboratory abnormalities, including urinary red cells and red cell casts, azotemia, decreased serum C3, and an increased titer of antistreptolysin O (ASO) as evidence of recent streptococcal infection.

—is characterized by an **intense inflammatory reaction** involving almost all glomeruli in both kidneys, resulting in:

a. Innumerable punctuate hemorrhages on the surface of both kidneys

b. Enlarged, hypercellular, swollen, bloodless glomeruli with proliferation of mesangial and endothelial cells and sometimes neutrophils

c. Glomerular basement membrane of normal thickness and uniformity in spite of the extensive inflammatory changes

d. Characteristic **electron-dense "humps"** on the epithelial side of the basement membrane (**subepithelial localization**)

e. "Lumpy-bumpy" immunofluorescence (extremely coarse granular immunofluorescence for IgG or C3)

3. Rapidly progressive (crescentic) glomerulonephritis

—is defined clinically as the nephritic syndrome, progressing rapidly to renal failure within weeks or months.

—is histologically defined by the formation of crescents between Bowman's capsule and the glomerular tuft, which result from deposition of fibrin in Bowman's space and from proliferation of parietal epithelial cells of Bowman's capsule; cells of monocytic origin often are involved.

—is of **poststreptococcal etiology** in approximately 50% of cases; an additional 40% are of diverse or unknown etiology.

—is characterized by anti-glomerular basement membrane antibodies (nonstreptococcal) in approximately 10% of cases; these cases often present clinically as Goodpasture's syndrome.

4. Goodpasture's syndrome

—is caused by antibodies directed against antigens in glomerular and pulmonary alveolar basement membranes.

—demonstrates linear immunofluorescence by fluorescent antibody studies for IgG.

—is manifest clinically by:

a. Glomerulonephritis

b. Pneumonitis with hemoptysis

c. Peak incidence in **men in the mid-20s age group**

5. Alport's syndrome

—is hereditary nephritis associated with nerve deafness.

—demonstrates glomerular basement membrane splitting by electron microscopy.

C. Other glomerular diseases

1. IgA nephropathy (Berger's disease)

—is an extremely common entity defined by deposition of IgA in the mesangium.

—is characterized by benign recurrent hematuria in children, usually following an infection, lasting 1 to 2 days, and most often of minimal clinical significance.

2. Membranoproliferative glomerulonephritis

—is characterized clinically by slow progression to chronic renal disease.

—is characterized histologically by both basement membrane thickening and cellular proliferation.

—is marked by reduplication of glomerular basement membrane into two layers due to expansion of mesangial matrix into the glomerular capillary loops; this results in a characteristic **tram-track appearance** best seen with silver stains.

—occurs in two forms:

a. Type I

—is an immune complex nephritis associated with an unknown antigen. It has a striking tram-track appearance.

b. Type II (dense deposit disease)

—has a tram-track appearance that is not as apparent as that of type I.

—is characterized by irregular electron-dense material deposited within the glomerular basement membrane; C3 is demonstrable adjacent to but not within the dense deposits; serum C3 is characteristically markedly reduced.

—is possibly caused by an IgG autoantibody (C3 nephritic factor) with specificity for the C3 convertase of the alternate complement pathway.

III. Urinary Tract Obstruction

—may occur anywhere in the urinary system.

—is most often congenital in children.

—is most often acquired in adults, usually occurring as a consequence of renal stones or benign prostatic hyperplasia.

—may be manifest clinically by:

A. Renal colic

—is excruciating pain caused by acute distention of the ureter, usually by the transit of a small stone.

B. Hydronephrosis

—is progressive dilatation of the renal pelvis and calyces.

C. Infection

—is localized proximal to the site of obstruction.

—may lead to infection of the renal parenchyma.

IV. Infection of the Urinary Tract and Kidney

A. General characteristics—infection

—is markedly increased in incidence in women, presumably because of the very short length of the female urethra; incidence is increased during pregnancy.

—can be caused by hematogenous bacterial dissemination to the kidney or by external entry of organisms through the urethra into the bladder; in the latter case infection can spread upward from the bladder into the ureters (vesicoureteral reflux) and through the ureters to the kidney (ascending infection).

—most frequently involves the normal flora of the colon, most often *Escherichia coli*.

B. Predisposing factors

1. Obstruction of urinary flow

2. Surgery on the kidney or urinary tract

3. Catheters inserted through the urethra into the bladder

4. Gynecologic abnormalities

C. Clinical manifestations

1. Urinary frequency—a compelling necessity to void small amounts of urine at frequent intervals

2. Dysuria—painful, burning sensation on urination

3. Pyuria—large numbers of neutrophils in the urine

4. **Hematuria**—blood in the urine; urinary red cells are a nonspecific finding in urinary tract infection.

5. **Bacteriuria**—usually defined as more than 10^5 organisms per milliliter of urine; must be distinguished from contamination of urine specimens by external flora.

D. **Additional diagnostically significant findings in acute pyelonephritis** (acute infection of the renal parenchyma)

   —include **fever, flank tenderness,** and **white cell casts in the urine** (this finding is pathognomonic of acute pyelonephritis).

V. Tubular and Interstitial Disorders of the Kidney

A. **Acute drug-induced interstitial nephritis**

   —is most often caused by penicillin derivatives, such as methicillin, and other drugs such as nonsteroidal anti-inflammatory drugs and diuretics.
   —is most likely of immune etiology.
   —is characterized by **acute interstitial renal inflammation.**
   —resolves on cessation of exposure to inciting drug.

B. **Renal papillary necrosis (necrotizing papillitis)**

   —is ischemic necrosis of the tips of the renal papillae.
   —is most often associated with **diabetes mellitus,** in which it is related to renal infection and coexisting vascular disease.
   —is occasionally a catastrophic consequence of **acute pyelonephritis.**
   —is also associated with long-term persistent use of **phenacetin,** most often in association with aspirin and other analgesics. This can lead to **chronic analgesic nephritis,** a chronic inflammatory change characterized by loss and atrophy of tubules and interstitial fibrosis and inflammation.

C. **Acute tubular necrosis**

   —is the most common cause of acute renal failure (acute renal shutdown).
   —is reversible. Proper medical management results in complete recovery; otherwise the syndrome is universally fatal.
   —can lead to death, most often during the **initial oliguric phase.**
   —is marked by complete return of renal function to normal within 10 to 21 days with appropriate therapy.
   —is most frequently precipitated by **renal ischemia,** which is frequently caused by prolonged hypotension or shock, most often induced by gram-negative sepsis, trauma, or hemorrhage.
   —is also associated with crush injury with myoglobinuria. Myoglobinuria also can be observed after intense exercise.
   —also may be caused by direct tubular injury from toxic substances such as mercuric chloride.

D. **Disorders of renal tubular function**

   1. **Fanconi's syndrome**

      —is a manifestation of generalized dysfunction of the proximal renal tubules.
      —may be hereditary or acquired.
      —is characterized by impaired reabsorption of glucose, amino acids, phosphate, and bicarbonate.

−is manifest clinically by **glycosuria; hyperphosphaturia and hypophosphatemia; aminoaciduria;** and **systemic acidosis**.

2. Cystinuria

−is genetically determined impaired tubular reabsorption of cystine.
−is manifest clinically by cystine stones.

3. Hartnup disease

−is genetically determined impaired tubular reabsorption of tryptophan.
−leads to pellagra-like manifestations.

E. Chronic pyelonephritis

−is marked by coarse, asymmetric corticomedullary scarring and deformity of the renal pelvis and calyces; these findings are essential to diagnosis.
−is characterized by interstitial inflammatory infiltrate in the early stages and later by interstitial fibrosis and tubular atrophy; atrophic tubules often contain eosinophilic proteinaceous casts, resulting in an appearance reminiscent of thyroid follicles (**thyroidization of the kidney**).
−is considered to be of probable infectious etiology, but the infectious agent is often not demonstrable.

VI. Diffuse Cortical Necrosis

−is acute generalized **ischemic infarction of the cortices** of both kidneys; the medulla is spared. Infarction is patchy in some instances, compatible with survival.
−is most often associated with **obstetric catastrophes** such as abruptio placentae or eclampsia.
−is also associated with **septic shock** and other causes of vascular collapse.
−is thought to be caused by a combination of end-organ vasospasm and disseminated intravascular coagulation.

VII. Urolithiasis

−is calculi (stones) in the urinary tract.
−is increased in incidence in men.

A. Calcium stones

−account for 80% to 85% of urinary stones.
−are composed of calcium oxalate or calcium phosphate, or both.
−are radiopaque.
−are associated with hypercalciuria, which is caused by:

1. Increased intestinal **absorption of calcium**

2. Increased primary renal **excretion of calcium**

3. **Hypercalcemia,** which may be caused by:

a. Hyperparathyroidism leads to nephrocalcinosis (calcification of the kidney) as well as urolithiasis.

b. Malignancy leads to hypercalcemia because of osteolytic metastases or ectopic production of parathyroid hormone (often by a squamous cell carcinoma of the lung).

    c. Other causes include sarcoidosis, vitamin D intoxication, and the milk–alkali syndrome (nephrocalcinosis and formation of calcium stones associated with self-treatment of peptic ulcer by milk and absorbable antacids).

B. Ammonium magnesium phosphate stones

    —are the second most common form of urolithiasis.

    —are radiolucent.

    —are facilitated by alkaline urine, which is most often caused by ammonia-producing organisms (urease-positive), such as *Proteus vulgaris* or *Staphylococcus*.

    —can form large **staghorn (struvite) calculi** (casts of renal pelvis and calyces).

C. Uric acid stones

    —are associated with hyperuricemia in approximately half of the patients; hyperuricemia can be secondary to gout or to increased cellular turnover as in the leukemias or myeloproliferative syndromes.

D. Cystine stones

    —are almost always associated with cystinuria or genetically determined aminoaciduria.

VIII. Cystic Diseases of the Kidney

A. Adult polycystic kidney disease

    —manifests clinically between the ages of 15 and 30.

    —the most common inherited disorder of the kidney, is characterized by **autosomal dominant** inheritance.

    —occurs bilaterally; the kidneys are markedly enlarged.

    —is characterized by the **partial replacement of renal parenchyma by cysts**.

    —is manifest clinically by:

1. Hypertension

2. Hematuria

3. Palpable renal masses

4. Progression to renal failure

    —frequently is associated with **berry aneurysm** of the circle of Willis.

    —is frequently associated with cystic disease of the liver or other organs.

B. Infantile polycystic kidney disease

    —is manifest clinically by multiple cysts evident at birth.

    —is an **autosomal recessive** disorder.

    —is marked by closed cysts that are not in continuity with the collecting system.

    —results in death shortly after birth.

C. Simple (solitary) renal cyst

    —is a common lesion that occurs in adults; it often is asymptomatic.

D. Medullary cystic disease

—is a very serious (but uncommon) form of cystic disease affecting older children.

—is characterized by cysts in the medulla that may result in renal failure.

E. Medullary sponge kidney

—is characterized by multiple small medullary cysts and impaired tubular function, usually without renal failure; renal stones may form in the dilated ducts.

—may be complicated by infection.

IX. Renal Failure

—can be acute or chronic and can result from any of the glomerular or tubulointerstitial lesions discussed in the preceding sections.

—is always associated with **azotemia** (increased serum creatinine and/or urea) **of renal origin**.

—in advanced stages results in uremia; the term **uremia** denotes the biochemical and clinical syndrome characteristic of symptomatic renal disease.

A. Major clinical characteristics of uremia

1. **Azotemia**

2. **Acidosis** resulting from the accumulation of sulfates, phosphates, and organic acids

3. **Hyperkalemia**

4. **Abnormal control of fluid volume**

—early characteristic is inability to concentrate urine; later manifestation is inability to dilute urine. Sodium and water retention can result in congestive heart failure.

5. **Hypocalcemia** caused by failure to synthesize the active form of vitamin D; hypocalcemia can lead to renal osteodystrophy.

6. **Anemia** caused by decreased secretion of erythropoietin

7. **Hypertension** caused by hyperproduction of renin

B. Other clinical characteristics of uremia

—include **anorexia,** nausea, and vomiting; **neurologic disorders,** ranging from diminished mental function to convulsions and coma; **bleeding** caused by disordered platelet function; **accumulation in the skin of urochrome** and other urinary pigments; and **fibrinous pericarditis.**

X. Nonrenal Causes of Azotemia

A. Prerenal azotemia

—results from **decreased renal blood flow** caused by blood loss, decreased cardiac output, systemic hypovolemia (as in massive burns), or peripheral pooling of blood due to marked vasodilatation (as in gram-negative sepsis).

—is characterized by increased tubular reabsorption of sodium and water, resulting in oliguria, concentrated urine, and decreased urinary sodium excretion.

1. Measurement of urinary sodium is diagnostically significant in the delineation of the **oliguria of shock**.

    a. Oliguria may be due to **decreased renal blood flow** with consequent decreased glomerular filtration rate, in which case tubular reabsorption of sodium is maximally increased and urinary sodium is low.

    b. Oliguria may be a manifestation of **acute tubular necrosis,** in which case tubular reabsorption is markedly impaired and urinary sodium is not decreased.

2. The **BUN:creatinine ratio is characteristically greater than 15** due to a combination of both decreased glomerular filtration and increased tubular reabsorption of urea.

B. Postrenal azotemia

—results from **mechanical blockage of urinary flow**.

XI. Tumors of the Kidney, Urinary Tract, and Bladder

A. Benign tumors of the kidney

1. Adenoma

—is most often small and asymptomatic.
—is derived from renal tubules.
—may be a precursor lesion to renal carcinoma.

2. Angiomyolipoma

—is a hamartoma consisting of fat, smooth muscle, and blood vessels.
—is often associated with the tuberous sclerosis syndrome.

B. Malignant tumors of the kidney

1. Renal cell carcinoma

—is the most common renal malignancy.
—occurs most often in men ages 50 to 70.
—has a higher incidence in cigarette smokers.
—is associated, in some instances, with gene deletions in chromosome 3; can also be associated with von Hippel-Lindau disease, which is caused by alterations in a gene localized to chromosome 3.
—originates in renal tubules.
—most often arises in one of the renal poles, frequently the upper pole.
—frequently invades renal veins or the vena cava, resulting in **hematogenous dissemination**.
—is characterized histologically by **polygonal clear cells,** sometimes with vestigial tubule formation.
—may be manifest clinically by any of the following findings:

    a. **Hematuria** (the most frequent presenting abnormality)

    b. **Palpable mass**

    c. **Flank pain**

    d. **Fever**

    e. **Secondary polycythemia** (results from erythropoietin production)

f. Ectopic production of a variety of hormones or hormone-like substances (e.g., ACTH, prolactin, gonadotropins, parathyroid-like hormone, and renin)

2. Wilms' tumor (nephroblastoma)

- —is the most common renal malignancy of early childhood.
- —has peak incidence in **children ages 2 to 4**.
- —most often presents with a **palpable flank mass** (often huge).
- —is characterized histologically by a varied picture, including immature stroma, primitive tubules and glomeruli, and mesenchymal elements, such as fibrous connective tissue, cartilage, bone, and, rarely, striated muscle.
- —is often associated with deletions of the short arm of chromosome 11, the WT-1 gene localized to this chromosome is a cancer suppressor gene.
- —can be part of AGR (or WAGR) complex (**W**ilms' tumor, **A**niridia, **G**enitourinary malformations, and mental–motor **R**etardation).
- —also can be associated with hemihypertrophy (gross symmetry due to unilateral muscular hypertrophy).

C. Transitional cell carcinoma

- —is the most common tumor of the urinary collecting system and can occur in renal calyces, pelvis, ureter, or bladder.
- —is likely to recur after removal.
- —most often presents clinically with **hematuria**.
- —tends to spread by local extension to surrounding tissues.
- —is associated with a number of toxic exposures, including

1. Industrial exposure to benzidine or beta-naphthylamine, an aniline dye

2. Phenacetin abuse

3. Cigarette smoking

4. Long-term treatment with **cyclophosphamide**

D. Squamous cell carcinoma

- —comprises a minority of urinary tract malignancies.
- —can result from chronic inflammatory processes such as chronic bacterial infection or schistosomiasis; can also be associated with renal calculi.

Review Test

Directions: Each of the numbered items or incomplete statements in this section is followed by answers or by completions of the statement. Select the **one** lettered answer or completion that is **best** in each case.

1. A renal biopsy was taken from a 20-year-old woman with the nephrotic syndrome and slowly progressive impairment of renal function. The patient's response to corticosteroid medication had been unimpressive. The appearance of the biopsy was similar to the illustration shown here. The most likely diagnosis is

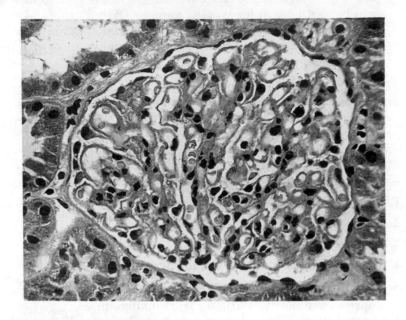

(Reprinted with permission from Golden A, Powell D, and Jennings C: *Pathology: Understanding Human Disease,* 2nd ed. Baltimore, Williams & Wilkins, 1985, p 216.)

(A) minimal change disease.
(B) focal and segmental glomerulosclerosis.
(C) membranous glomerulonephritis.
(D) poststreptococcal glomerulonephritis.
(E) rapidly progressive glomerulonephritis.

2. A renal biopsy was taken from a 50-year-old man with hypertension and the nephrotic syndrome. The appearance of the biopsy was similar to the illustration shown below. Of the following possible additional laboratory findings, which one is most characteristically associated with this lesion?

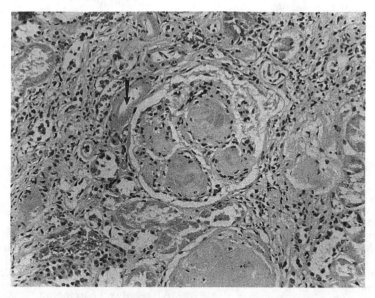

(Courtesy of JB Walter, M.D. Originally published in *Pathology of Human Disease*. Philadelphia, Lea & Febiger, 1989, p 349.)

(A) Hypocalcemia
(B) Hyperglycemia
(C) Decreased creatinine clearance
(D) Increased blood urea nitrogen
(E) Fixed specific gravity of urine

3. A 3-year-old girl presents with generalized edema shortly after recovery from an upper respiratory infection. Laboratory studies reveal marked albuminuria as well as hypoalbuminemia and hyperlipidemia. Prior similar episodes responded to adrenal steroid medication. The most likely diagnosis is

(A) minimal change disease.
(B) focal and segmental glomerulosclerosis.
(C) membranous glomerulonephritis.
(D) poststreptococcal glomerulonephritis.
(E) rapidly progressive glomerulonephritis.

4. A 22-year-old woman presents with fever, malaise, generalized arthralgias, and a skin rash over the nose and malar eminences. Which one of the following possible findings has the greatest relative significance in the overall prognosis for the patient?

(A) Immune complexes at the dermal–epidermal junction in skin
(B) Pleuritis
(C) Atypical verrucous vegetations of the mitral valve
(D) Perivascular fibrosis in the spleen
(E) Glomerular subendothelial immune complex deposition

Questions 5 and 6

5. Two weeks after recovery from a severe bout of pharyngitis, an 11-year-old girl is seen because of the acute onset of periorbital edema, hematuria, malaise, nausea, and headache. All of the following findings are expected in this patient EXCEPT

(A) oliguria.
(B) hypertension.
(C) marked hypoalbuminemia.
(D) increased antistreptolysin O titer.
(E) azotemia.

6. In the patient described in the previous question, expected findings on glomerular electron microscopic examination will demonstrate

(A) no changes except for fused epithelial foot processes.
(B) marked thickening of the glomerular basement membrane with numerous intra-membranous and epimembranous immune complex deposits.
(C) striking increase in thickness of glomerular basement membrane and diffuse increase in mesangial matrix material.
(D) marked subendothelial immune complex depositions.
(E) normal-appearing glomerular basement membrane with electron-dense "humps" in subepithelial location.

7. Crescent formation is characteristic of which one of the following glomerular diseases?

(A) Minimal change disease
(B) Focal and segmental glomerulosclerosis
(C) Membranous glomerulonephritis
(D) Rapidly progressive glomerulonephritis
(E) Poststreptococcal glomerulonephritis

8. A 28-year-old woman presented with fever, dysuria, urinary frequency, and flank tenderness. The urine contained numerous neutrophils and many white cell casts. Urine protein was moderately increased. A quantitative urine culture revealed more than 10^5 bacteria/ml. The most likely causative organism was

(A) *Pseudomonas aeruginosa.*
(B) *Proteus vulgaris.*
(C) *Haemophilus influenzae.*
(D) *Escherichia coli.*
(E) *Neisseria gonorrhoeae.*

9. Associations of renal papillary necrosis include all of the following EXCEPT

(A) impaired glucose tolerance.
(B) long-term use of phenacetin and aspirin compounds.
(C) myoglobinuria.
(D) fever and pyuria.

10. A kidney demonstrating coarse asymmetric renal corticomedullary scarring, deformity of the renal pelvis and calyces, interstitial fibrosis, and atrophic tubules containing eosinophilic proteinaceous casts is most suggestive of

(A) renal papillary necrosis.
(B) chronic pyelonephritis.
(C) chronic analgesic nephritis.
(D) membranoproliferative glomerulonephritis.
(E) Berger's disease.

Questions 11 and 12

11. A 2-year-old boy with visible abdominal distention is found to have an enormous left-sided flank mass apparently arising from, but dwarfing, the left kidney. The most likely diagnosis is

(A) renal cell carcinoma.
(B) polycystic kidney.
(C) transitional cell carcinoma.
(D) Wilms' tumor.
(E) angiomyolipoma.

12. Associations of the lesion described in the previous question include all of the following EXCEPT

(A) congenital aniridia.
(B) subtle or gross deletions of the short arm of chromosome 11.
(C) berry aneurysm of the circle of Willis.
(D) mental–motor retardation.
(E) "hemihypertrophy."

13. A 55-year-old man presents with painless hematuria. On cystoscopy, a papillary mass is found in the bladder. All of the following are characteristic of this lesion EXCEPT

(A) incidence is increased in cigarette smokers.
(B) the majority are adenocarcinomas.
(C) the incidence is increased in aniline dye workers.
(D) it is more likely to be malignant than benign.
(E) similar lesions with similar histology can occur throughout the urinary tract.

14. A glomerular immunofluorescent pattern for (IgG) similar to that shown in this illustration would be expected in which of the following patients?

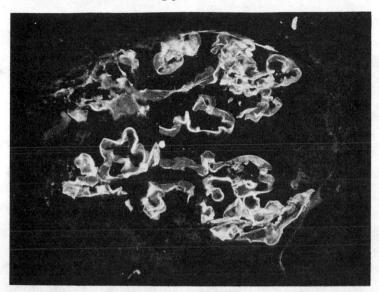

(Reprinted with permission from Walter JB: *An Introduction to the Principles of Pathology,* 2nd ed. Philadelphia, W. B. Saunders Co., 1992, p 490 [courtesy of Susan Ritchie, M.D., Department of Pathology, The General Division of the Toronto Hospital]).

(A) A 3-year-old girl with recurrent bouts of the nephrotic syndrome

(B) A 9-year-old boy with "smoky" urine 2 weeks after recovery from a streptococcal infection

(C) An 18-year-old woman with the nephrotic syndrome and progressive chronic renal disease

(D) A 25-year-old man with hemoptysis and hematuria

(E) A 26-year-old woman with a "butterfly" rash

15. An enormously enlarged kidney similar to that shown in the illustration below was found at autopsy in a 65-year-old man. Well-known associations or characteristics of this disease process include all of the following EXCEPT

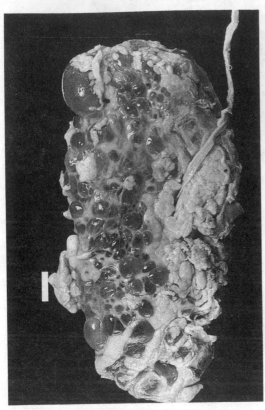

(Courtesy of JB Walter, M.D. Originally published in *Pathology of Human Disease.* Philadelphia, Lea & Febiger, 1989, p 700.)

(A) cysts in the liver.
(B) berry aneurysm of the circle of Willis.
(C) hypertension.
(D) autosomal dominant inheritance.
(E) polycythemia vera.

16. Characteristics or associations of the renal lesion shown below include all of the following EXCEPT

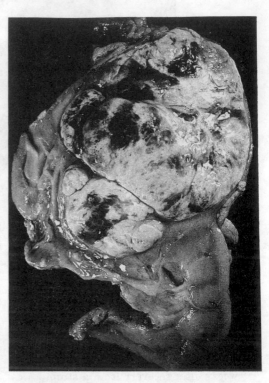

(Reprinted with permission from Golden A, Powell D, and Jennings C: *Pathology: Understanding Human Disease,* 2nd ed. Baltimore, Williams & Wilkins, 1985, p 225.)

(A) clear cell morphology.
(B) palpable mass.
(C) adrenal origin.
(D) hematuria.
(E) polycythemia.

17. Which of the following characteristics is LEAST frequently observed in renal cell carcinoma?

(A) Ectopic hormone production
(B) Fever
(C) Flank pain
(D) Hematuria
(E) Tumor cells in urine

Directions: Each group of items in this section consists of lettered options followed by a set of numbered items. For each item, select the **one** lettered option that is most closely associated with it. Each lettered option may be selected once, more than once, or not at all.

Questions 18 and 19

Match each predisposing factor with the appropriate type of renal stone.

(A) Calcium stones
(B) Ammonium magnesium phosphate stones
(C) Uric acid stones
(D) Cystine stones

18. *Proteus vulgaris* infection

19. Leukemias and myeloproliferative syndromes

Answers and Explanations

1–C. The diffuse thickening of the walls of the capillary loops seen in the illustration is characteristic of membranous glomerulonephritis, the most frequent cause of the nephrotic syndrome in young adults. Expected associated findings in this immune complex disease include granular immunofluorescence and a characteristic "spike and dome" appearance best visualized with special stains. Intramembranous and epimembranous electron-dense immune complex deposits are seen by electron microscopy.

2–B. The illustration shows nodular glomerulosclerosis (Kimmelstiel-Wilson nodules), the most characteristic glomerular finding in diabetes mellitus. The nodules are accumulations of mesangial matrix-like material.

3–A. The combination of generalized edema, massive proteinuria, hypoalbuminemia, and hyperlipidemia constitutes the nephrotic syndrome, the prototype of which is minimal change disease (lipoid nephrosis). This disorder characteristically occurs in very young children and demonstrates intracytoplasmic lipid in the proximal convoluted tubules, a paucity of glomerular abnormalities by light microscopy, and "fusing" (absence) of epithelial foot processes by electron microscopy.

4–E. The overall prognosis in systemic lupus erythematosus (SLE) is most closely related to the glomerular lesions in these patients. These renal lesions are highly variable. In the diffuse proliferative form, almost all of the glomeruli are involved in a marked inflammatory reaction to widespread subendothelial and mesangial immune complex deposition.

5–C. The combination of hematuria (with red cell casts), oliguria, azotemia, and hypertension constitutes the nephritic syndrome, the prototype of which is poststreptococcal glomerulonephritis. Fluid retention is usually minimal, often limited to periorbital edema, and the result of reduced renal excretion of salt and water, not hypoalbuminemia.

6–E. Characteristic electron-dense "humps" on the epithelial side of the basement membrane (subepithelial location) are an extremely important diagnostic feature of poststreptococcal glomerulonephritis. The basement membrane is not thickened in this acute, usually self-limited disorder.

7–D. Glomerular crescents are the hallmark of rapidly progressive (crescentic) glomerulonephritis, which is clinically characterized by progression to renal failure in weeks or months. The etiology is poststreptococcal in approximately 50% of the cases. Another 10% are due to anti-glomerular basement membrane antibodies and may present clinically as Goodpasture's syndrome.

8–D. Organisms involved in most urinary tract infections are most often normal flora of the colon, and the most frequent of these is *E. coli.*

9–C. Renal papillary necrosis (ischemic necrosis of the tips of the renal papillae) is most often a complication of diabetes mellitus, chronic analgesic nephritis, or acute pyelonephritis. It has no association with myoglobinuria.

10–B. The combination of coarse asymmetric corticomedullary scarring, deformity of the renal pelvis and calyces, and tubular atrophy is characteristic of chronic pyelonephritis. When the atrophic tubules contain eosinophilic proteinaceous casts, the resultant similarity in appearance to thyroid follicles is referred to as "thyroidization." Although an infectious etiology is assumed, the infectious agent is often not demonstrable.

11–D. Wilms' tumor is the most common renal neoplasm of children. The tumors are often huge and frequently cause abdominal distention. Renal cell carcinoma and adult polycystic kidney can also present as a large flank mass but not in a child.

12–C. Berry aneurysm of the circle of Willis is a frequent association and complication of adult polycystic kidney. Associations of Wilms' tumor notably include gene deletions localized to the short arm of chromosome 11 (11p13). In some instances, a "two-hit" mechanism of cancer suppressor gene inactivation, similar to that postulated for retinoblastoma, appears to be operative. Other associations of Wilms' tumor include congenital aniridia, genitourinary malformations, and mental–motor retardation (the AGR or WAGR complex). Another unusual association is "hemihypertrophy" (gross asymmetry of the body).

13–B. The majority of urinary tract tumors are transitional cell carcinomas. Adenocarcinomas are rare tumors of the lower urinary tract.

14–D. The illustration demonstrates linear immunofluorescence, which is characteristic of disease caused by anti-glomerular basement membrane antibodies. In Goodpasture's syndrome, antibodies directed against antigens in the basement membranes of the glomeruli as well as the pulmonary alveoli result in both hemorrhagic pneumonitis with hemoptysis and glomerular disease with hematuria.

15–E. Secondary polycythemia, not polycythemia vera, is a complication of adult polycystic disease and is due to increased secretion of erythropoietin.

16–C. The illustration demonstrates a renal cell carcinoma, which most often arises in one of the renal poles, frequently the upper pole. The tumor cells have a clear cell appearance, which led to an earlier erroneous concept that this tumor was of adrenal origin and to the older name "hypernephroma." The tumor is often quite large and may result in a palpable mass. Hematuria is the most frequent presenting sign. Polycythemia due to increased erythropoietin production may occur.

17–E. Malignant cells are only rarely detected in the urine in renal cell carcinoma.

18–B. The development of ammonium magnesium phosphate stones, the second most common form of urolithiasis, is facilitated by alkaline urine and most often by the growth of ammonia-producing (urea-splitting) organisms such as *P. vulgaris.* These stones are often large and account for the majority of staghorn calculi.

19–C. Hyperuricemia due to gout or increased urate excretion secondary to the increased cellular turnover of leukemias and myeloproliferative syndromes accounts for the presence of many uric acid stones.

18

Male Reproductive System

I. Diseases of the Penis

A. Congenital anomalies

1. Hypospadias

—is an anomaly in which the urethral meatus opens on the ventral surface of the penis.

2. Epispadias

—is an anomaly in which the urethral meatus opens on the dorsal surface of the penis.

—is less common than hypospadias.

B. Other abnormalities

1. Phimosis

—is an abnormally tight foreskin that is difficult or impossible to retract over the glans penis.

—may be congenital or result from inflammation or from trauma.

2. Peyronie's disease

—is subcutaneous fibrosis of the dorsum of the penis.

—occurs in the older age group.

—is of unknown etiology.

3. Priapism

—is an intractable, often painful erection.

—is sometimes associated with venous thrombosis of the corpora cavernosa.

C. Inflammatory disorders

—a number of infectious processes are sexually transmitted.

1. Balanitis

—is inflammation of the glans penis.

—is often associated with poor hygiene.

—is rare in circumcised individuals.

2. Syphilis (lues)

—is caused by spirochetes of *Treponema pallidum,* which are demonstrable by dark-field examination.

—manifests during the primary stage as **chancre,** an elevated, painless, superficially ulcerated, firm papule. This lesion is most commonly located on the glans penis or prepuce and ordinarily heals within 2 to 6 weeks. Without treatment, it is followed by secondary and tertiary lues.

3. Gonorrhea

—is caused by *Neisseria gonorrhoeae,* which appear as intracellular gram-negative diplococci.

—is manifest most often by acute purulent urethritis.

—can extend to prostate and seminal vesicles and can also involve the epididymis, but only rarely the testis.

4. Chlamydial infection

—is a common cause of nongonococcal urethritis.

—also can cause epididymitis.

—is sexually transmitted.

D. Neoplasms

1. Carcinoma in situ

a. Bowen's disease

—usually presents as a single erythematous plaque, most often on the shaft of the penis or on the scrotum.

—predominantly affects uncircumcised men.

—has peak incidence after the fifth decade.

—evolves into invasive carcinoma in less than 10% of cases.

—is associated with an increased risk of visceral malignancy.

b. Erythroplasia of Queyrat

—usually presents as a single erythematous plaque, most often involving the glans penis or prepuce.

—occurs predominantly in uncircumcised men.

—has a median incidence in the fifth decade.

—progresses to invasive squamous cell carcinoma in approximately 10% of cases.

—may be a variant of Bowen's disease.

—is not associated with visceral malignancies.

c. Bowenoid papulosis

—histologically resembles Bowen's disease and erythroplasia of Queyrat but is considered to be a distinct entity.

—differs from Bowen's disease and erythroplasia of Queyrat in clinical presentation, appearing as multiple verrucoid (wart-like) lesions often resembling condyloma acuminatum and containing human papillomavirus (HPV) type 16 viral sequences.

—affects younger age group than Bowen's disease and erythroplasia of Queyrat.

—is not known to progress to invasive carcinoma but is generally considered premalignant.

2. Carcinoma

—is most frequently squamous cell carcinoma.

—is rare in circumcised men.

—is markedly increased in incidence in the Far East, Africa, and Central America.

—is predisposed by poor personal hygiene and venereal disease.

—is often associated with HPV infection types 16 and 18.

II. Diseases of the Testes

A. Cryptorchidism

—is developmental failure of a testis to descend into the scrotum.

—is associated with a markedly increased incidence of germ cell tumors, especially seminoma and embryonal carcinoma.

—is associated with testicular atrophy and sterility.

B. Torsion of the spermatic cord

—compromises blood supply.

—may result in testicular gangrene.

C. Hydrocele

—is serous fluid filling and distending the tunica vaginalis.

—is most often idiopathic.

—is sometimes congenital in origin due to persistence of continuity of the tunica vaginalis with the peritoneal cavity.

—can be secondary to infection or to lymphatic blockage by tumor.

D. Hematocele

—is an accumulation of blood distending the tunica vaginalis.

—is most often due to trauma.

—is occasionally due to tumor.

E. Varicocele

—is a varicose dilatation of the veins of the spermatic cord.

F. Spermatocele

—is a sperm-containing cyst.

—is most often intratesticular.

G. Testicular atrophy

—is often of unknown cause.

—may be caused by or associated with:

1. Orchitis, especially mumps orchitis

2. Trauma

3. Hormonal excess or deficiency due to:

    a. Disorders of the hypothalamus or pituitary

    b. Hormonal therapy, especially with estrogens

    c. Cirrhosis of the liver

4. Cryptorchidism

5. Klinefelter's syndrome

6. Chronic debilitating disease

7. Old age

H. Inflammation

1. Orchitis

–when bacterial, is often associated with epididymitis.

–when viral, is most often due to mumps virus.

–may be caused by syphilis.

–when bilateral, may result in sterility.

2. Epididymitis

–is more common than orchitis.

–is most often caused by:

a. *Neisseria gonorrhoeae*

b. *Chlamydia trachomatis*

c. *Escherichia coli*

d. *Mycobacterium tuberculosis*

I. Testicular tumors (Table 18.1)

–are most often malignant; more than 90% are of germ cell origin.

1. Seminoma

–is a malignant germ cell tumor.

–is analogous to dysgerminoma, a tumor of the ovary.

–is the most frequently occurring germ cell tumor, accounting for 40%.

–has peak incidence in the mid-30s age group.

–presents as painless enlargement of the testis.

–is radiosensitive and often curable.

2. Embryonal carcinoma

–is a malignant germ cell tumor.

–is analogous to a similar tumor occurring in the ovary.

–accounts for 20% to 30% of germ cell tumors.

–often presents with pain or metastasis.

–has a much worse prognosis than seminoma.

3. Endodermal sinus (yolk sac) tumor

–is a malignant germ cell tumor.

–is analogous to endodermal sinus of the ovary.

–has peak incidence in infancy and early childhood.

–causes an **increase in serum alpha-fetoprotein,** the same tumor marker that is associated with hepatocellular carcinoma.

4. Teratoma

–is a germ cell tumor derived from two or more embryonic layers.

–is most frequently malignant.

–contains multiple tissue types, such as cartilage islands, ciliated epithelium, liver cells, neuroglia, embryonic gut, or striated muscle.

–can be subclassified into:

a. Mature teratoma

–is almost always malignant, while the corresponding ovarian tumor (dermoid cyst) is almost always benign.

Table 18.1. World Health Organization Classification of Testicular Tumors

Types	Comments
Germ cell tumors	More than 90% of testicular tumors are of germ cell origin
Tumors of one histologic type:	
Seminoma	Most frequently occurring germ cell tumor; peak incidence age 35
Spermatocytic seminoma	Older age group; more favorable prognosis
Embryonal carcinoma	Second most frequently occurring germ cell tumor; often presents with pain or metastasis; somewhat younger age incidence than seminoma
Yolk sac tumor (embryonal carcinoma, infantile type; endodermal sinus tumor)	Peak incidence infancy and early childhood
Polyembryoma	
Choriocarcinoma	
Teratoma	
Mature	Almost always malignant
Immature	
With malignant transformation	Malignant change of one of the tissues within a teratoma (e.g., development of squamous cell carcinoma within epidermoid component)
Tumors of more than one histologic type:	Combinations include mixes of seminoma, embryonal carcinoma, teratoma, and choriocarcinoma
Embryonal carcinoma and teratoma (teratocarcinoma)	
Choriocarcinoma and any other type (specify)	
Other combinations (specify)	
Stromal sex-cord tumors	
Well-differentiated forms:	
Leydig cell tumor	Usually benign; often causes precocious puberty
Sertoli cell tumor	Usually benign; usually no endocrine manifestations
Granulosa cell tumor	
Mixed forms (specify)	
Incompletely differentiated forms	

    b. Immature teratoma

    c. Teratoma with malignant transformation

        —contains malignant tissue such as squamous cell carcinoma.

   5. Choriocarcinoma

      —is a malignant germ cell tumor.

      —is analogous to choriocarcinoma of the ovary.

      —can occur as an element of other germ cell tumors.

      —has peak incidence in the second to third decades.

      —is characterized histologically by cells resembling syncytiotrophoblasts and cytotrophoblasts.

      —causes an increase in serum human chorionic gonadotropin (HCG), which is a diagnostically important marker.

6. Mixed germ cell tumors

–are composed of varying combinations of germ cell tumor types.

–can be teratocarcinoma, that is, a combination of teratoma and embryonal carcinoma, which is associated with poor prognosis.

–are of variable prognosis as determined by the least mature element.

–also can occur in other combinations, including:

a. Teratoma, embryonal carcinoma, and seminoma

b. Embryonal carcinoma and seminoma

7. Leydig cell (interstitial) tumor

–is a non-germ cell tumor derived from testicular stroma.

–is similar to the Sertoli-Leydig cell tumor of the ovary.

–is most often benign.

–is often characterized by intracytoplasmic Reinke crystals.

–is characteristically androgen-producing but sometimes produces both androgens and estrogens and sometimes corticosteroids.

–is most often associated with precocious puberty in children and with gynecomastia in adults.

8. Sertoli cell tumor (androblastoma)

–is a non-germ cell tumor derived from the sex cord–stroma.

–is also similar to the Sertoli-Leydig cell tumor of the ovary.

–is usually benign.

–is characterized by a paucity of endocrine manifestations.

III. Diseases of the Prostate

A. Anatomy of the prostate

–is a chestnut-sized and -shaped structure that surrounds the urethra at the base of the bladder.

–is comprised of two groups of glands.

1. The inner group of mucosal and submucosal glands draining via short ducts into the urethra is equivalent to the older designation of anterior, middle, and lateral lobes; it is often the site of benign prostatic hyperplasia (BPH).

2. The peripheral group of glands draining into ducts entering the urethral sinus close to the verumontanum is equivalent to the older designation of posterior lobe; it is the characteristic site for carcinoma.

B. Benign prostatic hyperplasia (benign nodular hyperplasia)

–is the most frequent cause of urinary tract obstruction.

–is extremely common (almost universal) in the older age group.

–may be due to an age-related increase in estrogens (estrogens promote expression of receptors for residual dihydrotestosterone, which promotes prostatic growth even though testosterone is decreased).

–is characterized by hyperplasia of both glandular and fibromuscular stromal elements.

–is characterized grossly by a rubbery, nodular enlargement of the gland, primarily affecting the **inner group of glands** (lateral and middle lobes).

–causes the urethra to be compressed side to side, resulting in a vertical slit.

−most characteristically results in **urinary obstruction,** which is manifest by:

1. Distention and muscular hypertrophy of the bladder; in cases of long duration, bands of enlarged bladder muscle form characteristic trabeculae.

2. Incomplete bladder emptying

3. Frequency, dysuria, hesitancy (difficulty in starting urination), and urinary tract infection

4. Hydroureter and hydronephrosis

C. Adenocarcinoma

−is extremely common.
−occurs in the older age group.
−arises most often from the peripheral group of glands (posterior lobe).
−is most often diagnosed by rectal examination.
−is characterized by increased serum prostatic acid phosphatase when the tumor penetrates the capsule into adjacent tissues. Another useful tumor marker is prostate-specific antigen.
−may frequently progress to bony osteoblastic metastasis, which, unfortunately, may be the presenting sign. In this instance, an increase in serum alkaline phosphatase is often an indicator of osteoblastic lesions.

Review Test

Directions: Each of the numbered items or incomplete statements in this section is followed by answers or by completions of the statement. Select the **one** lettered answer or completion that is **best** in each case.

1. All of the following penile lesions are correctly matched with the appropriate definition or association EXCEPT

(A) hypospadias—abnormal location of urethral meatus.
(B) phimosis—tight foreskin.
(C) priapism—intractable erection.
(D) balanitis—inflammation of glans penis.
(E) chancre—secondary syphilis.

2. All of the following testicular tumors are correctly matched with the appropriate definition or association EXCEPT

(A) seminoma—most common germ cell tumor.
(B) endodermal sinus (yolk sac) tumor—occurs in infancy and early childhood.
(C) teratoma—almost always malignant.
(D) choriocarcinoma—increased human chorionic gonadotropin.
(E) Sertoli cell tumor—frequent precocious sexual development.

Directions: Each group of items in this section consists of lettered options followed by a set of numbered items. For each item, select the **one** lettered option that is most closely associated with it. Each lettered option may be selected once, more than once, or not at all.

Questions 3 and 4

Match each of the following associations with the disease that is most closely linked to it.

(A) Bowen's disease of the penis
(B) Erythroplasia of Queyrat
(C) Carcinoma of the penis

3. Visceral malignancies

4. Human papillomavirus infection

Answers and Explanations

1–E. The chancre, an elevated, painless, superficially ulcerated papular lesion of the glans penis or prepuce, is a manifestation of primary, not secondary, syphilis.

2–E. The Sertoli cell tumor (androblastoma), a benign non-germ cell tumor of sex cord derivation, is most often associated with few, if any, clinically observable endocrine effects. This is in contrast to the Leydig cell (interstitial) tumor, another benign sex cord tumor, which is often associated with profound endocrine manifestations.

3–A. Bowen's disease of the penis is associated with an increased risk for visceral malignancy, in contrast to erythroplasia of Queyrat, a similar lesion that is not associated with visceral malignancy.

4–C. Carcinoma of the penis may be caused by human papillomavirus (HPV) infection (types 16 and 18), the same viral agents with a probable etiopathogenetic role in carcinoma of the cervix. HPV type 16 viral association is also noteworthy in bowenoid papulosis, one of the three forms of penile carcinoma in situ.

19

Female Reproductive System and Breast

I. Vulva and Vagina

A. Miscellaneous disorders

1. Bartholin's cyst

- —is due to **obstruction of Bartholin's ducts**.
- —can become secondarily infected, most often by *Neisseria gonorrhoeae* or, less often, by *Staphylococcus*.

2. Vulvar dystrophies

- —are a group of disorders of **epithelial growth** that often present with leukoplakia, a white, patch-like lesion.

a. Histologic forms

(1) **Lichen sclerosus** and **hyperplastic dystrophy,** which have no malignant potential

(2) **Atypical hyperplastic dystrophy,** a premalignant lesion

b. Clinical characteristics

- —include **pruritus** and **leukoplakia,** which can be a manifestation of several diverse processes and should be evaluated by biopsy.

B. Infectious disorders

1. Candidiasis (moniliasis)

- —is the **most common** form of vaginitis.
- —is caused by *Candida albicans,* a normal inhabitant of the vaginal flora.
- —is associated with diabetes mellitus, pregnancy, broad-spectrum antibiotic therapy, oral contraceptive use, and immunosuppression.
- —is characterized by a thick white discharge and vulvovaginal pruritus.

2. Trichomoniasis

- —is the second most common type of vaginitis.
- —is caused by *Trichomonas vaginalis*.
- —is most often transmitted by sexual contact.

3. Gardnerella vaginitis

- —is caused by *Gardnerella vaginalis*.

—accounts for many cases formerly classified as nonspecific vaginitis.

—is usually transmitted by sexual contact.

—is often discovered by finding characteristic "clue cells," epithelial cells containing dot-like organisms in Papanicolaou smear preparations.

4. Toxic shock syndrome

—was initially associated with the use of highly absorbent tampons.

—is caused by exotoxin produced by *Staphylococcus aureus,* which grows in the tampon.

—is characterized by fever, vomiting, and diarrhea, sometimes followed by renal failure and shock; generalized rash is followed by desquamation.

5. Gonorrhea

—is a frequent cause of pelvic inflammatory disease.

—is caused by *N. gonorrhoeae*.

—is transmitted by sexual contact.

—can be asymptomatic but infectious.

—is characterized by purulent acute inflammation, initially of the urethra, paraurethral and Bartholin's glands, and Skene's ducts.

—can ascend to infect the endocervix, uterine canal, and fallopian tubes.

—can result in extragenital infections, including:

a. Pharyngitis associated with orogenital sexual contact

b. Proctitis associated with anal intercourse

c. Purulent arthritis, which is most often monoarticular, involving a large joint, such as the knee, as a consequence of blood-borne infection

d. Ophthalmia neonatorum, a neonatal conjunctival infection acquired at delivery

6. Chlamydial infections

a. Chlamydial cervicitis

—is the **most common sexually transmitted disease**.

—is a frequent cause of pelvic inflammatory disease.

—is due to certain serotypes of *Chlamydia trachomatis*.

—is most often asymptomatic.

b. Lymphogranuloma venereum

—occurs primarily in the tropics.

—is caused by *C. trachomatis* L1, L2, or L3 serotypes.

—is manifest initially as a small papule or ulcer, followed by superficial ulcers and enlargement of regional lymph nodes, which become matted together.

—can lead to rectal stricture as a result of inflammatory reaction and scarring.

7. Herpes simplex virus (HSV) infections

—HSV type 2 infection accounts for the majority of genital herpes cases and is spread by sexual contact.

—produces small vesicles and shallow ulcers that can involve the cervix, vagina, clitoris, vulva, urethra, and perianal skin.

—multinucleated giant cells with viral inclusions are found in cytologic smears from lesions.

8. Syphilis

–is caused by *Treponema pallidum* and is transmitted by sexual contact.

–is manifest in the initial stage of primary syphilis by a firm, painless ulcer known as a chancre, which is usually not apparent clinically.

–is sometimes manifest during secondary syphilis as condyloma lata, which are gray, flattened wartlike lesions.

–is a hazard during pregnancy since spirochetes can cross the placenta and result in fetal malformation.

9. Chancroid

–is caused by *Haemophilus ducreyi.*

–is a sexually transmitted disease.

–is most common in tropical areas; it is rare in the United States.

–is characterized by a soft and painful ulcerated lesion in contrast to chancre of syphilis, which is firm and painless.

10. Granuloma inguinale

–is caused by *Calymmatobacterium (Donovania) granulomatis,* a gram-negative rod.

–is probably sexually transmitted.

–is characterized by **Donovan bodies,** multiple organisms filling large histiocytes, an important diagnostic histopathologic feature.

–appears initially as a papule, which becomes superficially ulcerated.

–progresses by adjacent lesions coalescing to form large genital or inguinal ulcerations, sometimes with lymphatic obstruction or genital distortion.

C. Neoplasms of the vulva (Table 19.1)

1. Papillary hidradenoma

–is the most common benign tumor of the vulva.

–originates from apocrine sweat glands.

–presents as a labial nodule; may ulcerate and bleed.

–is cured by simple excision.

2. Condyloma acuminatum

–is a benign squamous cell papilloma caused by **human papillomavirus (HPV),** most frequently HPV types 6 and 11.

–is transmitted by sexual contact.

–is manifest clinically by multiple wart-like lesions, **venereal warts,** in vulvovaginal and perianal regions, and sometimes on the cervix.

–is characterized histologically by **koilocytes,** expanded epithelial cells with perinuclear clearing.

3. Squamous cell carcinoma

–is the most common malignant tumor of the vulva.

–has its peak occurrence in older women.

–may be preceded by vulvar dystrophy.

–is often associated with HPV infection type 16 or 18.

4. Paget's disease of the vulva

–is similar to Paget's disease of the breast.

–is sometimes associated with underlying adenocarcinoma of apocrine sweat glands.

Table 19.1 Comparison of Tumors of the Female Reproductive System

Type	Behavior	Location	Comments
Condyloma acuminatum (venereal wart)	Benign	Vulvovaginal, perianal, sometimes cervical	Most often multiple; etiologic agent HPV (types 6 and 11)
Squamous cell carcinoma	Malignant	Vulva	May be preceded by atypical hyperplastic dystrophy
Clear cell adenocarcinoma	Malignant	Vagina	Peak incidence in teenagers and young women exposed in utero to DES
Squamous cell carcinoma	Malignant	Vagina	Uncommon location for primary squamous cell carcinoma; more often due to extension of squamous cell carcinoma of the cervix
Squamous cell carcinoma	Malignant	Uterine cervix	Squamocolumnar junction most frequent site of origin; often preceded by dysplasia; HPV (types 16 and 18) is suspected to be the etiologic agent
Leiomyoma	Benign	Uterine corpus	Most frequently occurring neoplasm of women; most often multiple; increases in size during pregnancy; regresses with menopause
Endometrial carcinoma	Malignant	Uterine corpus	Peak incidence in older age group; predisposed by estrogen stimulation; incidence increasing
Cystadenoma, serous or mucinous	Benign	Ovary	
Cystadenocarcinoma, serous or mucinous	Malignant	Ovary	Rupture of mucinous form can lead to pseudomyxoma peritonei
Mature teratoma (dermoid cyst)	Benign	Ovary	Most frequent ovarian tumor
Choriocarcinoma	Malignant	Ovary or gestational tissue	Increased HCG in serum and urine
Fibroma	Benign	Ovary	Can be associated with Meigs' syndrome (ovarian fibroma, ascites, and hydrothorax)
Granulosa cell tumor	Benign	Ovary	Estrogen-secreting
Krukenberg tumors	Malignant	Ovaries	Metastatic replacement of ovaries with signet-ring cells from primary malignant tumor elsewhere (often from stomach)

HPV = human papillomavirus; DES = diethylstilbestrol; HCG = human chorionic gonadotropin.

5. Malignant melanoma

—accounts for approximately 10% of malignant tumors of the vulva.

D. Neoplasms of the vagina

1. Squamous cell carcinoma

—is most often due to extension of squamous cell carcinoma of the cervix.
—infrequently involves the vagina as the primary site.

2. Clear cell adenocarcinoma

—is a rare malignant tumor.
—is markedly increased in incidence in daughters of women who received **diethylstilbestrol (DES)** therapy during pregnancy. Clear cell adeno-carcinoma of the cervix and vaginal adenosis also may occur in these patients. Vaginal adenosis, a benign condition characterized by mucosal columnar epithelial-lined crypts in areas normally lined by stratified squamous epithelium, is thought to be a precursor of clear cell adenocarcinoma.

3. Sarcoma botryoides

—is a rare variant of rhabdomyosarcoma.
—occurs in children younger than age 5.
—presents as multiple polypoid masses resembling a "bunch of grapes" projecting into the vagina, often protruding from the vulva.

II. Uterine Cervix

A. Non-neoplastic disorders

1. Erosion

—is characterized by columnar epithelium replacing squamous epithelium, grossly resulting in an erythematous area.
—is sometimes a manifestation of chronic cervicitis.

2. Cervicitis

—can be caused by staphylococci, enterococci, *Gardnerella vaginalis, Trichomonas vaginalis, Candida albicans,* and *Chlamydia trachomatis.*
—most often involves the endocervix.
—is often asymptomatic.
—may be manifest by cervical discharge.

3. Cervical polyps

—are inflammatory proliferations of cervical mucosa; they are not true neoplasms.

B. Dysplasia and carcinoma in situ

—**squamocolumnar junction** is the most frequent site.
—**HPV infection** plays a likely etiopathogenetic role; HPV types 16 and 18 genomic sequences are often demonstrable.

1. Dysplasia

—is characterized by disordered epithelial growth manifest by loss of polarity and nuclear hyperchromasia, beginning at the basal layer and extending outward.

   a. **Mild dysplasia** involves about one-third of the thickness of the epithelium.

   b. **Moderate dysplasia** involves about one-half of the thickness of the epithelium.

   c. **Severe dysplasia** involves about two-thirds of the thickness of the epithelium.

2. **Carcinoma in situ**
   —is characterized by atypical changes extending through the entire thickness of the epithelium.
   —is sometimes classified with dysplasia under the term **cervical intraepithelial neoplasia (CIN),** with subtypes of CIN 1, CIN 2, or CIN 3, depending on the extent of epithelial involvement.

C. **Invasive carcinoma**
   —has peak occurrence in **middle-age** groups.
   —is most often **squamous cell carcinoma;** adenocarcinoma accounts for approximately 5% of cases.
   —evolves through a series of increasing epithelial abnormalities proceeding from dysplasia to carcinoma in situ and then to invasive carcinoma.
   —has exhibited a striking decrease in mortality since the introduction of the Papanicolaou cytologic screening (**Pap test**).

1. **Epidemiologic factors** (probable spread by sexual contact)

   a. **Early sexual activity** and **multiple sexual partners** are associated with increased incidence.

   b. Incidence is high in **prostitutes,** rare in celibates, and rare in some Jewish populations; traditional belief that circumcision of male sexual partners exerts a protective effect has not been confirmed.

   c. Incidence is increased in the economically deprived.

   d. **HSV-2** infection is a frequently associated finding, although the relationship remains unclear; the virus may act as a cocarcinogen with **HPV infection**.

2. **Role of HPV**

   a. Dysplastic cells frequently demonstrate **koilocytosis** (as in HPV-induced condyloma acuminatum).

   b. HPV sequences are often integrated into genomes of dysplastic or malignant cervical epithelial cells; HPV types 16 and 18 are most common, as in the majority of malignant genital squamous cell tumors, and are associated with over 90% of cases.

III. Uterine Corpus

A. Endometritis

1. Acute endometritis
   —is most often related to intrauterine trauma from instrumentation, intrauterine contraceptive devices, or complications of pregnancy, such as postpartum retention of placental fragments.

—is most often caused by *Staphylococcus aureus* or *Streptococcus* species.

2. Chronic specific (granulomatous) endometritis

—is most often tuberculous in etiology.

B. Endometriosis

—is characterized by the presence and proliferation of ectopic, **non-neoplastic** endometrial tissue.

—may be due to retrograde dissemination of endometrial fragments through fallopian tubes during menstruation, with implantation on the ovary or other peritoneal structures, or to blood-borne or lymphatic-borne dissemination of endometrial fragments.

—is characteristically responsive to hormonal variations of the menstrual cycle.

—is characterized by menstrual-type bleeding into the ectopic endometrium, resulting in blood-filled, or so-called "chocolate," cysts

—occurs most often in the pelvic area; the ovary is the most common site, followed by the uterine ligaments, rectovaginal septum, pelvic peritoneum, and other sites.

—is manifest clinically by severe **menstrual-related pain**.

—often results in infertility.

C. Adenomyosis

—is characterized by islands of endometrium within myometrium.

D. Endometrial hyperplasia

—is an abnormal proliferation of endometrial glands.

—is usually caused by **excess estrogen stimulation,** which in turn may be caused by anovulatory cycles, estrogen-secreting ovarian tumors such as the granulosa cell tumor, and estrogen medication.

—is most often manifest clinically by **vaginal bleeding**.

—is sometimes a precursor lesion of endometrial carcinoma; **the risk for carcinoma varies with the degree of cellular atypia**.

E. Endometrial polyp

—is a **benign** lesion.

—usually occurs in **women older than age 40**.

—may result in uterine bleeding.

F. Leiomyoma (fibroid)

—is the **most common uterine tumor** and the most common of all tumors in women; incidence is increased in **blacks**.

—is a **benign** neoplasm; putative malignant transformation is extremely rare.

—occurs in multiple separate foci in most cases.

—is **estrogen-sensitive**. The tumor often **increases in size during pregnancy,** and it almost always **decreases in size following menopause**.

—may be within the myometrium (intramural) or in subendometrial (submucous) or subperitoneal (subserous) locations. Leiomyomas, especially if subendometrial, are often manifest clinically by **vaginal bleeding**.

G. Leiomyosarcoma

—is a tumor that occurs infrequently.

—arises de novo and is almost never due to malignant transformation of a leio-myoma.

H. Endometrial carcinoma

—is increasing in incidence, in contrast to carcinoma of the cervix.
—is the **most common gynecologic malignancy**.
—is increased in incidence in association with nulliparity.
—has peak occurrence in the **older age group**.
—is most often manifest clinically by **vaginal bleeding**.
—is often preceded by endometrial hyperplasia.
—is predisposed by **prolonged estrogen stimulation** as occurs with exogenous estrogen therapy or estrogen-producing tumors.
—is also predisposed by obesity, diabetes, and hypertension; the common factor may be **obesity** because estrone can be synthesized in peripheral adipose tissues.

IV. Fallopian Tubes

A. Salpingitis

—is most often associated with **inflammation of the ovaries and other adjacent tissue** (pelvic inflammatory disease).
—is most often due to *N. gonorrhoeae,* various anaerobic bacteria, *C. trachomatis,* streptococci, and other pyogenic organisms.
—can be caused by trauma such as surgical manipulation.
—can result in **pyosalpinx,** a tube filled with pus, or **hydrosalpinx,** a tube filled with watery fluid; it also may result in **tubo-ovarian abscess**.

B. Hematosalpinx

—is bleeding into the fallopian tube.
—is most often caused by **ectopic pregnancy**.

C. Fallopian tube tumors

1. Adenomatoid tumor

—is the most frequent benign tumor of the fallopian tubes.

2. Adenocarcinoma

—most often results from direct extension or metastasis from tumors originating elsewhere.

V. Ovaries

A. Ovarian cysts

1. Follicular cyst

—is due to distention of the unruptured graafian follicle.
—is sometimes associated with hyperestrinism and endometrial hyperplasia.

2. Corpus luteum cyst

—results from hemorrhage into a persistent mature corpus luteum.
—is symptomatically associated with menstrual irregularity, occasionally with intraperitoneal hemorrhage.

3. Theca-lutein cyst

    —results from **gonadotropin stimulation;** can be associated with chorio-carcinoma and hydatidiform mole.

    —is often multiple and bilateral.

    —is lined by luteinized theca cells.

4. Chocolate cyst

    —is a blood-containing cyst resulting from ovarian endometriosis with hemorrhage.

5. Polycystic ovary (Stein-Leventhal) syndrome

    —characteristically occurs in young women.

    —is an important cause of infertility.

    —is characterized clinically by **amenorrhea, infertility, obesity, and hirsutism**.

    —may be caused by **excess excretion of luteinizing hormone**.

    —is characterized morphologically by the following:

a. Markedly thickened ovarian capsule

b. Multiple small follicular cysts containing a granulosa cell layer and a luteinized theca interna

c. Cortical stromal fibrosis with islands of focal luteinization

B. Ovarian tumors

    —are categorized according to the World Health Organization (**WHO**) classification, which is based on the **site of origin** of the tumor. The tumors are divided as follows:

1. Tumors of surface epithelial origin

    —make up almost three-fourths of ovarian tumors.

    —occur in women older than age 20.

a. Serous tumors

    (1) Serous cystadenoma

        —is a benign cystic tumor lined with cells similar to fallopian tube epithelium.

        —accounts for approximately 20% of all ovarian tumors.

        —is frequently bilateral.

    (2) Serous cystadenocarcinoma

        —is malignant.

        —accounts for approximately **50% of ovarian carcinomas**.

        —is frequently bilateral.

b. Mucinous tumors

    (1) Mucinous cystadenoma

        —is a benign tumor characterized by multilocular cysts lined by mucus-secreting columnar epithelium and filled with mucinous material.

    (2) Mucinous cystadenocarcinoma

        —is a malignant tumor.

—can result through rupture or metastasis in **pseudomyxoma peritonei** with multiple peritoneal tumor implants, all producing large quantities of intraperitoneal mucinous material. Pseudomyxoma peritonei can also result from mucinous cystadenoma, carcinomatous mucocele of the appendix, and other mucinous tumors.

c. Endometrioid tumor
—histologically resembles endometrium.
—is usually malignant.

d. Clear cell tumor
—is a **rare** tumor that is almost always malignant.

e. Brenner tumor
—is a rare, benign tumor.
—is characterized by small islands of epithelial cells resembling bladder transitional epithelium interspersed within a fibrous stroma.

2. Tumors of germ cell origin
—make up one-fourth of ovarian tumors.
—account for most ovarian tumors occurring in women younger than age 20.

a. Dysgerminoma
—is homologous to testicular seminoma.
—is malignant.

b. Endodermal sinus (yolk sac) tumor
—resembles extraembryonic yolk sac structures.
—produces **alpha-fetoprotein**.
—is homologous to endodermal sinus tumor of the testis.

c. Teratomas
—characteristically demonstrate tissue elements derived from **two or three embryonic layers**.
—are observed in three distinct forms:

(1) Immature teratoma
—is an aggressive malignant tumor.
—includes immature cellular elements.

(2) Mature teratoma (dermoid cyst)
—accounts for approximately 20% of ovarian tumors and 90% of germ cell tumors.
—is the most frequent benign ovarian tumor.
—is lined by skin, including hair follicles and other skin appendages; other elements often include bone; tooth; cartilage; and gastrointestinal, neurologic, respiratory, and thyroid gland tissues.
—may arise by reduplication of meiotic maternal chromosomes.

(3) Monodermal teratoma
—contains only a single tissue element; for example, the most common is **struma ovarii,** which consists entirely of thyroid tissue and can be hyperfunctional, resulting in hyperthyroidism.

d. Ovarian choriocarcinoma
—is an aggressive malignant tumor.
—secretes **human chorionic gonadotropin (HCG)**.

3. Tumors of ovarian sex cord–stromal origin

—account for a small percentage of ovarian neoplasms. All age groups are affected.

a. Thecoma–fibroma group of tumors

(1) Fibroma

—is a solid tumor consisting of bundles of spindle-shaped fibroblasts.

—can be associated with **Meigs' syndrome,** a triad of ovarian fibroma, ascites, and hydrothorax.

(2) Thecoma

—demonstrates round lipid-containing cells in addition to fibroblasts.

—is occasionally estrogen-secreting.

b. Granulosa cell tumor

—is **estrogen secreting** and a cause of precocious puberty.

—in adults, is associated with **endometrial hyperplasia** or **endometrial carcinoma**.

—consists of small cuboidal, deeply staining granulosa cells arranged in anastomotic cords.

—is characterized by **Call-Exner bodies,** small follicles filled with eosinophilic secretion, an important diagnostic feature.

c. Sertoli-Leydig cell tumor (androblastoma, arrhenoblastoma)

—is **androgen-secreting**.

—is associated with masculinization.

4. Tumors metastatic to the ovary

—account for approximately 5% of all ovarian tumors.

—are frequently of gastrointestinal tract, breast, or uterine origin.

—are termed **Krukenberg tumors** when ovaries are replaced bilaterally by mucin-secreting **signet-ring cells;** site of origin is often the stomach.

VI. Disorders of Pregnancy

A. Abnormalities of placental attachment

1. Abruptio placentae (placental abruption)

—is premature separation of the placenta.

—is an important cause of antepartum bleeding and fetal death.

—is often associated with **disseminated intravascular coagulation (DIC).**

2. Placenta accreta

—is attachment of the placenta directly to the myometrium; the decidual layer is defective.

—is predisposed by endometrial inflammation and old scars from prior cesarean sections or other surgery.

—is manifest clinically by impaired placental separation after delivery, sometimes with massive hemorrhage.

3. Placenta previa

—is an attachment of the placenta to the lower uterine segment.

—may partially or completely cover the cervical os.

—may coexist with placenta accreta.

—is often manifest by bleeding.

B. Ectopic pregnancy

—most often occurs in the fallopian tubes.

—can also occur in the ovary, abdominal cavity, or cervix.

—is most frequently predisposed by chronic salpingitis, often gonorrheal.

—is also predisposed by endometriosis and postoperative adhesions.

—frequently has no obvious cause.

—is the most common cause of **hematosalpinx**.

—may lead to tubal rupture.

C. Toxemia of pregnancy

—is a disorder characterized by a severe hypertension most often occurring de novo during pregnancy or complicating preexisting hypertensive disease.

—characteristically occurs during the third trimester, most often in the first pregnancy.

—occurs in two forms:

1. Preeclampsia, a milder form of toxemia characterized by hypertension, albuminuria, and edema

2. Eclampsia, a severe form of toxemia characterized, in addition, by convulsions and DIC; reverses rapidly on termination of pregnancy, but can be fatal.

D. Gestational trophoblastic disease

—includes disorders characterized by degenerative or neoplastic changes of trophoblastic tissue.

1. Hydatidiform mole

—is manifest by enlarged, edematous placental villi resembling a bunch of grapes.

—is marked by a diagnostically significant increase in **human chorionic gonadotropin (HCG)**.

—characteristically occurs in early months of pregnancy.

—is characterized clinically by vaginal bleeding and rapid increase in uterine size; may be associated with toxemia of pregnancy.

—eventuates to **choriocarcinoma** in 2% to 3% of cases.

—occurs in two variants:

a. Complete hydatidiform mole

—no embryo is present; 46,XX karyotype, of exclusively **paternal derivation (androgenesis)**.

b. Partial hydatidiform mole

—embryo is present; triploidy and tetraploidy sometimes occur, thought due to fertilization of the ovum by two or more spermatozoa.

2. Gestational choriocarcinoma

—is more frequent than ovarian choriocarcinoma.

—is an aggressive malignant neoplasm.

—is preceded by:

a. Hydatidiform mole in 50% of cases

    b. Abortion of ectopic pregnancy in 20% of cases

    c. Normal-term pregnancy in 20% to 30% of cases

      –is characterized by increased serum concentration of **HCG**, an important diagnostic sign.

      –is characterized by **early hematogenous spread** to the lungs.

      –is **responsive to chemotherapy**.

      –is markedly increased in incidence in Asia and Africa.

VII. Breast

A. Fibrocystic disease

–is the most common disorder of the breast.

–is the most common cause of a palpable breast mass in patients between the ages of 25 and 50 years.

–is uncommon before adolescence or after menopause.

–is clinically characterized by lumpy breasts with midcycle tenderness.

–is postulated to be due to increased activity of, or sensitivity to, estrogen or to decreased progesterone activity.

–is usually bilateral.

–is associated with a slightly increased incidence of cancer when epithelial hyperplasia is marked; **risk of cancer is clear when hyperplastic epithelium demonstrates atypia;** risk of cancer is not increased in nonproliferative fibrocystic disease.

–is morphologically characterized by:

1. Fibrosis of varying extent

2. Cysts are grossly visible or may be evident only on histologic examination; thus may be filled with fluid, which may appear blue when seen through the cyst wall (**blue dome cyst**).

3. Epithelial changes

–lining of the epithelium may be flattened, may show apocrine metaplasia, or may be hyperplastic.

–hyperplastic epithelium may show varying degrees of cellular atypia: **adenosis,** is the proliferation of small ducts and myoepithelial cells; when combined with fibrosis, is termed **sclerosing adenosis**.

B. Tumors of the breast

1. Fibroadenoma

–is the **most common breast tumor in women younger than age 25**.

–is **benign**.

–presents as a firm, rubbery, painless, well-circumscribed lesion.

–is morphologically well-demarcated from adjacent breast tissue; delicate fibrous stroma encloses the epithelial component consisting of gland-like or duct-like spaces lined by cuboidal or columnar cells.

–is subclassified into:

a. Intracanalicular fibroadenoma: stroma compresses and distorts glands into slitlike spaces

b. Pericanalicular fibroadenoma: glands retain round shape

2. Phyllodes tumor

–is a large, bulky mass of variable malignancy with ulceration of overlying skin.

–is characterized by cystic spaces containing leaf-like projections from the cyst walls and myxoid contents.

3. Adenoma of the nipple

–presents with serous or bloody discharge and a palpable mass.

–can be mistaken for malignancy.

4. Intraductal papilloma

–is a benign tumor of the major lactiferous ducts.

–is clinically manifest by serous or bloody discharge.

–must be distinguished from carcinoma.

5. Carcinoma of the breast (Table 19.2)

–is the second most common malignancy of women (carcinoma of the lung is most common).

–is the most common cause of a breast mass in postmenopausal patients.

–occurs most frequently in the **upper outer quadrant** of the breast.

–occurs in a number of histologic types (see Table 19.2), most frequently as invasive duct carcinoma.

–demonstrates **estrogen and progesterone receptors** in some tumors but not in others; presence is correlated with better prognosis and is thought to be a predictor of the efficacy of antiestrogen therapy.

Table 19.2. Histologic Types of Carcinoma of the Breast

Types	Characteristics
Intraductal carcinoma in situ (comedocarcinoma)	Tumor cells fill ducts; tumor cell necrosis results in cheese-like consistency
Invasive duct carcinoma (scirrhous carcinoma)	Most common type; characterized by tumor cells arranged in cords, islands, and glands embedded in a dense fibrous stroma; abundant fibrous tissue results in firm consistency
Paget's disease of the breast	Eczematoid lesion of the nipple or areola; neoplastic Paget cells, characteristic large cells surrounded by a clear halo-like area, invade the epidermis; underlying duct carcinoma almost always present
Lobular carcinoma in situ	Clusters of neoplastic cells fill intralobular ductules and acini; may lead to invasive carcinoma (often many years later) in same or in contralateral breast
Infiltrating lobular carcinoma	Often multicentric or bilateral
Medullary carcinoma	Cellular with scant stroma; soft, fleshy consistency; characteristic lymphocytic infiltrate; prognosis better than invasive duct carcinoma
Mucinous (colloid) carcinoma	Pools of extracellular mucus surrounding clusters of tumor cells; gelatinous consistency; prognosis better than invasive duct carcinoma
Inflammatory carcinoma	Lymphatic involvement of skin by underlying carcinoma, causing red, swollen, hot skin resembling an inflammatory process; poor prognosis

—is not predisposed by current regimens of oral contraceptive therapy. Conflicting data from some studies indicate a slightly increased risk with high-dose postmenopausal estrogen therapy.

—is predisposed by:

a. **Age:** incidence increases with increasing age.

b. **Positive family history:** incidence markedly increased in **first-degree female relatives** of patients with carcinoma of the breast

c. **History of breast cancer in one breast:** associated with increased incidence in the opposite breast

d. **Early menarche and late menopause:** may be due to increased duration of reproductive life and associated hormonal activity

e. **Obesity:** possibly due to production of estrogens by adipose tissue

f. **Nulliparity**

g. **First pregnancy after age 30**

h. **High animal fat diet:** incidence is five times higher in the United States than in Japan

i. **Fibrocystic disease with atypical epithelial hyperplasia**

j. **Oncogene activation: amplification of HER-2/neu gene** is frequently observed and is apparently correlated with less favorable prognosis.

Review Test

Directions: Each of the numbered items or incomplete statements in this section is followed by answers or by completions of the statement. Select the **one** lettered answer or completion that is **best** in each case.

1. A 24-year-old woman is seen because of high fever, prostration, vomiting, and diarrhea. Her pulse is rapid and thready, and her blood pressure is recorded at 60/40. A diffuse generalized macular rash is noted. Culture of which of the following specimens will most likely lead to the correct diagnosis?

(A) Sputum
(B) Urine
(C) Stool
(D) Cervical secretions
(E) Cerebrospinal fluid

2. Which one of the following lesions of the vulva, vagina, or cervix is found in daughters of women who received DES therapy during pregnancy?

(A) Sarcoma botryoides
(B) Clear cell adenocarcinoma
(C) Squamous cell carcinoma
(D) Papillary hidradenoma
(E) Paget's disease of the vulva

3. All of the following conditions or findings are correctly matched with the appropriate etiologic agents EXCEPT

(A) cervicitis—*Chlamydia trachomatis*.
(B) condyloma lata—*Treponema pallidum*.
(C) condyloma acuminatum—human papillomavirus (HPV).
(D) multinucleated giant cells—herpes simplex virus (HSV).
(E) granuloma inguinale—*Haemophilus ducreyi*.

4. The combination of pelvic inflammatory disease and monoarticular arthritis is suggestive of which of the following conditions?

(A) Chlamydial infection
(B) Gonorrhea
(C) HSV infection
(D) HPV infection
(E) Syphilis

5. All of the following conditions are correctly matched with the appropriate association EXCEPT

(A) endometriosis—severe menstrual pain.
(B) endometrial hyperplasia—excess estrogen stimulation.
(C) leiomyoma—postmenopausal decrease in size.
(D) endometrial carcinoma—multiparity.
(E) ectopic pregnancy—hematosalpinx.

6. The most likely cause of a 1-cm mass in the upper outer quadrant of the breast of a 65-year-old woman is

(A) fibrocystic disease.
(B) acute mastitis.
(C) fibroadenoma.
(D) carcinoma.
(E) Paget's disease of the breast

7. All of the following are associated with carcinoma of the breast EXCEPT

(A) high-fat diet.
(B) positive family history.
(C) obesity.
(D) early menarche.
(E) multiparity.

8. A 20-year-old woman presents with a solitary discrete, freely movable, firm, rubbery, non-tender, well-circumscribed breast lesion. On resection biopsy, the lesion appears similar to that shown in the illustration below. The most likely diagnosis is

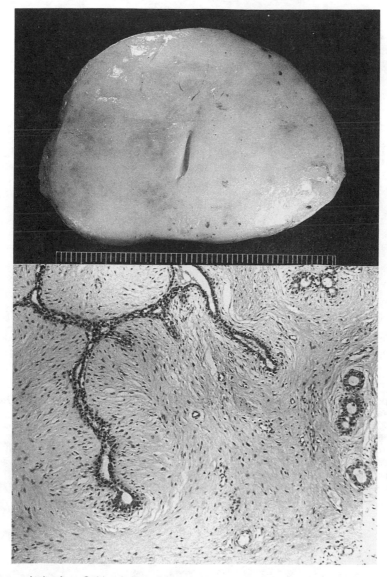

(Reprinted with permission from Golden A, Powell D, and Jennings C: *Pathology: Understanding Human Disease,* 2nd ed. Baltimore, Williams & Wilkins, 1985, p 447.)

(A) fibrocystic disease.
(B) fibroadenoma.
(C) medullary carcinoma.
(D) colloid carcinoma.
(E) intraductal carcinoma.

9. The cervical lesion shown in the illustration below is often characterized by

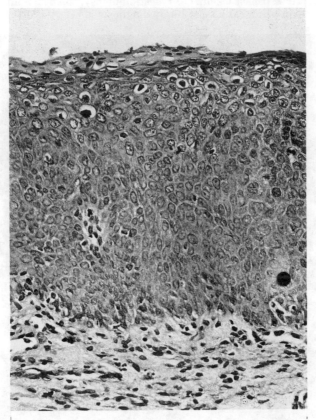

(Reprinted with permission from Golden A, Powell D, and Jennings C: *Pathology: Understanding Human Disease,* 2nd ed. Baltimore, Williams & Wilkins, 1985, p 413.)

(A) local invasion.
(B) penetration of the basement membrane.
(C) lymphatic spread.
(D) genomic integration of HPV viral seqences.
(E) hematogenous dissemination.

Directions: Each group of items in this section consists of lettered options followed by a set of numbered items. For each item, select the **one** lettered option that is most closely associated with it. Each lettered option may be selected once, more than once, or not at all.

Questions 10–13

Match each of the characteristics below with the condition with which it is associated.

(A) Dermoid cyst
(B) Struma ovarii
(C) Choriocarcinoma
(D) Fibroma

10. Hyperthyroidism

11. Fluid accumulations in serous cavities

12. Reduplication of meiotic chromosomes

13. Increased HCG

Questions 14–18

Match each of the characteristics below with the condition with which it is associated.

(A) Granulosa cell tumor
(B) Krukenberg tumor
(C) Abruptio placentae
(D) Preeclampsia
(E) Hydatidiform mole

14. Hypertension

15. Androgenesis

16. Signet-ring cells

17. Precocious puberty

18. DIC

Answers and Explanations

1–D. The association of a severe febrile illness with signs of gastrointestinal dysfunction and a diffuse macular rash is strongly suggestive of toxic shock syndrome. This diagnosis is especially likely if clinical abnormalities are associated with concomitant menstruation and the use of highly absorbent tampons. The clinical abnormalities are due to staphylococcal infection of the tampon, demonstrable in vaginal secretions, and the elaboration of staphylococcal exotoxins. The differential diagnosis includes streptococcal infection, usually in the throat, with a scarlatiniform eruption; meningococcemia; endotoxemia associated with a variety of gram-negative organisms; rickettsial infections, and so forth. Except for streptococcal infection, all of these conditions are less likely than toxic shock syndrome.

2–B. Clear cell adenocarcinoma of the vagina or cervix is found in daughters of women treated with DES therapy during pregnancy.

3–E. The etiologic agent of granuloma inguinale is *Calymmatobacterium granulomatis,* not *Haemophilus ducreyi,* which is the etiologic agent of chancroid, a sexually transmitted disease common in the tropics but rare in the U.S.

4–B. *N. gonorrhoeae,* the most frequent cause of PID, is sometimes complicated by purulent arthritis, which is often monoarticular, involving a large joint, such as the knee.

5–D. Endometrial carcinoma is associated with nulliparity, not multiparity. Other associations include obesity, diabetes, and hypertension, all predisposing conditions commonly associated with excess estrogen stimulation.

6–D. The location of the mass (the upper outer quadrant) and the age of the patient (65) suggest that the breast lesion is a carcinoma. A breast mass in a postmenopausal patient is most often a carcinoma.

7–E. Nulliparity, not multiparity, is an important association of breast cancer. Excess estrogen stimulation is common to long reproductive life, obesity, nulliparity or delayed first pregnancy, and exogenous estrogen therapy, all important associations of breast cancer. A history of breast cancer in first-degree female relatives and a diet high in animal fats are also epidemiologic factors.

8–B. Fibroadenoma is a benign tumor most often presenting as a single discrete, freely movable lesion, often demonstrating a pattern of compressed glands and young fibrous stroma similar to that shown in the illustration. Fibroadenoma is the most frequent cause of a palpable mass in the breast in women younger than age 25.

9–D. The illustration demonstrates dysplasia of the uterine cervix, which is characterized by disordered epithelial growth manifest by loss of polarity and nuclear hyperchromasia beginning at the basal layer and extending outward. In this illustration, the dysplastic changes involve about two-thirds of the epithelial thickness and would thus be classified as severe dysplasia (cervical intraepithelial neoplasia [CIN] grade 2 to 3). Although mild forms can be reversible, the principal significance of cervical dysplasia is its precursor role in the genesis of invasive cervical carcinoma. Invasion and metastases are not associated with dysplasia but only with fully developed invasive carcinoma. Genomic integration of HPV DNA sequences, most often types 16 and 18, is associated with cervical dysplasia as well as with frank malignant change.

10–B. The term struma is a synonym for goiter; struma ovarii is a form of teratoma in which thyroid tissue is prominent. The thyroid tissue may be hyperfunctional, resulting in hyperthyroidism.

11–D. The triad of hydrothorax, hydroperitoneum, and ovarian fibroma is known as Meigs' syndrome. The cause of this association is unknown.

12–A. All benign ovarian teratomas (dermoid cysts) are of 46,XX karyotype, and both isoenzyme and chromosome banding techniques suggest that these tumors are aberrant fetuses solely of maternal origin (parthenogenesis), arising after the first meiotic division.

13–C. Choriocarcinomas are functional tumors that secrete large amounts of HCG, a finding of major diagnostic significance.

14–D. Toxemia of pregnancy is characterized by severe hypertension often arising de novo during pregnancy; it characteristically occurs during the third trimester. Preeclampsia is a milder form of toxemia characterized by hypertension, albuminuria, and edema. Eclampsia, a more severe form of toxemia of pregnancy characterized, in addition, by convulsions and often by DIC, can be fatal.

15–E. Hydatidiform mole is thought to be a form of aberrant pregnancy in which the chromosomes are usually entirely of paternal origin (androgenesis). The chromosomes may be derived from fertilization of an ovum that has become devoid of maternal chromosomes.

16–B. Metastatic carcinoma to the ovary in which the ovary is replaced by metastatic mucus-secreting signet-ring cells is termed Krukenberg tumor. The site of origin is often the stomach.

17–A. The estrogen-secreting granulosa cell tumor is an important cause of precocious puberty.

18–C. Premature separation of the placenta is a well-known cause of DIC. Other obstetric difficulties associated with DIC are retained dead fetus and amniotic fluid embolism.

20

Endocrine System

I. Pituitary

A. Anterior pituitary (adenohypophysis) (Table 20.1)

1. **Cells and hormones**

a. **Somatotrophs**

—predominantly stain as **acidophils** with hematoxylin and eosin.
—secrete **growth hormone,** which stimulates production of somatomedins (a group of insulin-like growth factors synthesized in the liver and other tissues), which in turn stimulate growth in many tissues.

b. **Corticotrophs**

—predominantly stain as **basophils**.
—synthesize pro-opiomelanocortin (POMC), which then splits into:

(1) **Corticotropin (adrenocorticotropic hormone, or ACTH),** which controls adrenal glucocorticoid (mainly cortisol) and adrenal androgen secretion

(2) **β-lipotropin,** which is further split into **β-melanocyte-stimulating hormone (β-MSH), endorphins,** and **enkephalins**

c. **Thyrotrophs**

—vary in staining from basophilic to chromophobic.
—secrete **thyrotropin (thyroid-stimulating hormone, or TSH),** which stimulates growth of follicular cells of the thyroid and secretion of thyroid hormone.

d. **Gonadotrophs**

—vary in staining from basophilic to chromophobic.
—secrete **follicle-stimulating hormone (FSH)** and **luteinizing hormone (LH);** FSH stimulates production of ovarian graafian follicles; in females, LH is essential for ovulation and corpus luteum formation and function, and in males it stimulates production of testosterone by testicular interstitial cells.

Table 20.1. Pituitary Hyperfunction

Hormone	Lesion	Classic Staining of Tumor Cells	Manifestations
Prolactin	Prolactinoma	Chromophobic	Amenorrhea and galactorrhea in women; impotence and sometimes galactorrhea in men
Somatotropin (growth hormone)	Somatotropic adenoma	Acidophilic	Gigantism or acromegaly
Corticotropin (ACTH)	Corticotropic adenoma or multiple corticotropic microadenomas	Basophilic	Pituitary Cushing's syndrome
Antidiuretic hormone (ADH)	Nonpituitary lesions with ectopic hormone production (small cell carcinoma of the lung)		Water retention with dilutional hyponatremia

e. Lactotrophs
  —vary in staining from acidophilic to chromophobic.
  —secrete **prolactin (PRL),** which stimulates production of milk.

f. Nonsecretory cells
  —are probably resting forms of hormone-producing cells.
  —most often stain as chromophobes.

2. Anterior pituitary hyperfunction

a. Prolactinoma with hyperprolactinemia
  —is the **most common pituitary tumor** (30% of pituitary tumors).
  —staining is usually **chromophobic**.
  —in women, results in **amenorrhea** and **galactorrhea** (inappropriate milk secretion).
  —can be caused by hypothalamic lesions or by medications (methyldopa, reserpine) that interfere with dopamine (prolactin-inhibitory factor) secretion.
  —can also be associated with estrogen therapy.

b. Somatotropic adenoma with hypersecretion of growth hormone
  —is the second most common pituitary tumor.
  —staining is usually acidophilic (**acidophilic adenoma** is an older name for this tumor).
  —causes secondary hyperproduction of somatomedins by the liver. End-organ effects are caused by both growth hormone and somatomedins, especially somatomedin C (insulin-like growth factor-1, IGF-1).
  —results in **gigantism** if adenoma develops before epiphyseal closure.
  —results in **acromegaly** if adenoma develops after epiphyseal closure; acromegaly is characterized by overgrowth of the jaws, face, hands and feet, and generalized enlargement of viscera, along with hyperglycemia, osteoporosis, and hypertension.
  —can also result in local compression effects due to expansion of the tumor within the sella turcica.

c. Corticotropic adenoma and hypersecretion of ACTH

—results in increased production of adrenal cortical hormones (**hypercorticism**).

—is termed Cushing's syndrome or Cushing's disease (these terms are used in variable contexts by different authors).

(1) Cushing's disease

—classically refers to hypercorticism due to a corticotropic adenoma of the pituitary (most often a **basophilic adenoma**).

—also refers to hypercorticism associated with very small, sometimes multiple pituitary adenomas (**basophilic microadenomas**).

(2) Cushing's syndrome

—refers to hypercorticism regardless of cause.

—is most often of pituitary and less often of adrenal origin; some authors use the terms adrenal Cushing's syndrome and pituitary Cushing's syndrome for clarity.

—may be due to ectopic ACTH production by a variety of tumors (especially small cell carcinoma of the lung).

3. Anterior pituitary hypofunction

a. Pituitary cachexia (Simmonds' disease)

—is **generalized panhypopituitarism**.

—is characterized by marked wasting.

—can result from any process that destroys the pituitary.

—is most frequently caused by:

(1) Pituitary tumors

(2) Postpartum pituitary necrosis (Sheehan's syndrome)

—is due to ischemic necrosis of the pituitary gland, characteristically associated with hemorrhage and shock during childbirth.

—clinical manifestations are due at first to loss of gonadotropins, then to subsequent loss of TSH and ACTH.

b. Selective deficiency of one or more pituitary hormones

(1) Deficiency of growth hormone

—in children, results in growth retardation (**pituitary dwarfism**).

—in adults, may result in increased insulin sensitivity with hypoglycemia, decreased muscle strength, and anemia.

(2) Deficiency of gonadotropins

—in preadolescent children, results in retarded sexual maturation.

—in adults, results in loss of libido, impotence, loss of muscular mass, and decreased facial hair in men, and in amenorrhea and vaginal atrophy in women.

(3) Deficiency of TSH

—results in secondary hypothyroidism.

(4) Deficiency of ACTH

—results in secondary adrenal failure.

—does not result in hyperpigmentation of the skin, probably because of the lack of both ACTH and β-MSH; this is in contrast to primary adrenal failure (Addison's disease), in which ACTH is increased and hyperpigmentation is the rule.

B. Posterior pituitary (neurohypophysis)

1. Hormones

—are synthesized in the hypothalamus and transported via axons to the posterior pituitary.

a. Oxytocin

—induces uterine contraction during labor and ejection of milk from mammary alveoli.

b. Antidiuretic hormone (ADH, vasopressin)

—promotes water retention through action on the renal collecting ducts.

2. Inappropriate secretion of ADH

—is most commonly caused by ectopic production of ADH by a variety of tumors, such as **small cell carcinoma of the lung**.

—results in retention of water with consequent dilutional hyponatremia and inability to dilute the urine.

3. Deficiency of ADH

—results in **diabetes insipidus;** is characterized by polyuria, with consequent dehydration and insatiable thirst.

—can be caused by tumors, trauma, inflammatory processes, lipid storage disorders, and other conditions characterized by damage to the neurohypophysis or hypothalamus.

C. Nonfunctioning pituitary tumors

1. Nonsecreting pituitary adenomas

—are most often chromophobic.

—result in dysfunction because of local pressure phenomena.

—are clinically variable; manifestations include hypopituitarism, headache, visual disturbances (bilateral hemianopsia [loss of peripheral visual fields due to pressure on optic chiasm]), and palsies caused by cranial nerve damage.

2. Craniopharyngioma (adamantinoma)

—is a benign childhood tumor derived from Rathke's pouch.

—is not a true pituitary tumor.

—is similar to ameloblastoma of the jaw.

—is characterized by nests of squamous cells in a loose stroma, closely resembling the appearance of embryonic tooth bud enamel organ.

—is often cystic; lining epithelium of flat or columnar cells often expands into papillary projections.

—is often detected radiographically because of calcification.

II. Thyroid Gland

A. Thyroid hormones

—include **thyroxine (T_4)** and **triiodothyronine (T_3)**.

—synthesis depends upon sufficient quantities of iodine from dietary sources.

—the rate of extraction of iodine from the bloodstream and the rate at which T_4 and T_3 are synthesized and released from storage (as thyroglobulin) and secreted into the bloodstream are regulated by pituitary TSH.

—feedback mechanisms regulate pituitary production of TSH.

—serum T_3 and T_4 are bound to thyroid-binding globulin (TBG).

B. Congenital anomalies

1. Thyroglossal duct cyst

—is a remnant of the thyroglossal duct.

—is the most common thyroid anomaly.

2. Ectopic thyroid tissue

—may be found anywhere along the course of the thyroglossal duct.

C. Goiter

—is a general term for enlargement of the thyroid.

1. Causes

a. Physiologic enlargement

—is not uncommon in puberty and pregnancy.

b. Iodine deficiency

—occurs in geographic areas where diet is deficient in iodine.

c. Hashimoto's thyroiditis

d. Goitrogens

—are foods or drugs that suppress synthesis of thyroid hormones.

e. Dyshormonogenesis

—is partial or complete failure of thyroid hormone synthesis; can be caused by a variety of enzyme deficiencies.

2. Terminology

a. Simple goiter (nontoxic goiter)

—is goiter without thyroid hormone dysfunction.

b. Toxic goiter

—is goiter associated with hyperthyroidism; if the patient is euthyroid or hypothyroid, the term **nontoxic goiter** is appropriate.

c. Endemic goiter

—is goiter occurring with high frequency in iodine-deficient geographic areas; the term **sporadic goiter** is used for goiter caused by similar mechanisms in noniodine-deficient areas.

d. Nodular goiter

—is irregular enlargement of the thyroid, resulting in nodule formation.

—**nodular colloid goiter** refers to the late stage of simple goiter in which goiter is most often nodular; nodules may be single or multiple (multinodular goiter).

—most nodules are hypoplastic and do not take up radioactive iodine ("cold" nodules).

—occasionally nodules are hyperplastic and actively produce thyroid hormone and take up radioactive iodine ("hot" nodules).

D. Hypothyroidism

1. Laboratory abnormalities

a. Decreased serum T_3 and T_4, increased serum TSH

b. Increased serum cholesterol

c. Decreased T_3 resin uptake

—is also known as thyroid hormone-binding ratio (THBR).

—is inversely proportional to the number of unbound thyroid hormone binding sites on TBG; is measured by competitive uptake of radioactive T_3 by resin, which competes for unbound sites on TBG; T_3 resin uptake does not measure T_3.

2. Clinical syndromes

—hypothyroidism is manifest as myxedema in adults or as cretinism in children.

a. Myxedema

—is more common in women than in men.

(1) Causes

(a) Therapy for hyperthyroidism with surgery, irradiation, or drugs is the most common cause of myxedema in the U.S.

(b) Unknown cause—**primary idiopathic myxedema** is the second most common form of myxedema, which may be of autoimmune origin (TSH receptor-blocking antibodies have been identified).

(c) Hashimoto's thyroiditis

(d) Iodine deficiency is the most important cause in some geographic areas.

(2) Clinical characteristics

(a) Insidious onset

(b) Cold intolerance

(c) Tendency to gain weight because of low metabolic rate

(d) Lowered pitch of voice

(e) Mental and physical slowness

(f) Menorrhagia

(g) Constipation

(h) Abnormal physical findings:

(i) Puffiness of face, eyelids, and hands

(ii) Dry skin

(iii) Hair loss; coarse and brittle hair; scant axillary and pubic hair; thinning of the lateral aspect of the eyebrows

(iv) Increase in relaxation phase of deep tendon reflexes

b. Cretinism

(1) Causes

(a) Iodine deficiency

(b) Deficiency of enzymes necessary for the synthesis of thyroid hormones

(c) Maldevelopment of the thyroid gland

(d) Failure of the fetal thyroid to descend from its origin at the base of the tongue

(e) Transplacental transfer of antithyroid antibodies from a mother with autoimmune thyroid disease

(2) Characteristics

(a) Severe mental retardation

(b) Impairment of physical growth with retarded bone development and dwarfism

(c) Large tongue

(d) Protuberant abdomen

E. Hyperthyroidism (thyrotoxicosis)

1. Clinical features

a. Restlessness, irritability, fatigability

b. Tremor

c. Heat intolerance; sweating; warm, moist skin (especially of palms)

d. Tachycardia, often with arrhythmia and palpitation, sometimes with high-output cardiac failure

e. Muscle wasting and weight loss in spite of increased appetite

f. Fine hair

g. Diarrhea

h. Menstrual abnormalities; commonly amenorrhea or oligomenorrhea

i. Markedly increased T_3 and T_4; radioactive iodine uptake (RAIU) of thyroid increased; TSH markedly reduced

2. Graves' disease

a. General characteristics—Graves' disease

—is hyperthyroidism caused by diffuse toxic goiter.

—is often associated with striking exophthalmos (protrusion of the eyes), possibly due to autoimmune mechanisms and independent of thyroid hyperfunction.

—is manifest by the signs and symptoms of hyperthyroidism.

—occurs more frequently in women than in men.

—incidence is increased in HLA-DR3 and HLA-B8 positive individuals.

b. Mechanism

(1) Thyroid-stimulating immunoglobulin (TSI), an IgG antibody, reacts with thyroid follicle TSH receptors and stimulates thyroid hormone production.

(2) A similar reaction with **thyroid growth immunoglobulin (TGI)** stimulates glandular hyperplasia and enlargement.

(3) In addition to TSI and TGI, antimicrosomal and other autoantibodies are characteristic.

3. Other causes of hyperthyroidism

a. Plummer's syndrome

—hyperplastic nodules can result in hyperthyroidism without eye signs; the combination of hyperthyroidism, nodular goiter, and absence of exophthalmos is referred to as Plummer's disease. The nodules can be adenomas or non-neoplastic areas of nodular hyperplasia.

b. Pituitary hyperfunction

—can cause excess production of TSH and secondary hyperthyroidism.

c. Struma ovarii

—is an ovarian teratoma made up of thyroid tissue; can be hyperfunctional.

d. Exogenous administration of thyroid hormone

F. Thyroiditis

1. Hashimoto's thyroiditis

—is an **autoimmune disorder** that occurs more often in women than in men.

—is a common cause of hypothyroidism.

—is characterized clinically by a **slow, often inapparent course** and a modestly enlarged and nontender thyroid; the patient is euthyroid at first; transient hyperthyroidism may occur; hypothyroidism develops late when the gland is shrunken and scarred.

—is characterized histologically by **dense focal infiltrates of lymphocytes** with germinal center formation; thyroid follicles are atrophic.

—is associated with a variety of antithyroid antibodies, most prominently **anti-thyroglobulin and antimicrosomal antibodies;** may be associated with anti-TSH receptor antibodies, which may result in transient hyperthyroidism.

—may be associated with an increased incidence of other autoimmune disorders such as pernicious anemia, diabetes mellitus, and Sjögren's syndrome; incidence is increased in HLA-DR5 and HLA-B5 positive individuals.

2. Subacute (de Quervain's, granulomatous) thyroiditis

—is characterized by focal destruction of thyroid tissue and granulomatous inflammation.

—may be due to a variety of viral infections such as mumps or coxsackievirus.

—follows a self-limited course of several weeks' duration consisting of a flu-like illness along with pain and tenderness of the thyroid, sometimes with transient hyperthyroidism.

—is more common in women than in men.

3. Riedel's thyroiditis

—is characterized by thyroid replacement by fibrous tissue; it is of unknown origin.

—can clinically mimic carcinoma.

G. Benign tumors (adenomas) of the thyroid

—are most often solitary.

—present clinically as nodules.

—can occur in a variety of histologic patterns (follicular, Hürthle cell, and others).

—are most often nonfunctional but on occasion can cause hyperthyroidism.

H. Malignant tumors of the thyroid

1. Papillary carcinoma

—is the **most common thyroid cancer**.

—is characterized histologically by papillary projections into gland-like spaces; tumor cells have characteristic "ground-glass" nuclei; calcified spheres may be present (psammoma bodies).

—has a **better prognosis than other forms of thyroid cancer,** even when adjacent lymph nodes are involved.

2. Follicular carcinoma

—is characterized histologically by relatively uniform follicles.

—has a poorer prognosis than papillary carcinoma.

3. Medullary carcinoma

—is a form of APUDoma (amine precursor uptake and decarboxylation) originating from C cells of the thyroid.

—produces calcitonin, a calcium-lowering hormone.

—is characterized histologically by sheets of tumor cells in an amyloid-containing stroma.

—can be associated with multiple endocrine neoplasia (MEN) syndrome type IIa and type IIb.

4. Undifferentiated carcinoma

—tends to occur in older patients.

—has a very poor prognosis.

III. Parathyroid Glands

A. Parathyroid hormone (parathormone, PTH)

—secretion is not under pituitary control.

—is responsive to the plasma concentration of ionized calcium; decreased calcium concentration stimulates PTH production.

B. Hyperparathyroidism (Table 20.2)

1. Primary hyperparathyroidism

—is most often caused by **parathyroid adenoma;** a minority of cases are caused by primary **parathyroid hyperplasia;** carcinoma is rarely a cause.

Table 20.2. Hyperparathyroidism

Causes	Clinical Manifestations	Laboratory Abnormalities
Primary: Parathyroid adenoma, hyperplasia, or carcinoma; parathyroid hormone-like hormone production by tumors elsewhere; MEN type I and type IIa	Osteitis fibrosa cystica; metastatic calcification in many tissues; nephrocalcinosis and renal calculi	Increased PTH; hypercalcemia and hypercalciuria; hypophosphatemia and decreased tubular reabsorption of phosphorus; increased alkaline phosphatase
Secondary: Hypocalcemia (usually due to renal disease)	Diffuse osteoclastic bone disease; metastatic calcification	Increased PTH; hypocalcemia (may be slightly reduced); hyperphosphatemia; increased alkaline phosphatase

MEN = multiple endocrine neoplasia syndromes; PTH = parathyroid hormone.

—is less commonly caused by **production of PTH-like hormone by non-parathyroid malignant tumors** such as bronchogenic squamous cell carcinoma or renal cell carcinoma.

—can occur as part of MEN type I and type IIa.

a. Laboratory findings
   (1) Hypercalcemia and hypercalciuria
   (2) Decreased serum phosphorus, decreased tubular reabsorption of phosphorus, and increased serum alkaline phosphatase
   (3) Increased serum PTH

b. Clinical characteristics
   (1) **Osteitis fibrosa cystica,** cystic changes in bone due to osteoclastic resorption; it is also known as von Recklinghausen's disease of bone; fibrous replacement of resorbed bone may lead to formation of non-neoplastic tumor-like masses (**"brown tumor"**).
   (2) Metastatic calcification affecting various tissues, especially the kidneys (**nephrocalcinosis**)
   (3) **Renal calculi,** a frequent complication
   (4) Peptic duodenal ulcer; hypercalcemia predisposes to peptic ulcer

2. Secondary hyperparathyroidism

—is compensatory parathyroid hyperplasia in response to decreased concentration of serum ionized calcium.

—is **most commonly caused by hypocalcemia of chronic renal disease**. Vitamin D conversion by the kidney to biologically active 1,25-$(OH)_2D_3$ is impeded, resulting in decreased intestinal absorption of calcium; also, the increased serum phosphorus of renal disease induces a reciprocal decrease in serum calcium.

—is characterized by decreased serum calcium, increased serum phosphorus, and increased serum alkaline phosphatase; diffuse osteoclastic bone disease; and metastatic calcification. PTH is increased.

3. Tertiary hyperparathyroidism

—is persistent parathyroid hyperfunction in spite of correction of hypocalcemia and preexisting secondary hyperparathyroidism.

—is often caused by development of an adenoma in a previously hyperplastic gland.

C. Hypoparathyroidism

—is most commonly caused by accidental surgical excision during thyroidectomy.

—in rare instances is associated with congenital thymic hypoplasia (Di-George's syndrome).

—is characterized by severe hypocalcemia manifest clinically by increased neuromuscular excitability and tetany.

D. Pseudohypoparathyroidism

—is an autosomal recessive disorder.

—is characterized by renal end-organ unresponsiveness to PTH and by shortened fourth and fifth metacarpals and metatarsals, short stature, and other skeletal abnormalities.

—similar skeletal abnormalities, without parathyroid hormone dysfunction, characterize a rare entity termed pseudopseudohypoparathyroidism.

IV. Adrenal Glands (Table 20.3)

A. Cushing's syndrome (hypercorticism)

1. Causes

—results from increased circulating glucocorticoids, primarily cortisol.

a. Hyperproduction of ACTH by corticotrophs of the pituitary (most common)

b. Exogenous corticosteroid medication

c. Adrenal cortical adenoma or adrenal carcinoma (less common than adenoma)

d. Ectopic production of ACTH by nonpituitary carcinomas, especially small cell carcinoma of the lung

2. Morphologic changes in adrenal gland

a. Bilateral hyperplasia of the adrenal zone fasciculata

—occurs when the syndrome results from ACTH stimulation.

b. Adrenal cortical atrophy

—is seen when exogenous glucocorticoid medication is the cause.

c. Adrenal cortical adenoma or carcinoma

3. Clinical characteristics

a. Redistribution of body fat with round moon face, dorsal "buffalo hump,"

Table 20.3. Adrenal Endocrine Syndromes

Syndrome	Usual Anatomic Lesion	Comments
Cortex:		
Cushing's syndrome (hypercorticism)	Bilateral hyperplasia of adrenal zona fasciculata secondary to hyperactivity of pituitary corticotrophs or to ectopic ACTH-like production by a variety of tumors; adrenal cortical adenoma	May be of pituitary or adrenal origin; can also result from administration of exogenous hormone
Hyperaldosteronism (aldosteronism):		
Primary	Adenoma or hyperplasia of zona glomerulosa	Serum renin decreased
Secondary	Bilateral hyperplasia of zona glomerulosa caused by stimulation of renin-angiotensin system	Serum renin increased; frequently secondary to edema, regardless of cause
Adrenal virilism	Adenoma, carcinoma, or hyperplasia of zona reticularis	May be due to hyperplasia resulting from congenital enzyme deficiencies such as 21-hydroxylase and 11-hydroxylase
Hypocorticism	Idiopathic adrenal atrophy	Probable autoimmune etiology
	Tuberculosis	Most common cause of Addison's disease in prior years
	Infection	Waterhouse-Friderichsen syndrome most often associated with meningococcal infection
Medulla:		
Pheochromocytoma	Chromaffin cell tumor	Tumor secretes catecholamines (epinephrine and norepinephrine) and causes secondary hypertension

often with relatively thin extremities caused by muscle wasting; skin atrophy with easy bruising and purplish striae, especially over the abdomen; and hirsutism

b. Muscle weakness, osteoporosis, amenorrhea, hypertension, hyperglycemia, and psychiatric dysfunction

B. Hyperaldosteronism

1. Primary aldosteronism (Conn's syndrome)

—is caused by primary hyperproduction of adrenal mineralocorticoids.

—usually results from an aldosterone-producing adrenocortical adenoma (**aldosteronoma**).

—can also result from hyperplasia of the zona glomerulosa.

—rarely may be due to adrenocortical carcinoma.

—is characterized clinically by hypertension, sodium and water retention, and hypokalemia, often with hypokalemic alkalosis.

—demonstrates **decreased serum renin** due to negative feedback of increased blood pressure on renin secretion.

2. Secondary aldosteronism

—is secondary to renal ischemia, renal tumors, and edema (e.g., cirrhosis, nephrotic syndrome, cardiac failure).

—is caused by stimulation of the renin-angiotensin system.

—demonstrates **increased serum renin,** in contrast to primary aldosteronism.

C. Adrenal virilism (adrenogenital syndrome)

1. Causes

a. Congenital enzyme defects

—result in diminished cortisol production, compensatory increased ACTH, with resultant adrenal hyperplasia with androgenic steroid production.

(1) 21-hydroxylase deficiency, which is most common, results in salt loss and hypotension.

(2) 11-hydroxylase deficiency, a less common cause, results in salt retention and hypertension.

b. Tumors of the adrenal cortex

2. Clinical characteristics of adrenal virilism

—produces virilism in females and precocious puberty in males.

D. Hypocorticism (adrenal hypofunction)

—can be of primary adrenal cause or secondary to hypothalamic or pituitary dysfunction.

—is characterized by deficiency of glucocorticoids (primarily cortisol), often with associated mineralocorticoid deficiency.

1. Addison's disease (primary adrenocortical deficiency)

—is most commonly due to **idiopathic (probably autoimmune) adrenal atrophy**.

—can also be caused by tuberculosis, metastatic tumor, and a variety of infections.

—is characterized by hypotension; increased pigmentation of skin; decreased serum sodium, chloride, glucose, and bicarbonate; and increased serum potassium.

2. Waterhouse-Friderichsen syndrome

—is catastrophic adrenal insufficiency and vascular collapse due to hemorrhagic necrosis of the adrenal cortex.

—is often associated with disseminated intravascular coagulation.

—is characteristically due to **meningococcemia,** most often in association with meningococcal meningitis.

E. Tumors of the adrenal medulla

1. Pheochromocytoma

—is derived from **chromaffin cells of the adrenal medulla;** if derived from extra-adrenal chromaffin cells, it is termed paraganglioma.

—is most often **benign;** 10% are malignant.

—is an uncommon but important cause of surgically correctible hypertension resulting from hyperproduction of epinephrine and norepinephrine by the tumor; the hypertension is usually paroxysmal (episodic) but may be persistent.

—is characterized by **increased urinary excretion of catecholamines and their metabolites** (metanephrine, normetanephrine, and vanillylmandelic acid [VMA]).

—can be part of MEN type IIa or type IIb.

—can also be associated with neurofibromatosis or with von Hippel-Lindau disease.

2. Neuroblastoma

—is a highly **malignant** catecholamine-producing tumor of early childhood.

—usually originates in the adrenal medulla.

—occasionally converts into a more differentiated form termed ganglioneuroma.

—is characterized by **amplification** of the *N-myc* oncogene with thousands of gene copies per cell.

a. Amplification results in characteristic karyotypic changes (homogeneously staining regions or double minute chromosomes).

b. The number of *N-myc* gene copies is related to the aggressiveness of the tumor.

c. The malignant cells of neuroblastoma sometimes differentiate into benign cells, and this change is reflected by a marked reduction in gene amplification.

V. Endocrine Pancreas

A. Diabetes mellitus

1. Classification and general features

a. Type I (insulin-dependent diabetes mellitus [IDDM], juvenile or ketosis-prone diabetes mellitus)

—often **begins early in life,** usually before age 30.

—is less common than type II diabetes mellitus.

—is due to **failure of insulin synthesis** by β cells of pancreatic islets.

—may be caused by **genetic predisposition** complicated by **autoimmune inflammation** of islets (insulitis) triggered by a viral infection or environmental factors. Type I demonstrates a positive family history less frequently than does type II diabetes mellitus.

—has markedly increased incidence in individuals with a specific point mutation in the HLA-DQ gene. Incidence is markedly increased in HLA-DR3 and HLA-DR4 positive individuals.

—unless insulin is replaced, results in marked **carbohydrate intolerance with hyperglycemia,** leading to polyuria, polydipsia, weight loss in spite of increased appetite, **ketoacidosis,** coma, and death.

—ketoacidosis results from increased catabolism of fat, with production of "ketone bodies" (principally β-hydroxybutyric acid and acetoacetic acid along with small quantities of acetone). It is not limited to diabetic acidosis and, in a much milder form, is seen in starvation.

b. Type II (non–insulin-dependent diabetes mellitus [NIDDM], adult-onset, or ketosis-resistant diabetes mellitus)

—is much more common than type I diabetes mellitus.

—characteristically begins later in life, most often in **middle age**.

—is due to **increased insulin resistance** mediated by decreased cell membrane insulin receptors or post-receptor dysfunction; may also be associated with impaired processing of proinsulin to insulin, decreased sensing of insulin by β cells, or impaired function of intracellular carrier proteins.

(1) Etiologic factors

(a) Positive family history more frequent than in type I diabetes mellitus

(b) Most often associated with mild to moderate **obesity**

(2) Characteristics

(a) Normal, often increased, plasma insulin concentration

(b) Mild carbohydrate intolerance, most often managed by diet and oral antidiabetic agents; insulin therapy is not usually required.

(c) Ketoacidosis is unusual but does occur, characteristically precipitated by unusual stress such as infection or surgery

c. Secondary diabetes mellitus

—occurs as a secondary phenomenon in pancreatic and other endocrine diseases and pregnancy.

(1) Pancreatic disease

(a) Idiopathic hemochromatosis (bronze diabetes)

—is characterized by excess iron absorption and parenchymal deposition of hemosiderin, with reactive fibrosis in various organs, especially the pancreas, liver, and heart.

(b) Pancreatitis

—acute pancreatitis is characterized by hyperglycemia; chronic pancreatitis may result in islet cell destruction and secondary diabetes mellitus.

(c) Carcinoma of the pancreas
–diabetes mellitus may be the presenting sign.
(2) Other endocrine diseases
(a) Cushing's syndrome
–produces hyperglycemia as a result of increased gluconeogenesis and impaired peripheral utilization of glucose.
(b) Acromegaly
–produces hyperglycemia due to the anti-insulin-like effect of growth hormone.
(c) Glucagon hypersecretion
–promotes glycogenolysis; is characteristically caused by an islet α cell tumor (glucagonoma).
(d) Other endocrine disorders
–pheochromocytoma and hyperthyroidism are sometimes associated with hyperglycemia.
(3) Pregnancy
–may be associated with transient diabetes mellitus (**gestational diabetes**); overt nongestational diabetes sometimes develops later.
–is characteristically associated with **increased fetal birth weight** and increased fetal mortality, notably from neonatal respiratory distress syndrome (**hyaline membrane disease**).

2. Anatomic changes in diabetes mellitus

a. Pancreatic islets
(1) Type I diabetes
–islets are small and β cells are markedly decreased in number or are absent; **insulitis** maked by lymphocytic infiltration is highly specific for this form of diabetes mellitus.
(2) Type II diabetes
–focal islet fibrosis and hyalinization (due to deposits of **amylin**) are characteristic but not specific.
–amylin (also known as islet amyloid polypeptide, IAPP) deposition in the pancreatic islets is characteristic of type II diabetes mellitus and is thought to interfere either with the conversion of proinsulin to insulin or with the sensing of insulin by β cells.

b. Kidney
–diffuse glomerulosclerosis, nodular glomerulosclerosis (Kimmelstiel-Wilson disease), arteriolar lesions, exudative lesions such as the fibrin cap or capsular drop, and the Armanni-Ebstein lesion, are renal manifestations of diabetes mellitus.
–pyelonephritis is a frequent complication that may be compounded by renal papillary necrosis.

c. Cardiovascular system
(1) Incidence of **atherosclerosis** is markedly increased; clinically significant atherosclerotic complications occur at a much earlier age than in the nondiabetic population; incidence in women, both premenopausal and postmenopausal, is markedly increased.

(2) **Myocardial infarction** and **peripheral vascular insufficiency** (often with gangrene of the lower extremities) are frequent complications.

(3) **Capillary basement membrane thickening** occurs in multiple organs and is thought due to nonenzymatic glycosylation of membrane protein.

d. **Eye**

(1) **Cataract formation** is common.

(2) Diabetic retinopathy (retinal exudates, edema, hemorrhages, and microaneurysms of small vessels), can lead to blindness.

e. **Nervous system**

—changes include **peripheral neuropathy** and changes in the brain and spinal cord.

f. **Liver**

—fatty change is seen.

g. **Skin**

(1) **Xanthomas** (collections of lipid-laden macrophages in the dermis)

(2) **Furuncles** and **abscesses** because of increased propensity to **infection;** frequent **fungal** infections, especially with *Candida*

B. Endocrine tumors (islet cell tumors)

1. Insulinoma (β cell tumor)

—is the most common islet cell tumor.

—can be benign or malignant.

—is characterized by markedly increased secretion of insulin. The problem of distinguishing endogenous insulin production from exogenous insulin (therapeutically or surreptitiously administered) is solved by quantitation of C-peptide, a fragment of the proinsulin molecule split off during the synthesis of insulin. Circulating C-peptide is characteristically increased in patients with insulinoma. In contrast, C-peptide is not increased by exogenous insulin administration since it is removed during the purification of commercial insulin preparations.

—is clinically characterized by **Whipple's triad:**

a. Episodic hypoglycemia

b. Central nervous system (CNS) dysfunction temporally related to hypoglycemia (confusion, anxiety, stupor, convulsions, coma)

c. Dramatic reversal of CNS abnormalities by glucose administration

2. Gastrinoma

—is often a malignant tumor, sometimes occurring in extrapancreatic sites.

—results in gastrin hypersecretion and hypergastrinemia.

—is associated with **Zollinger-Ellison syndrome** (marked gastric hypersecretion of hydrochloric acid, recurrent peptic ulcer disease, and hypergastrinemia).

3. Glucagonoma (α cell tumor)

—is a rare tumor.

—results in **secondary diabetes mellitus** and a characteristic skin lesion termed necrolytic migratory erythema.

4. Vipoma

 —is a very rare tumor.

 —is marked by secretion of vasoactive intestinal peptide (VIP).

 —is associated with watery diarrhea, hypokalemia, and achlorhydria (WDHA) syndrome, also known as Verner-Morrison syndrome or pancreatic cholera.

VI. Multiple Endocrine Neoplasia (MEN) Syndromes

—are a group of autosomal dominant syndromes in which more than one endocrine organ is hyperfunctional.

—may be associated with hyperplasias or tumors.

A. MEN type I (Wermer's syndrome)

 —includes hyperplasias or tumors of the thyroid, parathyroid, adrenal cortex, pancreatic islets, or pituitary.

 —may manifest its pancreatic component by Zollinger-Ellison syndrome, hyperinsulinism, or pancreatic cholera.

B. MEN type IIa (Sipple's syndrome)

 —includes pheochromocytoma, medullary carcinoma of the thyroid, and hyperparathyroidism due to hyperplasia or tumor.

C. MEN type IIb or MEN type III

 —includes pheochromocytoma, medullary carcinoma, and multiple mucocutaneous neuromas.

 —in contrast to MEN type IIa, do not induce hyperparathyroidism.

Review Test

Directions: Each of the numbered items or incomplete statements in this section is followed by answers or by completions of the statement. Select the **one** lettered answer or completion that is **best** in each case.

1. All of the following characteristics are associated with prolactinoma EXCEPT

(A) inappropriate renal retention of water.
(B) amenorrhea.
(C) galactorrhea.
(D) chromophobic staining.
(E) most common pituitary tumor.

2. In addition to growth hormone, acromegaly is associated with an increased serum concentration of

(A) ACTH.
(B) FSH.
(C) prolactin.
(D) somatomedin C.
(E) TSH.

3. All of the following characteristics are associated with somatotropic adenoma EXCEPT

(A) gigantism.
(B) acromegaly.
(C) basophilic staining.
(D) hyperglycemia.
(E) hypertension.

4. Adrenal hypercorticism may be caused by all of the following EXCEPT

(A) adrenal cortical adenoma.
(B) adrenal cortical hyperplasia.
(C) pituitary basophilic microadenoma.
(D) pituitary basophilic hyperplasia.
(E) pituitary eosinophilic adenoma.

5. Hypersecretion of ADH is associated with all of the following EXCEPT

(A) inappropriate water retention.
(B) diabetes insipidus.
(C) dilutional hyponatremia.
(D) small cell carcinoma of the lung.
(E) inability to dilute urine.

6. A 35-year-old woman gave birth to a normal infant but suffered severe cervical lacerations during delivery, resulting in hemorrhagic shock. Following blood transfusion and surgical repair, her postpartum recovery was initially uneventful. She was seen six months later and complained of continued amenorrhea and loss of weight and muscle strength. Further investigation might be expected to demonstrate all of the following findings EXCEPT

(A) hyperglycemia.
(B) vaginal atrophy.
(C) loss of axillary and pubic hair.
(D) decreased serum T_4.
(E) decreased serum cortisol.

7. A 10-year-old boy presents with headache and bilateral hemianopsia as well as evidence of increased intracranial pressure and diabetes insipidus. Supersellar calcification is apparent on X-ray examination. Resection of the contents of the sella turcica and parasellar area yields a large tumor with histology closely resembling the enamel organ of the embryonic tooth. The most likely outcome of this lesion is

(A) local invasion and intracranial metastasis.
(B) hematogenous metastasis to distal sites.
(C) lymphatic spread to distal sites.
(D) possible local recurrence with continued pressure-related damage to adjacent structures.

8. Hypothyroidism is caused by all of the following EXCEPT

(A) autoimmune causes.
(B) surgery, radiation therapy, or both.
(C) iodine deficiency.
(D) thyroid adenoma.
(E) hereditary or developmental abnormalities.

9. During a yearlong training program, a 23-year-old Air Force officer fell from first place in her class to last place. She also noted a lower pitch to her voice and coarsening of her hair, along with an increased tendency toward weight gain, menorrhagia, and increasing intolerance to cold. All of the following laboratory abnormalities are expected EXCEPT

(A) decreased serum T_4.
(B) decreased serum T_3 resin uptake.
(C) decreased unbound thyroid hormone binding sites on TBG.
(D) increased serum TSH.
(E) increased serum cholesterol.

10. All of the following characteristics are associated with Hashimoto's thyroiditis EXCEPT

(A) diffuse lymphocytic infiltration with germinal center formation.
(B) component of Plummer's disease.
(C) anti-TBG and antimicrosomal antibodies.
(D) increased incidence in association with HLA-DR5 antigen.
(E) increased incidence in persons with pernicious anemia, diabetes mellitus, or Sjögren's syndrome.

11. A 35-year-old woman presents with amenorrhea and weight loss in spite of increased appetite. History and physical examination reveal exophthalmos, fine resting tremor, tachycardia, and warm, moist skin. All of the following laboratory abnormalities are expected EXCEPT

(A) increased T_4.
(B) increased T_3.
(C) increased T_3 resin uptake.
(D) increased radioactive iodine uptake (RAIU).
(E) increased TSH.

12. All of the following abnormalities in parathyroid function are matched with the appropriate association EXCEPT

(A) primary hyperparathyroidism—adenoma.
(B) secondary hyperparathyroidism—renal disease.
(C) tertiary hyperparathyroidism—shortened fourth and fifth metacarpals and metatarsals and other skeletal abnormalities.
(D) hypoparathyroidism—congenital T cell deficiency.
(E) pseudohypoparathyroidism—defective end-organ responsiveness.

13. Which of the following findings is not an association of primary hyperparathyroidism?

(A) "Brown tumor" of bone
(B) Dystrophic calcification
(C) Hypertension
(D) Peptic duodenal ulcer
(E) Multiple endocrine neoplasia (MEN) syndromes

14. Redistribution of body fat with round moon face, dorsal "buffalo hump," and relatively thin extremities suggests

(A) Addison's disease.
(B) Conn's syndrome.
(C) Cushing's syndrome.
(D) Sipple's syndrome.
(E) Waterhouse-Friderichsen syndrome.

15. Which one of the following findings distinguishes primary aldosteronism from secondary aldosteronism?

(A) Increased sodium retention
(B) Increased blood pressure
(C) Decreased serum potassium
(D) Decreased serum renin

16. Primary adrenocortical deficiency is most frequently caused by

(A) autoimmune mechanisms.
(B) tuberculosis.
(C) histoplasmosis.
(D) metastatic tumor.
(E) amyloidosis.

17. All of the following characteristics are associated with pheochromocytoma EXCEPT

(A) chromaffin cell origin.
(B) episodic hypoglycemia.
(C) episodic hypertension.
(D) urinary excretion of catecholamines.
(E) component of MEN syndromes.

18. A tumor similar to that shown in the illustration below was observed in a biopsy specimen from the thyroid of a 50-year-old woman. An adjacent lymph node was also involved. Which one of the following descriptions of this tumor is most appropriate?

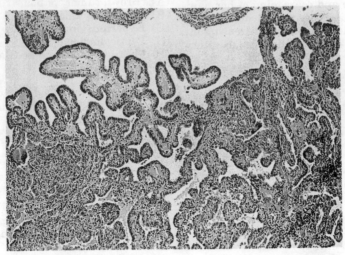

(Reprinted with permission from Golden A, Powell D, and Jennings C: *Pathology: Understanding Human Disease,* 2nd ed. Baltimore, Williams & Wilkins, 1985, p 388.)

(A) Functional tumor resulting in thyrotoxicosis
(B) Slow-growing lesion with relatively good prognosis
(C) APUDoma originating from C cells
(D) Calcitonin-producing tumor
(E) Tumor with amyloid-containing stroma

19. Type I diabetes mellitus is associated with all of the following characteristics EXCEPT

(A) focal islet cell fibrosis with amyloid deposits.
(B) linkage to HLA-D alleles.
(C) precipitation by viral infection.
(D) onset in childhood.
(E) propensity to ketoacidosis.

20. Type II diabetes mellitus is associated with all of the following characteristics EXCEPT

(A) normal or increased insulin synthesis.
(B) autoimmune origin.
(C) onset in adults.
(D) obesity.
(E) rare ketoacidosis.

21. After suffering a seizure, a 23-year-old woman is found to have profound hypoglycemia. Determination of which of the following would aid in differentiating exogenous hyperinsulinemia from endogenous hyperinsulinemia?

(A) C-peptide
(B) Gastrin
(C) Glucagon
(D) Proinsulin
(E) Vasoactive intestinal peptide

22. Which one of the following is most likely associated with an adrenal lesion such as that shown in the illustration below?

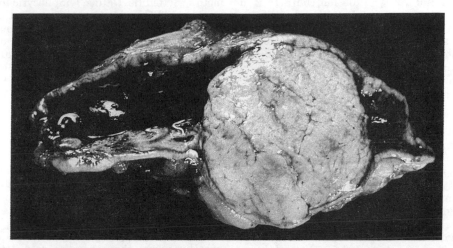

(Reprinted with permission from Golden A, Powell D, and Jennings C: *Pathology: Understanding Human Disease,* 2nd ed. Baltimore, Williams & Wilkins, 1985, p 396.)

(A) Hyperproduction of pituitary corticotropin
(B) Hyperproduction of adrenal glucocorticoids
(C) Adrenal (glucocorticoid) steroid therapy
(D) Ectopic ACTH production
(E) Hyperproduction of hypothalamic cortico-
    tropin-releasing factor

Answers and Explanations

1–A. Water retention is associated with inappropriate hyperactivity of antidiuretic hormone (ADH), not with prolactinoma. Inappropriate ADH secretion is most often a paraneoplastic syndrome. The tumor most often involved is small cell carcinoma of the lung, and the hormone is elaborated by the tumor itself, not the posterior pituitary.

2–D. In acromegaly, hypersecretion of growth hormone induces secondary hyperproduction of somatomedins by the liver. End-organ effects are caused by both growth hormone and somatomedins, especially somatomedin C (insulin-like growth factor-1, IGF-1).

3–C. Somatotropic adenoma most often exhibits eosinophilic staining. This growth hormone-secreting tumor results in gigantism if hypersecretion occurs before epiphyseal closure, or in acromegaly if hyperfunction begins in adolescence or adult life. In either case, hypersomatotropism is often complicated by hyperglycemia (sometimes by diabetes mellitus) and by hypertension.

4–E. Hypercorticotropic pituitary tumors (Cushing's disease) or hyperplasias are associated with basophilic, not eosinophilic, staining.

5–B. Diabetes insipidus is due to hypoactivity of ADH, not hyperactivity. It is associated with failure of renal water regulation, characterized by marked increase in urine volume and insatiable thirst. ADH hyperactivity is characteristically associated with ectopic hormone production from a tumor, most often small cell carcinoma of the lung, and is manifest by inappropriate water retention, dilutional hyponatremia, and inability to dilute the urine.

6–A. Hyperglycemia due to insulin-opposing effects of growth hormone is characteristic of hypersomatotropism and would be very unlikely in this patient. The history is suggestive of panhypopituitarism due to ischemic necrosis of the pituitary, occurring as a sequela to childbirth complicated by hemorrhagic shock (Sheehan's syndrome). This syndrome is clinically dominated by overt evidence of gonadotropin and corticotropin deficiencies along with laboratory evidence of these deficiencies and thyrotropin deficiency. Overt secondary hypothyroidism sometimes occurs.

7–D. The history is that of a craniopharyngioma (adamantinoma). Local effects of this tumor can be quite destructive, and recurrence due to incomplete resection is not uncommon. Local growth and tissue destruction result in both anterior and posterior pituitary dysfunction, and a patient often presents with signs of increased intracranial pressure, sometimes with hydrocephalus and frequently with bilateral hemianopsia (loss of peripheral visual fields) due to impingement on the optic chiasm. Diabetes insipidus is also frequent. Calcification apparent on X-ray is often prominent, facilitating diagnosis. Metastatic disease does not occur with this benign lesion.

8–D. Thyroid adenomas are most often nonfunctional and do not result in endocrine dysfunction. However, some are hormone-producing and can cause hyperthyroidism.

9–C. The history is strongly suggestive of idiopathic myxedema. Expected laboratory abnormalities include decreased serum T_3 and T_4, increased TSH, and increased cholesterol. Also, because hypothyroidism, with secretion of less thyroid hormone, results in less saturation of binding sites on TBG (or increased unbound binding sites), the T_3 resin uptake, which is inversely proportional to the number of unbound sites, will be decreased.

10–B. Plummer's disease, toxic nodular goiter without exophthalmos, is unrelated to Hashimoto's thyroiditis. Diffuse lymphocytic infiltration, anti-TBG and antimicrosomal antibodies, and increased incidence in association with HLA-DR5 antigen and in persons with autoimmune diseases such as pernicious anemia, insulin-dependent diabetes mellitus, or Sjögren's syndrome are all often cited as evidence of the autoimmune nature of Hashimoto's thyroiditis.

11–E. Graves' disease is characteristically associated with decreased TSH activity. Thyroid-follicle TSH receptors are stimulated by thyroid-stimulating immunoglobulin, an IgG autoantibody, not by TSH. Laboratory abnormalities in hyperthyroidism include increases in serum T_4, serum T_3, T_3 resin uptake, and RAIU.

12–C. Tertiary hyperparathyroidism is hyperparathyroidism that persists after definitive therapy for secondary hyperparathyroidism and is often due to the development of an adenoma in a persistently hyperplastic gland. Abnormalities, such as shortened fourth and fifth metacarpals and metatarsals, along with hypoparathyroidism in the face of normal concentration of parathyroid hormone, constitute pseudohypoparathyroidism, which may be caused by end-organ unresponsiveness in the kidney.

13–B. Dystrophic calcification occurs in previously damaged tissues and has no special association with hypercalcemia or primary hyperparathyroidism, in contrast to metastatic calcification, which is the most significant complication of the chronic hypercalcemia of primary hyperparathyroidism.

14–C. Cushing's syndrome is associated with redistribution of body fat, round moon face, dorsal "buffalo hump," and relatively thin extremities due to muscle wasting. In addition, muscle weakness, hirsutism, easy bruising, purplish abdominal striae, osteoporosis, amenorrhea, hypertension, hyperglycemia, and psychiatric disturbances may occur.

15–D. Serum renin is characteristically decreased in primary aldosteronism, in contrast to the increased renin observed in secondary aldosteronism. All forms of aldosteronism may be manifest by sodium and water retention, potassium loss (often with alkalosis), and hypertension.

16–A. Primary adrenocortical deficiency (Addison's disease) is most frequently caused by autoimmune mechanisms. Until recently, the most frequent cause was tuberculosis; approximately 70% of cases are now due to idiopathic (autoimmune) adrenal atrophy.

17–B. Episodic hypoglycemia is highly suggestive of insulinoma of the pancreas and is not a characteristic of pheochromocytoma.

18–B. The lesion shown is a papillary carcinoma of the thyroid, the most common form of thyroid cancer. This tumor most often remains localized to the thyroid and adjacent tissues for many years, even when local lymph nodes are involved. Papillary carcinoma is almost always nonfunctional.

19–A. Islet cell focal fibrosis with deposition of amyloid is characteristic of type II (noninsulin-dependent) diabetes mellitus. In type I (insulin-dependent) diabetes mellitus, the pancreatic islets are diffusely atrophic, β cells are markedly decreased, and insulitis marked by diffuse lymphocytic infiltration is prominent.

20–B. Autoimmune mechanisms are thought to play an important pathogenetic role in type I diabetes mellitus but not in type II diabetes.

21–A. Distinguishing endogenous insulin production from exogenous insulin (therapeutically or surreptitiously administered) is done by quantitation of C-peptide, a fragment of the proinsulin molecule split-off during the synthesis of insulin. Circulating C-peptide is characteristically increased in patients with insulinoma. C-peptide is not increased by exogenous insulin administration since it is removed during the purification of commercial insulin preparations.

22–B. The illustration demonstrates a well-circumscribed adrenal cortical adenoma. Cushing's syndrome is a manifestation of hyperproduction of adrenal glucocorticoids and when of adrenal origin, it is most often caused by adrenal cortical adenoma. Pituitary and hypothalamic causes of Cushing's syndrome result in bilateral adrenal cortical hyperplasia. In contrast, Cushing's syndrome caused by exogenous steroid medication results in adrenal atrophy.

21
Skin

I. Terminology Relating to Skin Diseases

—see Table 21.1 for terms and definitions relating to diseases of the skin.

II. Inflammatory and Vesicular Lesions

A. Eczematous dermatitis

—is a heterogeneous group of pruritic inflammatory disorders.

1. Etiology

a. Infection

b. Chemicals (contact dermatitis). Chemicals can directly injure skin or may act as antigens in type IV cell-mediated hypersensitivity reactions, resulting from cooperation of skin macrophages (Langerhans' cells) and T-helper lymphocytes.

c. Atopy (allergy). Eczematous dermatitis frequently occurs in persons with type I anaphylactic-type hypersensitivities, such as hay fever or bronchial asthma; however, the skin manifestations in these atopic patients are most often caused by type IV rather than type I hypersensitivity.

2. Morphologic findings

—vary depending on the stage of the disorder.

a. Acute stage—spongiosis with vesicle formation

b. Chronic stage—acanthosis, hyperkeratosis, and lichenification; focal lymphocytic dermal infiltrates

c. Subacute stage—intermediate changes between acute and chronic; less spongiosis and vesiculation than in acute; less acanthosis and hyperkeratosis than in chronic eczematous dermatitis

B. Neurodermatitis (lichen simplex chronicus)

—is clinically indistinguishable from chronic eczematous dermatitis.

—produces anatomic changes entirely secondary to scratching. The cause of the pruritus is unknown but may be psychogenic.

Table 21.1. Terms and Definitions Applied Specifically to Skin Disorders

Term	Definition
Macule	Flat, nonpalpable lesion of a different color than the surrounding skin; less than 1 cm in diameter
Patch	Similar to macule; larger than 1 cm in diameter
Papule	Small, palpable, elevated skin lesion less than 1 cm in diameter
Plaque	Similar to papule; larger than 1 cm in diameter
Vesicle	Small fluid-containing blister
Bulla	Large fluid-containing blister; 0.5 cm or more in diameter
Pustule	Blister containing pus
Crust	Dried exudate from vesicle, bulla, or pustule
Hyperkeratosis	Increased thickness of the stratum corneum
Parakeratosis	Hyperkeratosis with retention of nuclei of keratinocytes
Acanthosis	Thickening of the epidermis
Spongiosis	Epidermal intercellular edema with widening of intercellular spaces
Acantholysis	Separation of epidermal cells one from the other; cells appear to float within extracellular fluid
Lichenification	Accentuation of skin markings caused by scratching

Terms are arranged in loosely related groups, generally in order of increasing severity.

C. Psoriasis

- is a chronic inflammatory process characterized by erythematous papules and plaques with characteristic silvery scaling; lesions are sharply demarcated.
- most often involves the extensor surfaces of the elbows and knees as well as the scalp and sacral area.
- is most often nonpruritic.
- demonstrates histologic epidermal proliferation with acanthosis and highly characteristic parakeratosis; minute neutrophilic abscesses (Munro abscesses) may be found within the parakeratotic stratum corneum.
- may be of autoimmune etiology.
- can be associated with severe destructive rheumatoid arthritis-like lesions (**psoriatic arthritis**) that most commonly affect the fingers.

D. Varicella (chickenpox)

- is a viral infection of childhood characterized by fever and a generalized vesicular eruption; immune individuals may develop herpes zoster (shingles) in adult life.
- the varicella-zoster virus may remain latent for years in dorsal root ganglia.
- the painful skin eruption of herpes zoster has a characteristic distribution along the dermatomes corresponding to the affected dorsal root ganglia.

E. Pemphigus vulgaris

- occurs most often in persons ages 30 to 60.

—is an acantholytic disorder characterized by formation of severe intraepidermal bullae. First lesions often occur in oral mucosa, and extensive skin involvement follows. Lesions often rupture, leaving large denuded surfaces subject to secondary infection.

—is characterized by prominent intraepidermal acantholysis and sparing of the basal layer.

—is an autoimmune disorder characterized by IgG autoantibodies directed against the epidermal intercellular cement substance; antibodies can be demonstrated in serum or by characteristic immunofluorescence encircling the individual epidermal cells.

—can be fatal.

F. Bullous pemphigoid

—resembles pemphigus vulgaris but is clinically much less severe.

—is characterized by subepidermal bullae, with characteristic inflammatory infiltrate by eosinophils in the surrounding dermis.

—is an autoimmune disorder characterized by IgG autoantibodies directed against epidermal basement membrane; antibodies can be demonstrated in serum or by a characteristic linear band of immunofluorescence along the basement membrane.

G. Dermatitis herpetiformis

—has its greatest incidence in persons 20 to 40 years old.

—is a recurrent pruritic blistering disorder, usually of the extensor surfaces of the knees and elbows, scalp, upper back, and sacral area; blisters tend to occur in groups.

—is characterized by dermal microabscesses with neutrophils and eosinophils at the tips of dermal papillae, which become subepidermal blisters.

—demonstrates deposits of IgA at the tips of dermal papillae.

—commonly is associated with gluten-sensitive enteropathy; both skin lesions and enteropathy improve when patients are placed on gluten-free diets.

III. Disorders of Pigmentation

A. Albinism

—is a failure of pigment production by otherwise intact melanocytes.
—occurs as two variants.

1. **Ocular albinism** is a melanin dysfunction that is limited to the eyes. This condition is an X-linked disorder.

2. **Oculocutaneous albinism** is a melanin synthetic defect that involves the eyes, skin, and hair; it **predisposes to actinic keratosis, basal and squamous cell carcinoma, and malignant melanoma** because of sensitivity of skin to sunlight. Inheritance is most often autosomal recessive. Oculocutaneous albinism is often subclassified as:

   a. **Tyrosinase-negative albinism** is failure of conversion of tyrosine to dihydroxyphenylalanine (DOPA), an intermediary in melanin synthesis.

   b. **Tyrosinase-positive albinism.** The mechanisms of deficient melanin synthesis are unknown.

B. Vitiligo

—is an acquired loss of melanocytes in discrete areas of skin that appear as depigmented white patches.

—may be of autoimmune etiology; is associated with other autoimmune disorders, such as Graves' disease and Addison's disease; antimelanocyte antibodies are sometimes demonstrable.

—may be caused by destruction of melanocytes by toxic intermediates of melanin production or by neurochemical factors.

C. Freckle (ephelis)

—is produced by an increase of melanin pigment within basal keratinocytes.

D. Lentigo

—is a pigmented macule caused by melanocytic hyperplasia in the epidermis.

E. Pigmented nevi

1. Nevocellular nevus (common mole)

—is variably classified as a benign tumor or hamartoma; nevus cells are derived from melanocytes and ordinarily occur in clusters or nests.

—the three most common types are:

a. Junctional nevus—nevus cells confined to the epidermal–dermal junction

b. Compound nevus—nevus cells both at the epidermal–dermal junction and in the dermis

c. Intradermal nevus—nevus cells confined to clusters within dermis (these cells are often nonpigmented)

2. Blue nevus

—is present at birth.

—is characterized by nodular foci of dendritic, highly pigmented melanocytes in dermis; blue external appearance results from dermal location.

3. Spitz nevus (juvenile melanoma)

—most often occurs in children.

—is always benign. (The term juvenile melanoma is misleading and falling into disuse.)

—is often characterized by spindle-shaped cells; it can be confused with malignant melanoma.

4. Dysplastic nevus

—is an atypical, irregularly pigmented lesion with disorderly proliferation of melanocytes, dermal fibrosis, and often subjacent dermal lymphocytic infiltration.

—**may transform into malignant melanoma.**

—is familial in some cases (dysplastic nevus syndrome); these cases exhibit autosomal dominant inheritance and a marked tendency toward conversion to malignant melanoma.

5. Lentigo maligna (Hutchinson freckle)

—is a nonfamilial **precursor to lentigo maligna melanoma**.

—is an irregular macular pigmented lesion on sun-exposed skin.

—is characterized by atypical melanocytes at the epidermal–dermal junction.

IV. Disorders of Viral Origin

A. Molluscum contagiosum
—is a contagious viral disorder occurring most often in children and adolescents; it is transmitted by direct contact.
—is due to a DNA poxvirus.
—demonstrates umbilicated, dome-shaped papules.

B. Verruca vulgaris (common wart)
—is a benign papilloma.
—is caused by certain strains of human papillomavirus (HPV), which are distinct from those associated with gynecologic neoplasms.
—is characterized by vacuolated cells (koilocytes) in the granular cell layer of the epidermis.

V. Miscellaneous Skin Disorders

A. Acrochordon (fibroepithelial polyp, skin tag)
—is an extremely common lesion, most often occurring on the face near the eyelids, neck, trunk, or axilla.
—consists of a central connective tissue core covered by stratified squamous epithelium.

B. Epidermal inclusion cyst
—is lined by stratified squamous epithelium and is filled with keratinous material.
—manifests clinically as a dome-shaped nodule that is filled with soft gray-white material.
—has erroneously been termed sebaceous cyst; sebaceous glands are not involved.

C. Dermatofibroma
—is a benign neoplasm.
—presents as a firm nodule, sometimes with pigmented acanthosis.
—is characterized by intertwining bundles of collagen and fibroblasts.
—is termed fibrous histiocytoma when histiocytes are prominent.

D. Dermatofibrosarcoma protuberans
—is a slowly growing, well-differentiated malignant neoplasm histologically resembling dermatofibroma.
—rarely metastasizes.

E. Seborrheic keratosis
—is an extremely common benign neoplasm of older persons; it is also called senile keratosis.
—is manifest by sharply demarcated raised papules or plaques with a typical pasted-on appearance; lesions occur on the head, trunk, and extremities.

F. Keratoacanthoma
—is generally considered to be a benign neoplasm.
—closely resembles squamous cell carcinoma.
—regresses spontaneously without therapy.

G. Actinic keratosis

—is a **premalignant** epidermal lesion caused by excessive chronic exposure to sunlight.

—is characterized by rough, scaling, poorly demarcated plaques on the face, neck, upper trunk, or extremities.

H. Acanthosis nigricans

—is sometimes a **marker of visceral malignancy** (stomach, lung, breast, uterus).

—is characterized by acanthosis and hyperpigmentation, most often involving flexural areas.

I. Xanthoma

—is most often associated with hypercholesterolemia.

—is characterized by yellowish papules or nodules composed of focal dermal collections of lipid-laden histiocytes.

—occurs most frequently on the eyelids (xanthelasma); it can also occur as nodules over tendons or joints.

J. Hemangioma

—is sometimes considered to be a hamartoma rather than a neoplasm.

1. Major forms

a. **Capillary hemangioma**—small, blood-filled capillaries lined with a single layer of endothelium. Capillary hemangioma occurs in three variants:

(1) **Port-wine stain**—purple-red area on the face or neck

(2) **Strawberry hemangioma**—bright-red raised lesion

(3) **Cherry hemangioma**—small, dome-shaped red papule

b. **Cavernous hemangioma**—large, endothelial-lined spaces in the dermis and subdermis

2. Other manifestations

—hemangiomas occur rarely as part of:

a. **Sturge-Weber syndrome**

—is a port-wine stain of the face, ipsilateral glaucoma, vascular lesions of ocular choroidal tissue, and extensive hemangiomatous involvement of meninges.

—manifests clinically by convulsions, mental retardation, and retinal detachment.

b. **Von Hippel-Lindau disease**

—is multiple vascular tumors and other tumors and cysts that are widely scattered throughout many organ systems.

K. Granuloma pyogenicum

—is a vascular pedunculated lesion.

—is characterized by numerous capillaries and edematous stroma.

—often develops following trauma.

—is common in skin or mucous membranes.

L. Keloid

—is an abnormal proliferation of the connective tissue of skin scars that results in large, raised, tumor-like lesions.

–often follows trauma to the skin, such as ear-piercing or surgical wounds.

–occurs in genetically susceptible individuals.

–occurs frequently in blacks.

VI. Skin Malignancies

A. Squamous cell carcinoma

–is a common skin tumor.

–is most often locally invasive; less than 5% metastasize.

–is most frequently associated with excessive exposure to sunlight; it occurs most frequently in sun-exposed areas such as the face and back of the hands.

–frequently originates in a preexisting actinic keratosis.

–is also associated with chemical carcinogens, such as arsenic, and radiation or x-ray exposure.

–most often presents as a scaling, indurated, ulcerated nodule.

–is characterized by invasion of dermis by **sheets and islands of neoplastic epidermal cells,** often with **keratin "pearls."**

B. Basal cell carcinoma

–is the most common of all skin tumors.

–tends to involve sun-exposed areas, most frequently the head and neck.

–grossly presents as a pearly papule.

–is characterized by clusters of darkly staining cells with a typical **palisade arrangement of the nuclei** of the cells at the periphery of the tumor cell clusters.

–can be locally aggressive; however, it almost never metastasizes.

–is almost always cured by surgical resection.

C. Malignant melanoma

–is increasing in incidence.

–is most common in fair-skinned persons.

–arises from melanocytes or nevus cells.

–is most often associated with **excessive exposure to sunlight**.

1. Growth phases

a. Radial (initial phase)

(1) Growth occurs in all directions but is predominantly lateral within the epidermis and papillary zone of the dermis.

(2) Lymphocytic response is prominent.

(3) Melanomas in the radial growth phase do not metastasize; clinical cure is frequent.

b. Vertical (later phase)

(1) Growth extends into the reticular dermis or beyond.

(2) Prognosis varies with thickness of the lesion.

(3) Lymphatics or hematogenous metastasis may occur.

2. Clinical variants

–malignant melanomas have a better prognosis when characterized by a long period of radial growth than when associated with an early vertical growth phase. The most important clinical variants include:

a. **Lentigo maligna melanoma** occurs on sun-exposed skin. The radial growth phase predominates initially; most often develops from preexisting lentigo maligna (Hutchinson freckle).

b. **Superficial spreading melanoma** is the most common of the variants. The lesion is irregularly bordered with variegated pigmentation; most frequent locations are the trunk and extremities. Radial growth phase predominates.

c. **Nodular melanoma** begins with the vertical growth phase. It has the **poorest prognosis** of the clinical variants.

d. **Acral-lentiginous melanoma** most often appears on the hands and feet of dark-skinned persons.

Review Test

Directions: Each of the numbered items or incomplete statements in this section is followed by answers or by completions of the statement. Select the **one** lettered answer or completion that is **best** in each case.

1. All of the following findings are frequently associated with oculocutaneous albinism EXCEPT

(A) autosomal recessive inheritance.
(B) involvement of the eyes, skin, and hair.
(C) tyrosinase deficiency.
(D) loss of melanocytes.
(E) increased incidence of skin malignancy.

2. All of the following characteristics apply to the lesion illustrated below EXCEPT

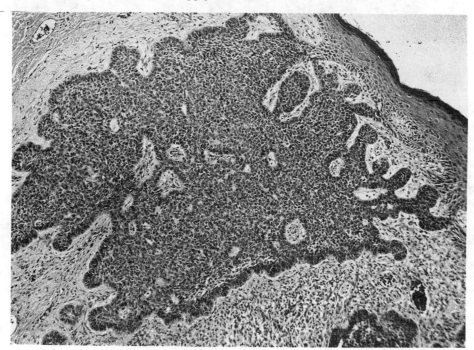

(Reprinted with permission from Golden A, Powell D, and Jennings C: *Pathology: Understanding Human Disease,* 2nd ed. Baltimore, Williams & Wilkins, 1985, p 508.)

(A) it often occurs on sun-exposed areas.
(B) distal metastases almost never occur.
(C) it is a common skin tumor.
(D) it frequently originates in preexisting actinic keratosis.

3. All of the following characteristics are applicable to the lesion shown in the figure EXCEPT

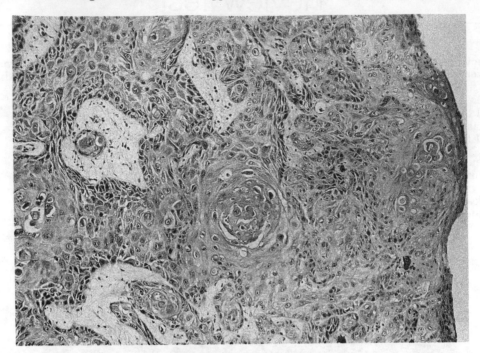

(Reprinted with permission from Golden A, Powell D, and Jennings C: *Pathology: Understanding Human Disease,* 2nd ed. Baltimore, Williams & Wilkins, 1985, p 506.)

(A) predilection for sun-exposed areas.
(B) distal metastases almost never occur.
(C) common skin tumor.
(D) frequent origin in preexisting actinic keratosis.

4. Which of the following pigmented lesions is associated with the poorest prognosis?

(A) Lentigo maligna melanoma
(B) Superficial spreading melanoma
(C) Nodular melanoma
(D) Juvenile melanoma

5. All of the following skin lesions are correctly paired with the appropriate association or descriptive phrase EXCEPT

(A) verruca vulgaris—human papillomavirus.
(B) seborrheic keratosis—benign neoplasm of old age.
(C) actinic keratosis—premalignant lesion.
(D) granuloma pyogenicum—frequent metastases.
(E) keloid—more frequent in blacks.

Directions: Each group of items in this section consists of lettered options followed by a set of numbered items. For each item, select the **one** lettered option that is most closely associated with it. Each lettered option may be selected once, more than once, or not at all.

Questions 6–9

Match each description with the appropriate type of nevus.

(A) Nevocellular nevus
(B) Blue nevus
(C) Spitz nevus
(D) Dysplastic nevus
(E) Lentigo maligna

6. Familial premalignant condition
7. Intradermal nodular foci of dendritic melanocytes
8. Childhood lesion with spindle-shaped cells
9. Nonfamilial malignant precursor lesion

Answers and Explanations

1–D. Loss of melanocytes is characteristic of vitiligo but not of oculocutaneous albinism, which is caused by failure of melanin synthesis. This autosomal recessive disorder, which manifests by lack of pigmentation of the eyes, skin, and hair, occurs in two variants, tyrosinase negative and tyrosinase positive. Oculocutaneous albinism is characterized by increased actinic sensitivity of the skin with increased incidence of actinic keratosis, basal and squamous cell carcinoma, and malignant melanoma.

2–D. The illustration shows a basal cell carcinoma with typical palisading of the nuclei of the cells at the periphery of the tumor cell clusters. Unlike squamous cell carcinoma, this tumor does not originate in preexisting actinic keratosis.

3–B. The lesion shown is a well-differentiated squamous cell carcinoma demonstrating sheets of neoplastic epidermal cells with keratin "pearls." Although most of these lesions are discovered early and are cured by ablative therapy, metastasis does occur in a significant number of cases.

4–C. Nodular melanoma, which begins with a vertical growth phase, has the poorest prognosis of all the clinical variants of malignant melanoma. Lentigo maligna melanoma and superficial spreading melanoma are all associated with a prolonged initial radial growth phase, a characteristic that correlates with a better prognosis. Juvenile melanoma, a misleading term formerly applied to the Spitz nevus, is a benign tumor most often seen in children.

5–D. Granuloma pyogenicum is most often a posttraumatic reactive lesion and is not a malignant neoplasm.

6–D. Some cases of dysplastic nevus occur as part of the dysplastic nevus syndrome, an inherited autosomal-dominant condition in which there is a markedly increased incidence of malignant melanoma.

7–B. The blue nevus, a lesion present at birth, appears blue because of the presence of foci of highly pigmented dendritic melanocytes deep in the dermis.

8–C. The Spitz nevus, formerly called juvenile melanoma, is a benign lesion most frequently seen in children. It is often characterized by spindle-shaped cells.

9–E. Lentigo maligna, or Hutchinson freckle, is characterized by atypical melanocytes at the epidermal-dermal junction and is considered to be a precursor lesion to lentigo maligna melanoma, a form of malignant melanoma.

22
Musculoskeletal System

I. Diseases of Skeletal Muscle

A. Muscle atrophies

1. Denervation atrophy

–is associated with muscle denervation.

–involves both type I (red) and type II (white) fibers, which may appear small and angular on cross section.

–may demonstrate **target fibers** (fibers that on cross section have a central darker area reminiscent of the bull's-eye of a target).

–after reinnervation may be characterized by **fiber-type grouping,** a cluster of type I fibers adjacent to a cluster of type II fibers, in contrast to the mix of individual type I and type II fibers characteristic of normal muscle.

2. Disuse atrophy

–is associated with prolonged immobilization.

–is characterized histologically by **angular atrophy,** primarily of type II fibers.

B. Muscular dystrophies

–are a group of genetically determined, progressive disorders characterized by degeneration of skeletal muscle and profound wasting and weakness.

–are differentiated by age of onset, muscle groups involved, and mode of inheritance.

–are characterized by increased serum activities of creatine phosphokinase (CPK) and other muscle enzymes derived from degenerating muscle fibers.

–are also characterized by nonspecific degenerative changes on muscle biopsy; although nonspecific, the muscle biopsy findings are helpful in distinguishing dystrophies from abnormalities secondary to denervation or from entities characterized by specific morphologic changes.

1. Duchenne muscular dystrophy

–is the most common and most severe of the muscular dystrophies.

–occurs almost entirely in male children.

–begins with weakness commencing at about 1 year of age, progressing to immobilization, wasting, muscle contracture, and death in early teens, most often due to pneumonia caused by weakness of respiratory muscles.

–is characterized histologically by random variation in muscle fiber size, necrosis of individual muscle fibers, and replacement of necrotic fibers by fibrofatty tissue.

–is further characterized by **increased serum CPK**.

–presents initially in proximal muscles of extremities.

–is characterized later by **compensatory hypertrophy** of distal sites, such as the calf muscles, followed eventually by **pseudohypertrophy** (increased fibrous tissue and adipose tissue).

–is caused by deficiency of **dystrophin,** a trace protein of unknown function.

–exhibits **X-linked inheritance,** with up to one-third of cases resulting from de novo mutation. A variety of deletions occur involving segments of the dystrophin gene, which is located on the short arm of the X chromosome. The deletions are variable, but are constant within families and characteristically lead to a DNA coding frame-shift, with resultant formation of stop codons and total failure of dystrophin synthesis.

2. Becker's muscular dystrophy

–is clinically similar to, but less severe than, Duchenne muscular dystrophy.

–is also caused by an abnormality in dystrophin; the molecule is truncated and presumably less functional; the dystrophin abnormality is caused by segmental deletions within the gene that do not cause a coding frame-shift.

3. Facioscapulohumeral muscular dystrophy

–demonstrates autosomal dominant inheritance.

–is associated with a slowly progressive, nondisabling course and an almost normal life expectancy.

–sequentially involves the muscles of the face, scapular area, and humerus.

4. Limb-girdle dystrophy

–demonstrates autosomal recessive inheritance.

–involves the proximal muscles of the shoulder, pelvic girdle, or both.

5. Myotonic dystrophy

–demonstrates autosomal dominant inheritance.

–is characterized by weakness associated with myotonia (inability to relax muscles once contracted).

–is associated with cataracts as well as with testicular atrophy and baldness in men.

C. Congenital myopathies with specific histologic changes

–are often characterized by floppy infant syndrome, marked hypotonia at birth.

–can be distinguished from dystrophies by the combination of specific histologic changes, often with normal serum creatine kinase.

1. Central core disease
   —demonstrates loss of mitochondria and other organelles in the central portion of type I muscle fibers.
   —is characterized by muscle weakness and hypotonia, but infants with this disease eventually become ambulatory.

2. Nemaline myopathy
   —demonstrates tangles of small rod-shaped granules predominantly in type I fibers.
   —varies clinically from a mild, nonprogressive disease to severe weakness ending in death from respiratory failure.

3. Mitochondrial myopathies
   —demonstrate non-Mendelian inheritance.
   —are mediated by maternally transmitted mitochondrial DNA abnormalities (most often deletions).
   —may be characterized by a ragged red appearance of muscle fibers and by a variety of mitochondrial enzyme or coenzyme defects. For example, the Kearns-Sayre syndrome is characterized by ophthalmoplegia, pigmentary retinopathy, heart block, cerebellar ataxia, and an exclusively **maternal mode of transmission**.

D. Myasthenia gravis
   —is an autoimmune disorder caused by **autoantibodies to acetylcholine receptors** of the neuromuscular junction.
   —is characterized by muscle weakness that is intensified by muscle use, with recovery on rest.
   —is manifest clinically by effort-associated weakness involving the extraocular and facial muscles, muscles of the extremities, and other muscle groups.
   —frequently presents with ptosis or diplopia, or with difficulty in chewing, speaking, or swallowing.
   —can be complicated by respiratory failure.
   —dramatically improves with administration of drugs with anticholinesterase activity, an important diagnostic finding.
   —is frequently associated with tumors of the thymus or with thymic hyperplasia.
   —is three times more frequent in women than in men.

II. Diseases of Bone

A. Metabolic bone disease
   —is usually characterized by osteopenia (diffuse radiolucency of bone) or alterations in serum calcium, phosphorus, and alkaline phosphatase (Table 22.1).

1. Osteoporosis
   —is characterized by a **decrease in bone mass**.
   —can be caused by impaired synthesis or increased resorption of bony matrix protein.
   —results in bony structures inadequate for weight bearing; fractures commonly result, especially compression fractures of the vertebrae that cause spinal deformity (most typically kyphosis) and shortened stature.

Table 22.1. Blood Chemistries in Metabolic Bone Disease

Bone Disease	Blood Chemistries		
	Calcium	**Phosphorus**	**Alkaline Phosphatase**
Osteoporosis	Normal	Normal	Normal or decreased
Von Recklinghausen's disease of bone	Increased	Decreased	Increased
Osteomalacia and rickets	Decreased or normal	Variable	Increased or normal
Paget's disease of bone	Normal	Normal	Markedly increased

—is radiographically characterized by diffuse radiolucency of bone.

—is clinically associated with:

a. Postmenopausal state (estrogen deficiency is a presumptive cause)

b. Physical inactivity

c. Hypercorticism

d. Hyperthyroidism

e. Calcium deficiency

2. Von Recklinghausen's disease of bone (osteitis fibrosa cystica)

—is caused by primary or secondary **hyperparathyroidism**.

—is characterized by widespread osteolytic lesions.

—may manifest as **"brown tumor"** of bone, cystic spaces that are lined by multinucleated osteoclasts and filled with vascular fibrous stroma, often with brown discoloration resulting from hemorrhage.

—may sometimes be manifest by diffuse radiolucency of bone mimicking osteoporosis.

—is accompanied by laboratory manifestations of hyperparathyroidism, high serum calcium, low serum phosphorus, and high serum alkaline phosphatase.

3. Osteomalacia

—is caused by **vitamin D deficiency in adults**.

—is characterized by defective calcification of osteoid matrix.

—is characterized radiographically by diffuse radiolucency, which can mimic osteoporosis.

—when secondary to renal disease is termed **renal osteodystrophy**.

4. Rickets

—is caused by **vitamin D deficiency in children**.

—is characterized by inadequate calcification and increased thickness of epiphyseal growth plates with resultant skeletal deformities.

—is manifest clinically by:

a. Craniotabes: thinning and softening of occipital and parietal bones

b. Late closing of fontanelles

c. Rachitic rosary: thickening of the costochondral junctions that results in a string-of-beads-like appearance

d. Harrison's groove: depression along the line of insertion of the diaphragm into the rib cage

e. Pigeon breast: caused by protrusion of the sternum

f. Decreased height: caused by spinal deformity

5. Paget's disease of bone (osteitis deformans)

—is most common in the elderly.

—is of unknown etiology; a viral etiology is suggested by ultrastructural intranuclear inclusions in osteoclasts; studies suggest a possible role of measles or respiratory syncytial virus.

—is characterized by **abnormal bony architecture** caused by increases in both osteoblastic and osteclastic activity.

—most commonly involves the spine, pelvis, calvarium of the skull, femur, and tibia.

—may manifest clinically by a marked increase in serum alkaline phosphatase and normal serum calcium and phosphorus.

—can be **monostotic** (involving only one bone) or **polyostotic** (involving multiple bones).

a. Morphologic phases

(1) Osteolytic phase: osteoclastic resorption predominates.

(2) Mixed osteoblastic and osteolytic phase: new bone formation leads to a characteristic **mosaic pattern**.

(3) Late phase: bone density is increased, trabeculae are thick, and mosaic pattern is prominent.

b. Complications

(1) Bone pain resulting from fractures: although bone is thick, it lacks strength; fractures can lead to deformity.

(2) High output cardiac failure can result from multiple functional arteriovenous shunts within highly vascular early lesions.

(3) Hearing loss is caused by narrowing of the auditory foramen or direct involvement of the bones of the middle ear.

(4) Osteosarcoma occurs in approximately 1% of cases.

B. Other non-neoplastic diseases of bone

1. Scurvy

—is caused by **ascorbic acid (vitamin C) deficiency**.

—is characterized by bony lesions caused by impaired osteoid matrix formation, which in turn is caused by the failure of proline and lysine hydroxylation required for collagen synthesis.

—is manifest by the following bony changes:

a. Subperiosteal hemorrhage (often painful)

b. Osteoporosis (especially at the metaphyseal ends of bone)

c. Epiphyseal cartilage not replaced by osteoid

2. Achondroplasia

—is one of the most common causes of dwarfism.

—is an autosomal dominant disorder characterized by short limbs with normal-sized head and trunk.

—is characterized by narrow epiphyseal plates and bony sealing off of the area between the epiphyseal plate and the metaphysis; the failure of elongation results in short, thick bones.

3. Fibrous dysplasia

—is characterized by replacement of portions of bone with fibrous tissue.

—is of unknown etiology.

—is of three main types:

a. Monostotic fibrous dysplasia: solitary lesions that are often asymptomatic but can result in spontaneous fractures with pain, swelling, and deformity.

b. Polyostotic fibrous dysplasia: multiple sites are involved; it can be associated with severe deformity.

c. Albright's syndrome: polyostotic fibrous dysplasia, precocious puberty, café-au-lait spots on skin, and short stature, occurring in very young girls.

4. Aseptic (avascular) necrosis

—is most often of unknown etiology.

—most often results from infarction caused by interruption of arterial blood supply.

—can be secondary to trauma or to embolism of diverse types, such as thrombosis, decompression syndrome or "the bends," and sickle cell anemia.

—in growing children, may involve a variety of characteristic sites, including the head of the femur (**Legg-Calvé-Perthes disease**), the tibial tubercle (**Osgood-Schlatter disease**), or the navicular bone (**Köhler's bone disease**).

5. Osteogenesis imperfecta

—is characterized by multiple fractures occurring with minimal trauma (brittle bone disease).

—is caused by a group of specific gene mutations, all resulting in defective collagen synthesis, which results in generalized connective tissue abnormalities affecting the teeth, skin, eyes, and bones.

—is often accompanied by blue sclerae from translucency of thin connective tissue overlying the choroid.

—occurs in a variety of clinical types varying greatly in severity; in the most common type, an autosomal dominant variant, blue sclerae and multiple childhood fractures are prominent clinical findings.

6. Osteoporosis (marble bone disease, Albers-Schönberg disease)

—is characterized by markedly increased density of the skeleton.

—is caused by failure of osteoclastic activity.

—is associated with multiple fractures in spite of increased bone density.

—is also associated with anemia as a result of decreased marrow space, and with blindness, deafness, and cranial nerve involvement because of narrowing and impingement of neural foramina.

—occurs in two major clinical forms, an autosomal recessive variant that is usually fatal in infancy and a less severe autosomal dominant variant.

7. Pyogenic osteomyelitis

   a. Incidence

   (1) Children

   —occurs most often as a result of blood-borne spread from an infection located elsewhere. *Staphylococcus aureus* is the most common organism; group B β-streptococci or *Escherichia coli* are frequent in newborns; *Salmonella* is frequent in association with sickle cell anemia.

   (2) Adults

   —occurs usually as a complication of compound fracture or a sequela of surgery.

   (3) Intravenous drug users

   —is frequently a result of *Pseudomonas* infection.

   b. Characteristics—osteomyelitis

   —is an acute pyogenic infection of bone.

   —most often initially involves the metaphysis; the distal end of the femur, proximal end of the tibia, and proximal end of the humerus are the most common sites.

   c. Course—osteomyelitis

   —in the acute stage, may resolve with antibiotic therapy.

   —may compress vasculature with pyogenic exudate, resulting in ischemic necrosis of bone and marrow; necrotic bone (**sequestrum**) acts as a foreign body and as a locus for persistent infection.

   —subperiosteal dissection by pyogenic exudate may further impair blood supply; pus can rupture into surrounding tissues and form sinuses draining through skin.

   —a sleeve of new bone formation (**involucrum**) may surround the infected necrotic area.

   —may be localized by a surrounding wall of granulation tissue (Brodie's abscess).

   —may be complicated by secondary (reactive systemic) amyloidosis.

8. Tuberculous osteomyelitis

   —is secondary to tuberculous infection located elsewhere.

   —characteristically occurs in:

   a. Vertebrae (Pott's disease); vertebral collapse can lead to spinal deformity.

   b. Hip

   c. Long bones, especially the femur and tibia

   d. Bones of the hands and feet

9. Histiocytosis X

   —can occur in a variety of sites, including bone.

   —is a group of disorders characterized by proliferation of histiocytic cells that closely resemble the Langerhans' cells of the epidermis; **Birbeck granules,** tennis racket-shaped cytoplasmic structures, are characteristic markers of these cells; distinctive surface antigens also characterize these Langerhans'-like cells.

−includes the following variants:

a. Letterer-Siwe disease (acute disseminated Langerhans' cell histiocytosis)

−is an aggressive, usually fatal, disorder of infants and small children.

−is characterized by hepatosplenomegaly, lymphadenopathy, pancytopenia, pulmonary involvement, and recurrent infections as a result of widespread histiocytic proliferation.

b. Hand-Schüller-Christian disease (chronic progressive histiocytosis)

−has a better prognosis than Letterer-Siwe disease.

−usually presents before age 5 years.

−is characterized by histiocytic proliferation mixed with inflammatory cells in bone, especially the skull; liver; spleen; and other tissues.

−is clinically manifest by the classic triad of skull lesions, diabetes insipidus, and exophthalmos caused by involvement of the orbit.

c. Eosinophilic granuloma

−has the best prognosis within the group; fatalities are rare, and lesions sometimes heal without treatment.

−can present as solitary bone lesion; extraskeletal involvement is most often limited to the lung.

−is characterized by histiocytic proliferation mixed with inflammatory cells, including ordinary macrophages, lymphocytes, and many eosinophils.

C. Bone tumors

−see Table 22.2 for a comparison of several important bone tumors.

−the most frequently occurring benign tumors of bone are **osteochondroma and giant cell tumor;** the most frequently occurring malignant tumors of bone are osteosarcoma, chondrosarcoma, and Ewing's sarcoma; this excludes metastatic carcinoma and multiple myeloma, which are more common than primary bone tumors.

1. Benign bone tumors

a. Osteochondroma (exostosis)

−is a bony growth covered by a cap of cartilage projecting from the surface of a bone.

−is the most common benign tumor of bone.

−is most common in men younger than age 25.

−may be a hamartoma rather than a true neoplasm.

−most often originates from the metaphysis of long bones, with the lower end of the femur or the upper end of the tibia being favored locations.

−rarely undergoes transition to chondrosarcoma; malignant transformation is more frequent in multiple familial osteochondromatosis, the rare hereditary variant characterized by multiple lesions.

b. Giant cell tumor

−is characterized by oval or spindle-shaped cells intermingled with numerous multinuclear giant cells.

Table 22.2. Notable Features of Selected Bone Tumors

Type	Description	Most Frequent Location	Incidence
Benign:			
Osteochondroma (exostosis)	Cartilage-capped subperiosteal bony projection from bone surface	Lower end of femur and upper end of tibia	Males under age 25
Giant cell tumor	Tumor characterized by multinucleated giant cells and fibrous stroma	Epiphyses of long bones, especially at lower end of femur and upper end of tibia	Females ages 20–40
Enchondroma	Intramedullary cartilaginous neoplasm	Bones of hands and feet	No special age or sex incidence
Osteoma	Tumor of dense mature bone	Skull or facial bones; often protrudes into a paranasal sinus	Males of any age
Osteoid osteoma	Neoplastic proliferation of osteoid and fibrous tissue	Near end of diaphysis of femur or tibia	Males under age 25
Osteoblastoma	. . .	Within vertebrae	. . .
Malignant:			
Osteosarcoma (osteogenic sarcoma)	Osteoid- and bone-producing neoplasm	Tibia and femur near knee	Males ages 10–20
Chondrosarcoma	Cartilaginous tumor	Pelvic bones, proximal and distal femur, proximal tibia, ribs, vertebrae	Males ages 30–60
Ewing's sarcoma	Undifferentiated round cell tumor	Long bones, pelvis, scapulae, ribs	Males under age 15

—occurs most often on the epiphyseal end of long bones; more than 50% occur about the knee.

—has a characteristic "soap bubble" appearance on X-ray.

—has its peak incidence in persons aged 20 to 40 years.

—is somewhat more common in women than in men.

—although benign, is a locally aggressive tumor that frequently recurs after local curettage.

2. Malignant bone tumors

a. Osteosarcoma (osteogenic sarcoma)

—is the most common primary tumor of bone.

—has a peak incidence in men aged 10 to 20 years.

—occurs most frequently in the metaphysis of long bones; the proximal portion of the tibia and most distal portion of the femur are preferred sites (about the knee).

(1) **Clinical characteristics**
    (a) Pain and swelling and occasionally pathologic fracture
    (b) A two- to threefold increase of serum alkaline phosphatase
    (c) Lifting of the periosteum by the expanding tumor, which creates a characteristic radiologic appearance known as **Codman's triangle**
    (d) Early hematogenous spread to the lungs, liver, and brain
(2) **Predisposing factors**
    (a) Paget's disease of bone
    (b) Ionizing radiation
    (c) Bone infarcts
    (d) Familial retinoblastoma (in these patients, surgical cure of the primary ocular tumor is often followed by the later development of osteosarcoma, presumably due to loss of the rb suppressor gene locus on chromosome 13)

b. Chondrosarcoma
    —is a **malignant cartilaginous tumor**.
    —has its peak incidence in men aged 30 to 60.
    —may arise as a primary tumor or from transformation of preexisting cartilaginous tumors, especially multiple familial osteochondromatosis or multiple enchondromatosis.
    —has characteristic **sites of origin,** including the pelvis, spine, or scapula; the proximal humerus or proximal femur; and femur or tibia near the knee.

c. Ewing's sarcoma
    —is an extremely anaplastic **small-cell malignant tumor** with a morphologic resemblance to malignant lymphoma.
    —occurs most often in long bones, ribs, pelvis, and scapula.
    —has a peak incidence in boys under age 15.
    —follows an extremely malignant course with early metastases.
    —is responsive to chemotherapy.
    —in early stages, may clinically mimic acute osteomyelitis.
    —is characterized by 11;22 chromosomal translocation identical to that found in highly undifferentiated neuroectodermal tumors (soft-tissue lesions of neural crest origin) and olfactory neuroblastoma, and is most likely closely related to this group.

III. Diseases of Joints (Table 22.3)

A. Arthritides of probable autoimmune origin

1. Rheumatoid arthritis
    —is a chronic inflammatory disorder primarily affecting synovial joints.
    —is most common in women aged 20 to 50.

a. Pathogenetic factors—rheumatoid arthritis
    —is likely of **autoimmune origin,** with interplay of genetic and environmental factors.
    —is often characterized by the presence of serum **rheumatoid factor,** an immunoglobulin (most often IgM) with anti-IgE Fc specificity, which is highly characteristic of but not specific for rheumatoid arthritis.
    —occurs most often in HLA-DR4 positive individuals.

Table 22.3. Distinctive Features of Selected Arthritides and Related Disorders

Type	Etiology	Incidence	Most Frequent Site	Notable Features
Rheumatoid arthritis	Autoimmune	Women ages 20–50	Joints of hands, knees, and feet; proximal interphalangeal and metacarpophalangeal joints	Subcutaneous nodules; rheumatoid factor (anti-IgG)
Ankylosing spondylitis	Probably autoimmune; may have genetic component	Young men	Spine and sacroiliac joints	Vast majority of patients positive for HLA-B27 antigen
Osteoarthritis (degenerative joint disease)	Mechanical injury ("wear-and-tear"); may have a genetic component	After age 50; somewhat more frequent in women	Weight-bearing joints; distal and proximal interphalangeal joints	Osteophytes; Heberden's and Bouchard's nodes; joint mice
Gout	Hyperuricemia with deposition of urate crystals in multiple sites	Men older than age 30	Metatarsophalangeal joint of great toe	Tophi; kidney damage; urate nephrolithiasis
Gonococcal arthritis	Infection with *Neisseria gonorrhoeae*	Variable	Knee, wrist, small joints of hands	Often monoarticular
Hypertrophic osteoarthropathy	Secondary manifestation of chronic lung disease, cyanotic heart disease, and various nonpulmonary systemic disorders	Variable, depending on primary disorder	Fingers, radius, and ulna	Clubbing of fingers; periostitis

b. Morphology—rheumatoid arthritis

—manifests most characteristically by **synovitis**.

—progresses as follows:

(1) Earliest changes include an **acute inflammatory reaction** with edema and an inflammatory infiltrate, beginning with neutrophils and followed by lymphocytes and plasma cells.

(2) Hyperplasia and hypertrophy of the synovial lining cells eventuate into numerous finger-like villi.

(3) Granulation tissue (**pannus**) extends over articular cartilage; extension of pannus to subchondral bone results in erosion and cyst formation, leading to deformities of both cartilage and bone.

(4) Scarring, contracture, and deformity result from destructive inflammation of ligaments, tendons, and bursae.

(5) Subcutaneous **rheumatoid nodules** develop in approximately one-third of patients.

c. Clinical course

(1) Episodic changes

(a) Fatigue, malaise, anorexia, weight loss, fever, and myalgia

      (b) Swelling of the joints and stiffness, especially in the morning or after inactivity

      (c) Polyarticular and symmetric joint involvement

  (2) Chronic joint changes

      (a) Proximal interphalangeal and metacarpophalangeal joints of the hands are frequent sites.

      (b) Ulnar deviation of fingers results from synovitis of ligaments.

      (c) Minimal radial deviation of the wrist may occur.

  (3) Extra-articular manifestations

      (a) Pleural and pericardial effusions

      (b) Anemia of chronic disease

      (c) Vasculitis

      (d) Lymphadenopathy

      (e) Pulmonary involvement

      (f) Neurologic abnormalities

      (g) Secondary reactive amyloidosis

d. Variants of rheumatoid arthritis

  (1) Sjögren's syndrome with rheumatoid arthritis

  (2) Felty's syndrome: splenomegaly, neutropenia, and rheumatoid arthritis

  (3) Still's disease (juvenile rheumatoid arthritis), often preceded or accompanied by generalized lymphadenopathy and hepatosplenomegaly and an acute onset marked by fever.

2. Seronegative arthritis (spondyloarthropathies)

a. Characteristics

  (1) Absence of rheumatoid factor

  (2) Extremely high incidence in **HLA B27**-positive individuals

  (3) Peripheral arthritis

  (4) Sacroiliitis

b. Types

  (1) Ankylosing spondylitis: HLA-B27 association is most striking with this entity (up to 90% of patients). This chronic condition affects the spine and sacroiliac joints and can lead to rigidity and fixation of the spine as a result of bone fusion (ankylosis).

  (2) Reiter's syndrome: urethritis, conjunctivitis, and arthritis is often associated with venereal or intestinal infection.

  (3) Psoriatic arthritis occurs in approximately 10% of patients with psoriasis.

  (4) Arthritis associated with inflammatory bowel disease: peripheral arthritis or ankylosing spondylitis complicating ulcerative colitis or Crohn's disease.

B. Osteoarthritis (degenerative joint disease)

  —is a chronic noninflammatory joint disease characterized by degeneration of articular cartilage accompanied by new bone formation subchondrally and at the margins of the affected joint.

  —is the most common form of arthritis.

—has a higher incidence in women, most often beginning after age 50.

—is most often related to mechanical trauma to the affected joints ("wear-and-tear" arthritis).

1. **Characteristic morphologic changes**

   a. Loss of elasticity, pitting, and fraying of cartilage; fragments may separate and float into synovial fluid.

   b. **Eburnation:** polished, ivory-like appearance of bone, resulting from erosion of overlying cartilage

   c. **Cystic changes** in subchondral bone

   d. **New bone formation,** resulting in:

      (1) Increased density of subchondral bone

      (2) **Osteophyte** (bony spur) formation at the perimeter of the articular surface and at points of ligamental attachment to bone

   e. **Osteophytes fracturing** and floating into synovial fluid (along with fragments of separated cartilage; these particles are termed **joint mice**).

   f. **Heberden's nodes:** osteophytes at distal interphalangeal joints of fingers

   g. **Bouchard's nodes:** osteophytes at the proximal interphalangeal joints of the fingers

2. **Types**

   a. **Primary osteoarthritis**

      —occurs without known cause.

      —may result from a complex interplay of genetic predisposition with a variety of mechanical or inflammatory mechanisms.

   b. **Secondary osteoarthritis**

      —occurs in joints damaged by known mechanisms, including mechanical factors, metabolic disorders such as ochronosis, and inflammatory disorders.

C. **Arthritides of metabolic origin**

   1. **Gout**

      a. **General characteristics—gout**

         —is characterized by **deposition of urate crystals** in a number of tissues, especially the joints, as a result of **hyperuricemia**.

         —is marked by an intense inflammatory reaction beginning with opsonization of crystals by IgG, followed by phagocytosis by neutrophils, and eventuating in the release of proteolytic enzymes and inflammatory mediators from the phagocytic cells.

         —is manifest by an inflammatory response that leads to extremely painful acute arthritis and bursitis.

         —occurs most frequently in the metatarsophalangeal joint of the great toe. Acute gouty arthritis in this characteristic location is known as **podagra**.

–is often precipitated by a large meal or alcohol intake, both of which may increase hyperuricemia.

–eventually leads to the formation of nodular **tophi,** which are located about joints, in the helix and the antihelix of the ear, in the Achilles' tendon, and in other sites. Tophi are composed of urate crystals in a protein matrix surrounded by fibrous connective tissue, all demonstrating a foreign body giant cell reaction.

–often leads to **renal damage** characterized by interstitial deposition of urate crystals and obstruction of collecting tubules by urate crystals and by formation of urate and calcium stones.

–is diagnosed by findings of hyperuricemia along with urate crystals in synovial fluid or with biopsy evidence of tophaceous deposits; urate crystals are negatively birefringent under polarized light.

b. Types

(1) Primary gout

–is characterized by hyperuricemia without evident cause.

–is the most common form of gout.

–is most common in middle-aged men.

–tends to be familial.

(2) Secondary gout

–is much less common.

–is characterized by hyperuricemia with evident cause, such as:

(a) Myeloproliferative syndromes, with increased cellular turnover

(b) Decreased urate excretion because of chronic renal disease or intake of a variety of drugs

(c) Lesch-Nyhan syndrome: hyperuricemia with severe neurologic manifestations, including self-mutilation, due to X-linked hypoxanthine-guanine phosphoribosyltransferase (HGPRT) deficiency

2. Chondrocalcinosis (pseudogout)

–is caused by calcium pyrophosphate dihydrate crystal deposition, which elicits inflammatory reaction in cartilage.

–clinically resembles gout.

D. Infective arthritis

–is characterized by purulent synovial fluid.

1. Gonococcal arthritis

–is the most common form of bacterial arthritis.

–is most often **monoarticular**.

–most frequently involves the **knee;** other favored sites are the wrist and small joints of the hand.

2. Lyme disease

–is caused by infection by the spirochete *Borrelia burgdorferi,* most often transmitted by *Ixodes dammini,* a tick.

–demonstrates a characteristic skin lesion, erythema chronicum migrans, a slowly spreading lesion with prominent erythematous margins and central fading ("bull's-eye" lesion).

—most characteristically leads to polyarticular arthritis as a late sequela; typically involves the knees and other large joints.

—can also lead to myocardial, pericardial, or neurologic changes as late sequelae.

—is diagnosed by demonstration of IgM serum antibodies to *B. burgdorferi*.

—responds well if treated early with antibiotics.

E. Miscellaneous joint diseases

1. Hypertrophic osteoarthropathy

—is associated with systemic disorders such as chronic lung disease, congenital cyanotic heart disease, cirrhosis of the liver, and inflammatory bowel disease.

—is a chronic condition that may manifest as **clubbing of the fingers** (the most obvious abnormality) and, more frequently, as associated **periostitis** at the distal end of the radius and ulna.

—may also present as painful swelling and tenderness of the peripheral joints.

2. Ganglion cyst

—is a small cystic nodule arising in the tendon sheath or the joint capsule of the wrist.

—is thought to be caused by myxoid degeneration of connective tissue.

IV. Soft-tissue Tumors

A. General characteristics

1. Tumors originate in fibrous connective tissue, adipose tissue, skeletal muscle, joint tissue, and the peripheral nervous system.

2. Tumors most often require diagnostic adjuncts such as special stains, electron microscopy, or immunohistochemistry (studies for S-100, desmin, vimentin, and cytokeratin are most commonly employed).

B. Examples of soft-tissue tumors

1. Rhabdomyosarcoma

—is a malignant tumor of skeletal muscle.

—may arise in other soft tissues.

—has several variants, including pleomorphic rhabdomyosarcoma, embryonal rhabdomyosarcoma, and alveolar rhabdomyosarcoma.

2. Synovial sarcoma

—is a highly malignant soft-tissue tumor.

—most often originates in tissue adjacent to a joint rather than in a joint cavity.

—often occurs in the lower extremities.

—is characterized by a biphasic growth pattern in which both epithelial and spindle cells are seen.

3. Fibrous histiocytoma

—is a benign tumor consisting of a mix of fibroblasts and histiocytes.

4. Malignant fibrous histiocytoma

—is the most common soft-tissue sarcoma of late middle and old age.

5. Fibrosarcoma

—is a malignant tumor of fibroblasts.

—is characterized by spindle-shaped cells demonstrating a herringbone pattern.

6. Lipoma

—is the most common soft-tissue tumor.

—is a benign tumor of mature adipose tissue.

7. Liposarcoma

—is a malignant tumor of adipose tissue.

Review Test

Directions: Each of the numbered items or incomplete statements in this section is followed by answers or by completions of the statement. Select the **one** lettered answer or completion that is **best** in each case.

1. Which of the following histologic patterns is most characteristic of disuse atrophy?

(A) Angular atrophy predominantly involving type I muscle fibers
(B) Angular atrophy predominantly involving type II muscle fibers
(C) Angular atrophy equally involving type I and type II muscle fibers
(D) Target fibers
(E) Fiber-type grouping

2. Duchenne muscular dystrophy is characterized by all of the following EXCEPT

(A) progressive muscular wasting beginning in proximal muscles.
(B) autosomal recessive inheritance.
(C) absence of muscle dystrophin.
(D) pseudohypertrophy.
(E) partial or segmental gene deletion mutations.

3. All of the following types of muscular dystrophy are matched with the appropriate characteristic or association EXCEPT

(A) Duchenne muscular dystrophy—dystrophin abnormality.
(B) Becker's muscular dystrophy—autosomal dominant inheritance.
(C) facioscapulohumeral muscular dystrophy—nondisabling course.
(D) limb-girdle dystrophy—autosomal recessive inheritance.
(E) myotonic dystrophy—testicular atrophy.

4. All of the following muscular disorders are correctly paired with the appropriate phrase EXCEPT

(A) central core disease—loss of mitochondria and other organelles.
(B) nemaline myopathy—tangles of small rod-shaped granules.
(C) mitochondrial myopathies—X-linked inheritance.
(D) Duchenne muscular dystrophy—frameshift mutations.
(E) myasthenia gravis—thymic tumor.

5. A 40-year-old woman presents with ptosis, diplopia, and dysarthria that fluctuate in intensity and tend to worsen as the day progresses. All of the following are well-known features, associations, or complications of the illness suggested by these findings EXCEPT

(A) thymoma.
(B) antiacetylcholine receptor antibodies.
(C) respiratory failure.
(D) tangles of small rod-shaped granules in type I muscle fibers.
(E) improvement with cholinesterase inhibitor drugs.

6. Characteristics of pyogenic osteomyelitis include all of the following EXCEPT

(A) in children, it most often is caused by blood-borne spread from infection elsewhere.
(B) in adults, it often is a complication of trauma or surgery.
(C) it can lead to bone necrosis.
(D) it can lead to draining sinuses.
(E) it is almost never amenable to antibiotic therapy.

7. Birbeck granules in histiocytic cells are ultrastructural markers of

(A) monocytic leukemia.
(B) histiocytosis X.
(C) Gaucher's disease.
(D) Niemann-Pick disease.
(E) histiocytic lymphoma.

8. Characteristics of osteosarcoma include all of the following EXCEPT

(A) highest incidence occurs in teenagers with preexisting Paget's disease of bone.
(B) high incidence occurs following surgical cure of familial retinoblastoma.
(C) it is the most common malignant primary tumor of bone.
(D) it is more common in males.
(E) early hematogenous spread is to the lungs, liver, and brain.

9. All of the following characteristics are associated with rheumatoid arthritis EXCEPT

(A) serum anti-IgG antibodies.
(B) subcutaneous rheumatoid nodules.
(C) osteophyte formation.
(D) fatigue, malaise, anorexia, weight loss, fever, and myalgia.
(E) symmetric polyarthritis.

10. Which of the following disorders is most closely associated with HLA-B27 positivity?

(A) Rheumatoid arthritis
(B) Sjögren's syndrome
(C) Felty's syndrome
(D) Ankylosing spondylitis
(E) Osteoarthritis

11. All of the following features are characteristics of osteoarthritis EXCEPT

(A) eburnation of bone.
(B) joint mice.
(C) pannus formation.
(D) Heberden's nodes.
(E) Bouchard's nodes.

12. Acute monoarticular purulent arthritis of the knee with purulent synovial fluid is most likely a manifestation of

(A) rheumatoid arthritis.
(B) Felty's syndrome.
(C) Osgood-Schlatter disease.
(D) gonorrhea.
(E) chondrocalcinosis.

13. All of the following are characteristic of gout EXCEPT

(A) higher incidence in women.
(B) hyperuricemia.
(C) involvement of great toe.
(D) tophi.
(E) urate urolithiasis.

Directions: Each group of items in this section consists of lettered options followed by a set of numbered items. For each item, select the **one** lettered option that is most closely associated with it. Each lettered option may be selected once, more than once, or not at all.

Questions 14–16

Match each bone disease with its blood chemistry profile.

(A) High serum calcium, low serum phosphorus, high serum alkaline phosphatase
(B) Low calcium, normal phosphorus, high alkaline phosphatase
(C) Normal calcium, normal phosphorus, normal alkaline phosphatase
(D) Normal calcium, normal phosphorus, markedly increased alkaline phosphatase

14. Osteoporosis

15. Von Recklinghausen's disease of bone

16. Paget's disease of bone

Answers and Explanations

1–B. Disuse atrophy is histologically characterized by angular atrophic changes predominantly involving type II muscle fibers. Similar changes involving both type I and type II fibers, fiber-type grouping, and target fibers are all associated with denervation atrophy.

2–B. Duchenne muscular dystrophy is an X-linked disorder characterized by progressive muscular wasting beginning in proximal muscles and by the late development of pseudohypertrophy. The disorder is due to partial or segmental deletion of the dystrophin gene, leading to essentially total absence of dystrophin.

3–B. Becker's muscular dystrophy is caused by a deletion abnormality of the dystrophin gene, which is located on the X chromosome, and is thus characterized by X-linked inheritance. In this disorder, segmental deletion does not interrupt the coding reading frame, and the resultant dystrophin protein is shortened and presumably less functional. This is in contrast to the total failure of dystrophin synthesis in Duchenne muscular dystrophy.

4–C. Mitochondrial myopathies are caused by abnormalities (most often deletions) of mitochondrial DNA and are associated with an exclusively maternal mode of transmission. This mode of inheritance should be distinguished from X-linked inheritance.

5–D. The history of this patient strongly suggests myasthenia gravis, a disorder of the neuromuscular junction that is not associated with any morphologic abnormalities of skeletal muscle. Patients often present with ptosis and diplopia resulting from ocular muscle weakness, with frequent progression to difficulty in chewing, speaking, or swallowing, or weakness of muscles of the extremities. Thymoma or thymic hyperplasia is frequent. The disorder is caused by antiacetylcholine receptor antibodies. Respiratory failure from diaphragmatic weakness can occur. Marked improvement with cholinesterase inhibitors is characteristic.

6–E. Pyogenic osteomyelitis may resolve with antibiotic therapy in early stages of the infection. However, after sequestrum, abscess, or draining sinus formation, surgical intervention is required.

7–B. Birbeck granules, ultrastructural tennis racket-shaped inclusions, are markers of Langerhans' cells of the skin and of the closely related cells of histiocytosis X. This marker and other antigenic determinants distinguish these cells from other histiocytes and from unrelated histiocytic proliferative disorders, such as Gaucher's disease.

8–A. While the incidence of osteosarcoma is generally higher in teenagers, osteosarcoma secondary to Paget's disease of bone usually occurs in the elderly.

9–C. Osteophyte (bony spur) formation is a cardinal feature of osteoarthritis, not rheumatoid arthritis. Serum anti-IgG antibodies (rheumatoid factor), subcutaneous rheumatoid nodules, systemic symptoms and signs (fatigue, malaise, anorexia), and symmetric polyarthritis are all well-known characteristics of rheumatoid arthritis.

10–D. The association with HLA-B27 positivity is most striking in ankylosing spondylitis, with as many as 90% of patients exhibiting this finding. A less frequent association of HLA-B27 is noted with Reiter's syndrome (urethritis, conjunctivitis, and arthritis), with psoriatic arthritis, and with the arthritis associated with inflammatory bowel disease.

11–C. Pannus formation, the extension of granulation tissue over damaged articular cartilage, is a characteristic of rheumatoid arthritis, not osteoarthritis. Joint mice, eburnation, Heberden's nodes, and Bouchard's nodes are all characteristics of osteoarthritis.

12–D. Purulent synovial fluid suggests a diagnosis of infective arthritis, and gonococcal arthritis is the most frequently occurring of the bacterial arthritides. It is often monoarticular, and the knee is the most frequently involved site.

13–A. Gout is most typically seen in adult men, with a much lower incidence in women.

14–C. Osteoporosis is caused by a loss of bony matrix unassociated with abnormalities in mineral metabolism. Serum calcium and phosphorus are characteristically normal as is serum alkaline phosphatase.

15–A. Von Recklinghausen's disease of bone is caused by hyperparathyroidism and is characterized by increased serum calcium, decreased phosphorus, and increased alkaline phosphatase.

16–D. Paget's disease of bone is unaccompanied by changes in serum calcium or phosphorus, but striking elevation of serum alkaline phosphatase is characteristic.

23

Nervous System

I. Congenital Disorders

A. Neural tube defects

—are characteristically associated with increased concentration of maternal serum **alpha-fetoprotein,** a finding of diagnostic value.

—are a group of disorders characterized by failure of closure of the neural tube. The resulting defects can involve the vertebrae or skull with or without involvement of the underlying meninges, spinal cord, or brain. These disorders include:

1. **Spina bifida:** failure of posterior vertebral arches to close

2. **Spina bifida occulta:** spina bifida with no clinically apparent abnormalities; vertebral arch defect most often limited to one or two vertebrae

3. **Spina bifida cystica:** spina bifida complicated by herniation of meninges through a defect

4. **Meningocele:** herniated membranes consisting of meninges only

5. **Meningomyelocele:** portion of spinal cord included in herniated tissue

6. **Anencephaly:** marked diminution (sometimes absence) of fetal brain tissue; usually associated with absence of overlying skull.

B. Hydrocephalus

—denotes increased volume of cerebrospinal fluid (CSF) within the cranial cavity.

—occurs in these variants:

1. **Internal hydrocephalus:** increased volume of CSF is entirely within ventricles

2. **External hydrocephalus:** increased volume of CSF is confined to subarachnoid space

3. **Communicating hydrocephalus:** free flow of CSF between ventricles and subarachnoid space

4. Noncommunicating hydrocephalus: obstructed flow of CSF from ventricles to subarachnoid space

—in infants is associated with (sometimes marked) enlargement of the skull.

—is most often caused by obstruction to the CSF circulation by mechanisms such as congenital malformations, inflammation, and tumors.

—can also result from overproduction of CSF by choroid plexus papilloma (very rare).

—can also occur as **hydrocephalus ex vacuo** without obstruction or increased CSF production in disorders characterized by decreased cerebral mass, such as ischemic brain atrophy or advanced Alzheimer's disease.

C. Arnold-Chiari malformation

—is a herniation of the posterior cerebellum and medulla through the foramen magnum.

—results in pressure atrophy of herniated brain tissue.

—causes hydrocephalus as a result of obstruction of the CSF outflow tract.

—is almost always characterized by the presence of a thoracolumbar meningomyelocele.

D. Agenesis of the corpus callosum

—can be asymptomatic.

—is often found in association with other abnormalities.

E. Fetal alcohol syndrome

—is associated with excessive maternal alcohol intake during pregnancy.

—is characterized by facial abnormalities and developmental defects such as microcephaly, atrial septal defect, mental and growth retardation, and other anomalies.

F. Tuberous sclerosis syndrome

—includes autosomal dominant nodular proliferation of multinucleated atypical astrocytes forming tubers (small white nodules scattered in the cerebral cortex and periventricular areas).

—also includes adenoma sebaceum of the skin and angiomyolipoma of the kidney.

—is characterized by seizures and mental retardation beginning in infancy.

II. Cerebrovascular Disease (Table 23.1)

—is the most common group of central nervous system (CNS) disorders; it ranks after heart disease and cancer as the third major cause of death in the United States.

A. Infarction

—is more frequent than hemorrhage.

—is caused by arterial occlusion from:

1. Thrombosis, most often caused by atherosclerosis

2. Embolism, from cardiac mural thrombi, vegetations of infected endocarditic valves, clumps of tumor cells, bubbles of air, or droplets of fat. Embolism is much less common than thrombosis.

—results in clinical manifestations that depend on the site of vascular obstruction and extent of collateral circulation; the middle cerebral artery is the most frequent site of embolic occlusion. Arterial obstruction in this site causes contralateral paralysis as well as motor and sensory defects and aphasias.

Table 23.1. Cerebrovascular Disease

Type	Principal Predisposing Factors	Common Sites
Infarction: Thrombosis	Atherosclerosis	Arterial obstruction of internal and external carotid arteries at origin in neck, vertebral and basilar arteries, and vessels branching from circle of Willis, especially middle cerebral artery
Embolism	Cardiac mural thrombi, valvular vegetations, fat emboli	Middle cerebral artery most frequent site of embolic occlusion
Hemorrhage: Intracerebral	Hypertension, coagulation disorders, hemorrhage within a tumor	Can result from rupture of Charcot-Buchard aneurysms, which result from long-standing hypertension
Subarachnoid	Rupture of congenital berry aneurysm; likelihood of rupture compounded by hypertension	Circle of Willis and bifurcation of middle cerebral artery

—when due to obstruction of small vessels, can result in small lesions that upon healing are recognizable as lacunae (small pits). Clinical manifestations of **lacunar strokes** are focal and are most often purely sensory or motor. Pure motor lacunar stroke most often results from lesions affecting the internal capsule. Pure sensory lacunar stroke most often results from lesions affecting the thalamus.

B. Hemorrhage

1. Intracerebral hemorrhage

—consists of bleeding into the brain substance.
—is most frequently caused by **hypertension**.
—most often occurs in the basal ganglia; other favored sites include the pons, frontal lobe, and cerebellum.

2. Subarachnoid hemorrhage

—consists of bleeding into the subarachnoid space.
—is frequently associated with **berry aneurysm** of the circle of Willis.
—is also caused by arteriovenous malformations, trauma, or hemorrhagic diatheses.

C. Transient ischemic attacks (TIAs)

—are brief episodes of impaired neurologic function caused by temporary disturbance of cerebral circulation.
—are not associated with permanent damage but are considered precursors to more serious occlusive events.

III. Head Injuries

—result from **penetrating wounds,** which, in addition to brain damage, can predispose to infection.
—also result from **nonpenetrating injuries;** brain injury at the site of impact is referred to as **coup** injury; injury on the opposite side of the brain from the site of impact is **contrecoup** injury; contusions characterize both coup and contrecoup injuries.

A. Epidural hematoma

–is an arterial hemorrhage associated with skull fracture and most often with laceration of branches of the **middle meningeal artery**.

–is characterized clinically by a short period of consciousness (lucid interval) followed by rapidly developing signs of cerebral compression.

–is amenable to emergency surgical intervention because bleeding into the brain substance itself does not occur.

B. Subdural hematoma

–is caused by venous bleeding, most often from **bridging veins** joining the cerebrum to venous sinuses within the dura.

–is characterized clinically by gradual signs of cerebral compression occurring hours to days or even weeks after head injury; venous hemorrhage typically arrests early, but the volume of the hematoma gradually increases as a result of osmotic imbibement of water, resulting in a slowly enlarging tumor-like mass.

IV. Infections

A. Pyogenic meningitis

1. General features—pyogenic meningitis

–is manifest clinically by fever, headache, prostration, and nuchal rigidity.

–can lead to arachnoiditis, with scarring and consequent hydrocephalus.

–can also lead to vasculitis, with consequent infarction or brain abscess.

–has its peak incidence in children (nearly 75% of cases), with a second high incidence peak in the elderly.

–is characterized by purulent exudate in the subarachnoid space. **CSF findings** of diagnostic significance include:

a. Numerous neutrophils

b. Decreased glucose (less than two-thirds of the serum glucose concentration)

c. Increased protein

2. Etiology—pyogenic meningitis

–in newborns, is most frequently caused by *Escherichia coli*.

–in older infants and young children, is most frequently caused by *Haemophilus influenzae*.

–in young adults, is most frequently caused by *Neisseria meningitidis;* its occurrence may be sporadic or epidemic and may be accompanied by meningococcemia secondary to a primary infection in the nasopharynx.

–meningococcemia is sometimes associated with Waterhouse-Friderichsen syndrome (hemorrhagic destruction of the adrenal cortex, acute hypocorticism with circulatory collapse, and disseminated intravascular coagulation).

–in older adults, is most frequently caused by *Streptococcus pneumoniae* (pneumococcus).

B. Cerebral abscess

–can result from penetrating skull injuries or from spread of infection originating elsewhere; sources of infection include the sinuses or middle ear (the most common source), bronchopulmonary infections, infective endocarditis, and other sites.

C. Tuberculosis

—occurs as tuberculosis of the brain substance or as tuberculous meningitis.

—is secondary to tuberculous infection occurring elsewhere in the body.

D. Fungal infection

—is caused most often by *Cryptococcus neoformans, Coccidioides immitis, Aspergillus,* or *Histoplasma.*

—can involve the brain substance or the meninges.

—is often associated with impaired resistance to infection.

E. Toxoplasmosis

—is a parasitic infection of the brain.

—is caused by *Toxoplasma gondii.*

—in neonates, is **transmitted transplacentally** from the infected mother.

—is also spread by ingestion of foods contaminated by animal urine or feces; household pets, especially cats, are frequent reservoirs.

—in newborns, results in hydrocephalus, mental retardation, and other **neurologic abnormalities;** characteristic **periventricular calcifications** are demonstrable radiographically; cerebral cortex, basal ganglia, and retinae as well as heart, lungs, and liver are sites of involvement.

—in adults, is most often manifest as lymphadenitis; CNS involvement may occur in immunosuppressed persons.

F. Viral infection

1. General features—viral infection

—can be limited to the meninges or can involve the brain or spinal cord.

a. Viral meningitis (lymphocytic or aseptic meningitis)

—is caused by a variety of viral agents.

—is manifest clinically by fever, headache, and nuchal rigidity; CSF demonstrates an increase in lymphocytes, moderately increased protein, and normal glucose concentration.

b. Meningoencephalitis and encephalitis

—demonstrates the following morphologic changes in the brain substance:

(1) Perivascular cuffing (infiltrate of mononuclear cells within Virchow-Robin spaces)

(2) Inclusion bodies in neurons or glial cells (a frequent but not invariable finding)

(3) Glial nodules as a result of nonspecific proliferation of microglia

—can present as brain stem disease (e.g., poliomyelitis, which even more characteristically exhibits prominent involvement of the spinal cord).

2. Examples of viral infection

a. Arbovirus encephalitides

(1) St. Louis encephalitis: reservoir, horses and birds; mosquito vector; disease varies from an asymptomatic state to severe meningoencephalitis.

(2) Eastern equine encephalitis: associated with a high mortality rate; reservoir, horses and birds.

(3) **Western equine encephalitis:** less severe than Eastern equine encephalitis.

b. Herpes simplex encephalitis

–is most common in teenagers and young adults.

–is an uncommon complication of herpes simplex virus infection but is nonetheless the most common agent of severe viral encephalitis.

c. Poliomyelitis

–is characterized by degeneration and necrosis of anterior horn cells of the spinal cord.

d. Rabies

–is spread by the bite of dogs, raccoons, foxes, squirrels, skunks, bats, and so forth; saliva contains the virus.

–results in severe encephalitis with increased excitability of the CNS; it is characterized by violent muscle contractions and convulsions after minimal stimuli.

–is aborted by active immunization during the interval between the bite and the projected onset of clinical manifestations; it is usually fatal once clinical signs develop.

–is histologically characterized by neuronal degeneration, perivascular accumulations of mononuclear cells in the brain stem and spinal cord, and characteristic eosinophilic intracytoplasmic inclusions (**Negri bodies**) in the hippocampus and Purkinje cells of the cerebellum.

e. Cytomegalovirus infection

–generally affects immunosuppressed persons.

–results in encephalomyelitis as well as in lesions of the kidneys, liver, lungs, and salivary glands.

–is characterized by giant cells with **eosinophilic inclusions** involving both the nucleus and cytoplasm.

–in infants, may be characterized in severe cases by mental retardation, microcephaly, chorioretinitis, and hepatosplenomegaly; periventricular calcification within the brain is demonstrable.

f. Human immunodeficiency virus (HIV) infection

–can cause nervous system dysfunction prior to onset of immunodeficiency.

–may affect the brain, spinal cord, or peripheral nervous system by direct HIV infection. Cells of monocyte–macrophage origin are vehicles for viral entry into the nervous system and may serve as the viral reservoir.

–may facilitate opportunistic infection or tumor development within the nervous system, both mediated by immunodeficiency.

–most often results in AIDS dementia complex, although other clinical syndromes also occur; difficulty concentrating, memory impairment, slowness of thinking, depression, personality changes, lethargy, and difficulty with balance, coordination, and motor function are all frequently seen; downhill course with progressive dementia is characteristic.

G. Other entities of viral or suspected viral etiology (slow virus infections)

—are characterized by a long incubation period, lack of conventional inflammatory response, and a progressive course. Spongiosis (spongiform change or spongiform encephalopathy) often can be demonstrated. Numerous clusters of small cysts can be found in CNS gray matter. For example:

1. Kuru

—is caused by an unknown infectious agent.

—is transmitted by ingestion of human brain by cannibals of New Guinea.

—manifests by loss of neurons, gliosis, and striking spongiosis in the cerebrum, cerebellum, and spinal cord; cerebellar atrophy is often present.

—is characterized by cerebellar degeneration with marked tremor, ataxia, slurred speech, and progressive mental deficiency, followed by death within a few months.

2. Creutzfeldt-Jakob disease

—exhibits morphologic changes similar to kuru; spongiosis is prominent.

—the viral nature of the infectious agent is speculative; the infectious role of prions is questionable; prions are presumably self-replicating, nonnucleotide-containing protein particles.

—is believed to be a hazard to health workers who work with brain specimens; however, the mode of transmission is unknown.

—is characterized by ataxia, rapidly progressive dementia, and early death.

3. Subacute sclerosing panencephalitis

—is caused by persistent infection with **measles virus;** patients are infected in infancy but an asymptomatic interval of several years is followed by neurologic manifestations in late childhood or the early teenage years.

—is slowly progressive; is usually fatal.

—is characterized by lack of M component of measles virus, a protein required for extracellular spread of virus; this deficiency may explain the slow nature of infection. CSF contains oligoclonal immunoglobulins against viral proteins but lacks "anti-M."

4. Progressive multifocal leukoencephalopathy

—is most often caused by the JC polyoma type of **papovavirus**.

—is characterized by rapidly progressive multiple foci of demyelination in the brain, and it is associated with abnormal oligodendrocytes and astrocytes.

—is often associated with **leukemia or lymphoma** or with immunodeficiency.

V. Demyelinating Diseases

—are characterized by destruction of myelin with relative preservation of axons.

A. Multiple sclerosis

1. Incidence—multiple sclerosis

—is by far the most common of the demyelinating diseases.

—most often begins between ages 20 and 30 years.

—is slightly more common in women.

2. Etiology—multiple sclerosis

—is of unknown etiology; immune or viral factors are suspected but un-proven causes; multiple sclerosis is thought to be multifactorial in origin, with both **environmental and genetic factors** playing a role, a view supported by the following:

a. Frequent occurrence of increased CSF immunoglobulin, often manifest as multiple oligoclonal bands on electrophoresis, suggests that viral or immune factors may play a role.

b. Increased incidence in association with certain HLA haplotypes (A3, B7, DR2, and DW2) suggests that immune factors may play a role.

c. Highest incidence occurs in persons of northern European ancestry.

d. Incidence is directly proportional to the geographic distance from the equator; predisposition remains when persons move to a low-incidence geographic site if the move is made after age 15.

3. Morphologic changes—multiple sclerosis

—is characterized by multiple focal areas of demyelination (plaques) that are irregularly scattered in the brain and spinal cord; the optic nerve, brain stem, and paraventricular areas are favored sites; helper CD4 + and cytotoxic CD8 + lymphocytes and macrophages infiltrate plaques; reactive gliosis occurs later.

4. Clinical manifestations—multiple sclerosis

—follows a highly variable clinical course depending on the site of involvement.

—is characterized by exacerbations with long asymptomatic remissions and often a progressive course, leading to invalidism with mental deterioration.

—manifests by early findings: weakness of the lower extremities, visual disturbances and retrobulbar pain, sensory disturbances, and possible loss of bladder control.

—may be manifest with the classic Charcot triad (nystagmus, intention tremor, and scanning speech), which is significant for diagnosis.

B. Acute disseminated encephalomyelitis

—follows viral illnesses such as measles, mumps, rubella, and chicken pox and is often known as **postinfectious encephalitis**.

—may be a manifestation of a delayed hypersensitivity reaction.

—varies in course from complete recovery to fatal outcome.

—is characterized by widespread demyelination.

C. Guillain-Barré syndrome (acute idiopathic polyneuritis)

—is an acute inflammatory demyelinating disease primarily involving **peripheral nerves**.

—has its highest incidence in young adults.

—is often preceded by viral infection, immunization, or allergic reactions.

—is generally considered to be of autoimmune etiology.

–is manifest clinically by **ascending muscle weakness and paralysis** beginning in the lower part of the lower extremities and ascending upward; respiratory failure and death can occur but most patients recover.

–causes **albumino-cytologic dissociation** of CSF, a markedly increased protein concentration with only modest increase in cell count, which is an important diagnostic finding.

VI. **Degenerative Diseases** (Table 23.2)

A. **Alzheimer's disease**

–is the most important cause of dementia.

–was formerly viewed as premature senility occurring in middle-aged persons (presenile dementia); the entity now includes dementia at any age if associated with characteristic clinical and pathologic findings.

Table 23.2. Degenerative Brain Disease

Type	Clinical Presentation	Occurrence	Anatomic Changes
Alzheimer's disease	Progressive dementia	Sporadic form presents at age 60 or older; familial form may present as early as age 40	Generalized cerebral atrophy; neurofibrillary tangles, neuritic (senile) plaques, granulovacuolar degeneration, Hirano bodies; decreased number of neurons in nucleus basalis of Meynert
Pick's disease	Progressive dementia	More frequent in women	Cerebral atrophy with gliosis and loss of cortical neurons, especially affecting temporal and frontal lobes; Pick bodies within some neurons, especially in Ammon's horn
Huntington's disease	Chorea and athetoid movements, progressive motor deterioration, wasting	Autosomal dominant disorder with delay of onset of clinical abnormalities until age 30–40	Atrophy, neuronal depletion, and gliosis of caudate nuclei, putamen, and frontal cortex
Idiopathic Parkinson's disease (paralysis agitans)	Parkinsonism	Usually presents after age 50	Neuronal depletion and depigmentation of cells of substantia nigra and locus ceruleus; Lewy bodies
Amyotrophic lateral sclerosis (ALS)	Rapidly progressive upper and lower motor neuron failure, leading to death, most often from respiratory failure	Middle-aged men	Degeneration of lateral corticospinal tracts and anterior motor neurons of spinal cord

1. Clinical findings

a. Slow, progressive intellectual deterioration during the course of several years, including:

   (1) Loss of recent memory, the most frequent early sign

   (2) Loss of long-term memory and other intellectual functions, leading to inability to read, count, or speak

b. Motor problems, contractures, and paralysis, which are sometimes terminal events

2. Morphologic abnormalities

a. **Neurofibrillary tangles:** intracytoplasmic bundles of filaments, derived in part from microtubules and neurofilaments, occur within neurons, especially in the cerebral cortex.

b. **Neuritic (senile) plaques:** swollen eosinophilic nerve cell processes occurring in spherical focal collections within the cerebral cortex, hippocampus, and amygdala. A central amyloid core with a distinctive peptide structure is characteristic.

c. **Granulovacuolar degeneration:** intraneuronal cytoplasmic granule-containing vacuoles occurring within the pyramidal cells of the hippocampus.

d. **Hirano bodies:** intracytoplasmic proximal dendritic eosinophilic inclusions consisting of actin.

e. **Generalized cerebral atrophy with moderate neuronal loss** is most prominent in frontal and hippocampal areas; sulci are widened because of narrowing of gyri.

3. Lack of specificity of morphologic abnormalities

a. Similar morphologic changes are associated with aging.

b. Patients with Down's syndrome who survive to age 40 and older often exhibit Alzheimer-like findings.

c. Neurofibrillary tangles are observed in postencephalitic Parkinson's disease.

4. Etiology—Alzheimer's disease

—is of unknown etiology; possible etiologic mechanisms include:

a. **Choline acetyltransferase deficiency:** the brain content of the enzyme and its product, acetylcholine, is decreased, especially in the cerebral cortex and hippocampus. Acetylcholine plays a role in learning, and drugs that block its action adversely affect short-term memory.

b. **Alterations in nucleus basalis of Meynert:** marked reduction in the number of neurons within the nucleus; neuritic plaques may represent degenerating neuronal processes from this site.

c. **Abnormal amyloid gene expression**

   —is the most favored etiologic concept today.

   (1) Gene for amyloid peptide of neuritic plaques and nearby cerebral vessels codes for an amyloid protein referred to as A4 amyloid, or amyloid β-protein, which differs from other amyloid proteins.

(2) Gene has been localized by restrictive fragment length polymorphism (RFLP) studies to chromosome 21; gene for familial form of
Alzheimer's disease has been similarly localized to chromosome 21;
increased gene copy number has been demonstrated in some patients with the sporadic form of Alzheimer's disease; Alzheimer-like
abnormalities occur in trisomy 21 (Down's syndrome).

5. Other causes of dementia

a. Multi-infarction dementia is the second most frequent cause of dementia after Alzheimer's disease; it is caused by cerebral atherosclerosis.

b. Chronic alcoholism

c. Binswanger's disease (subcortical leukoencephalopathy) is associated with hypertension; it is characterized by the presence of multiple
lacunar infarcts and progressive demyelination limited to the subcortical area, with characteristic sparing of cortex.

d. Pick's disease

B. Pick's disease

—clinically resembles Alzheimer's disease.
—is more frequent in women.
—is characterized by marked cortical atrophy, especially of the temporal and
frontal lobes, by swollen neurons, and by Pick bodies, round intracytoplasmic inclusions consisting of neurofilaments.

C. Huntington's disease

—is an autosomal dominant, fatal, **progressive degeneration and atrophy of the caudate nucleus, putamen, and frontal cortex** with neuronal depletion and gliosis.
—is characterized by the **delay of clinical abnormalities until age 30 to
40;** course extends 15 to 20 years, beginning with athetoid movements, followed by progressive deterioration leading to hypertonicity, fecal and urine
incontinence, anorexia and weight loss, and eventually dementia and
death.
—is caused by a mutant gene that has been localized to the short arm of chromosome 4; the **abnormal gene can be detected by RFLP studies** prior
to onset of clinical abnormalities.
—especially affects cholinergic and GABA-ergic neurons; it is possibly mediated by a receptor defect.

D. Idiopathic Parkinson's disease (paralysis agitans)

—appears clinically most often after age 50.
—is manifest histologically by depigmentation of cells of the substantia nigra
and locus ceruleus; damaged cells contain highly characteristic eosinophilic
intracytoplasmic inclusions (**Lewy bodies**).
—damages neuronal pathways from the substantia nigra to the corpus striatum, resulting in dopamine depletion of the corpus striatum; therapy with
L-dopa, a dopamine precursor, is often effective.
—is the most common cause of **parkinsonism,** a group of disorders characterized by resting pill-rolling tremor, masked (expressionless) facies, slowness of movements, muscular rigidity, and festinating (shuffling) gait.
Other causes of parkinsonism include:

1. **Von Economo's encephalitis,** an infectious disorder that appeared transiently from 1915 to 1918 concurrent with the influenza pandemic, causes **postencephalitic parkinsonism,** most often in older persons affected by that pandemic.

2. **Trauma,** especially repeated trauma as may occur in boxers

3. **Drugs and toxins,** especially dopamine antagonists such as MPTP (methyl-phenyl-tetrahydropyridine), a contaminant in illicit street drugs

4. **Shy-Drager syndrome,** parkinsonism with autonomic dysfunction and orthostatic hypotension

E. **Motor neuron disease**

1. **Amyotrophic lateral sclerosis (ALS, Lou Gehrig's disease)**
   —is characterized by **degeneration of upper and lower motor neurons**.
   —is morphologically marked by degeneration and atrophy of the lateral corticospinal tracts as well as of the anterior motor neurons of the cord.
   —results in denervation atrophy of musculature.
   —is manifest clinically by symmetric atrophy and fasciculation (lower motor neuron signs) as well as by hyperreflexia, spasticity, and pathologic reflexes (upper motor neuron signs).
   —has its clinical onset in early middle age, with a **rapid course leading to death** (most often from respiratory failure) in 1 to 6 years.
   —is the most common form of motor neuron disease.

2. **Other forms of motor neuron disease**

   a. **Progressive bulbar palsy:** brain stem and cranial nerve involvement predominate; characteristic findings include difficulty in swallowing and speaking and termination in respiratory failure.

   b. **Werdnig-Hoffmann syndrome (infantile progressive spinal muscular atrophy)** is an autosomal recessive lower motor neuron disease that manifests clinically in infancy.

VII. Tumors (Table 23.3)

A. **General characteristics**

1. Most tumors are intracranial; tumors of the spinal cord are much less frequent.

2. In adults, the majority of intracranial tumors are supratentorial.

3. In children, the majority of intracranial tumors are infratentorial.

4. CNS tumors are the second most common form of malignancy in children (only leukemia is more frequent).

5. Primary malignant CNS tumors rarely metastasize.

6. Benign intracranial tumors can result in devastating clinical consequences due to compression phenomena.

7. In order of frequency, the most common intracranial tumors are glioblastoma multiforme, metastatic tumors, meningioma, and acoustic neuroma.

Table 23.3. Selected Central Nervous System Tumors

Type	Predominant Incidence	Most Frequent Site	Characteristics
Astrocytoma, grade IV (glioblastoma multiforme)	Older persons	Cerebral hemispheres	Highly malignant, rapidly growing tumor; most common primary intracranial neoplasm
Meningioma	Middle and later life; more frequent in women	Convexities of cerebral hemispheres, parasagittal region, falx cerebri, sphenoid ridge	Benign tumor external to brain and usually resectable; second most common primary intracranial neoplasm
Medulloblastoma	Young children	Cerebellum	Highly malignant tumor; most common intracranial tumor of children
Neuroblastoma	Children	Cerebral hemispheres	Less common than adrenal and other peripheral neuroblastomas; linked to marked amplification of *N-myc* oncogene
Retinoblastoma	Young children; occurs in familial and sporadic forms	Retina; bilateral and multifocal in familial form; unilateral and unifocal in sporadic form	Most common eye tumor of young children; linked to rb gene deletion or inactivation
Neurilemmoma (schwannoma)	Middle and later life	Eighth cranial nerve (when schwannoma is intracranial)	Acoustic schwannoma, common intracranial tumor, ranking third after glioblastoma multiforme and meningioma; most often benign and usually resectable
Metastatic tumors	Variable	From primary sites in lung, breast, skin, kidney, gastrointestinal tract, and thyroid	Almost equal in incidence to glioblastoma multiforme

B. Astrocytomas

1. **Grade I** is the least aggressive type; cells closely resemble normal astrocytes.

2. **Grade II** is similar to grade I but with some pleomorphism and vascular changes.

3. **Grade III** (anaplastic astrocytoma) exhibits more marked pleomorphism, prominent mitoses, hyperplastic vasculature with endothelial hyperplasia, and some tissue necrosis.

4. **Grade IV (glioblastoma multiforme)**
   —is the **most common primary intracranial neoplasm**.

—has a peak occurrence in the late middle-age group.

—is associated with marked anaplasia and pleomorphism; pronounced vascular changes with endothelial hyperplasia occur. Areas of necrosis and hemorrhage are surrounded by **"pseudopalisade" arrangement** of tumor cells.

—originates most often in the cerebral hemisphere.

—has a very poor prognosis, with death in less than 1 year.

C. Oligodendroglioma

—presents as a slow-growing tumor in the middle-age group.

—is morphologically characterized by:

1. Closely packed cells with large round nuclei surrounded by a clear halo of cytoplasm ("fried egg" appearance)

2. Site of origin in the cerebral hemispheres

3. Tumor divided into groups of cells by delicate capillary strands

4. Foci of calcification

D. Ependymoma

—most frequently occurs in the fourth ventricle.

—has its peak incidence in childhood and adolescence.

—is characterized histologically by tubules or rosettes with cells encircling vessels or pointing toward a central lumen; tumor cells characteristically demonstrate blepharoplasts, rod-shaped structures near the nucleus representing basal bodies of cilia.

—may result in papillary growths that obstruct flow of CSF and lead to hydrocephalus.

E. Meningioma

—is the **second most common primary intracranial neoplasm**.

—is a **benign, slowly growing tumor**.

—originates in arachnoidal cells of the meninges; the tumor is external to the brain and often can be removed surgically.

—occurs most frequently in the convexities of the cerebral hemispheres and the parasagittal region; other common locations include the falx cerebri, sphenoid ridge, olfactory area, and suprasellar region.

—is characterized histologically by a whorled pattern of concentrically arranged spindle cells and laminated calcified psammoma bodies.

—occurs more frequently in women than in men.

—most often occurs after age 40.

F. Medulloblastoma

—has its peak incidence in young children.

—is a highly **malignant tumor of the cerebellum**.

—is characterized histologically by sheets of closely packed cells with scant cytoplasm arranged in a rosette or perivascular pseudorosette pattern.

G. Neuroblastoma

—is closely related to neuroblastoma of the adrenal medulla or sympathetic ganglia.

—is much less common than peripheral neuroblastoma.

—is characterized by amplification of the *N-myc* oncogene (multiple copies demonstrable either as homogeneously staining regions or as extrachromosomal double minute chromatin bodies); a greater degree of amplification correlates with worse prognosis.

H. Retinoblastoma

—is a malignant retinal tumor of childhood.

—is sporadic in approximately 60% of cases; sporadic cases are unilateral and monocentric in origin.

—is familial in approximately 40% of cases; familial cases are frequently bilateral and multicentric in origin.

—demonstrates homozygous deletion of the rb gene (located on chromosome 13 at band q14).

—supports the "two-hit" hypothesis of genetically determined carcinogenesis.

1. First deletion ("hit") is inherited in germ line cells in familial cases, or occurs as a somatic mutation in sporadic cases.

2. Second deletion ("hit") results from somatic mutation in both familial and sporadic cases.

3. Both deletions are required for tumor development; persistence of heterozygosity for the rb gene prevents retinoblastoma development (antioncogene activity).

I. Hemangioblastoma

—occurs most frequently in the cerebellum.

—may be associated with similar lesions in the retina and other organs as part of von Hippel-Lindau disease.

—sometimes produces erythropoietin, leading to secondary polycythemia.

J. Neurilemmoma (schwannoma)

—is a benign, slowly growing encapsulated tumor arising from Schwann cells.

—when intracranial, is most frequently localized to the eighth cranial nerve (**acoustic neuroma,** acoustic schwannoma); acoustic neuroma is the **third most common primary intracranial neoplasm**.

—also originates frequently in posterior nerve roots and peripheral nerves.

—is characterized histologically by one of two patterns:

1. Antoni A: interlacing bundles of elongated cells with palisading nuclei

2. Antoni B: looser, less cellular pattern than Antoni A

K. Neurofibroma

—occurs as solitary or multiple tumors of peripheral nerves derived from Schwann cells.

—may be part of von Recklinghausen's neurofibromatosis.

L. Metastatic tumors

—are almost as common as glioblastoma multiforme among intracranial neoplasms.

—originate most frequently from primary sites in lung, breast, skin, kidney, gastrointestinal tract, and thyroid.

Review Test

Directions: Each of the numbered items or incomplete statements in this section is followed by answers or by completions of the statement. Select the **one** lettered answer or completion that is **best** in each case.

1. All of the following statements concerning cerebrovascular disease are true EXCEPT

(A) most common cause is embolization from cardiac mural thrombi.
(B) infarction is more frequent than hemorrhage.
(C) hemorrhage is frequently associated with hypertension.
(D) subarachnoid hemorrhage is frequently associated with berry aneurysm of the circle of Willis.
(E) atherosclerosis is the most frequent underlying basis of arterial thrombosis and occlusion.

2. Which one of the following is a well-known association or characteristic of subdural hematoma?

(A) Bleeding from arteries of the circle of Willis
(B) Rapidly progressive cerebral compression
(C) Characteristically caused by venous hemorrhage
(D) Laceration of branches of middle meningeal artery
(E) Causally associated with hypertension

3. A 2-year-old child presents with fever, headache, prostration, and nuchal rigidity. The CSF is cloudy, and microscopic examination reveals innumerable neutrophils. The CSF protein is increased, and glucose is decreased. The most likely etiologic agent is

(A) *Escherichia coli.*
(B) *Haemophilus influenzae.*
(C) *Neisseria meningitidis.*
(D) *Streptococcus pneumoniae.*
(E) *Staphylococcus aureus.*

4. All of the following characteristics are associated with infantile toxoplasmosis EXCEPT

(A) periventricular calcifications demonstrable by X-ray.
(B) common occurrence of hydrocephalus, mental retardation, and other neurologic abnormalities.
(C) favored sites of involvement include the cerebral cortex, basal ganglia, retinae, heart, lungs, and liver.
(D) characteristically spread by a child ingesting foods contaminated by the urine of household pets.
(E) cats are a frequent reservoir.

5. All of the following viral diseases or viruses are correctly matched with the appropriate association or characteristic EXCEPT

(A) St. Louis encephalitis—reservoir is horses and birds.
(B) Herpes simplex encephalitis—common complication of herpes simplex virus (HSV) infection.
(C) poliomyelitis—degeneration and necrosis of anterior horn cells of spinal cord.
(D) rabies—Negri bodies.
(E) cytomegalovirus infection—immunosuppressed persons.

6. All of the following diseases of viral or suspected viral etiology are correctly matched with the appropriate association or characteristic EXCEPT

(A) AIDS—CD4 + T lymphocytes probable vehicle for viral entry into the CNS.
(B) kuru—ingestion of human brain.
(C) Creutzfeldt-Jakob disease—possible danger to health workers.
(D) subacute sclerosing panencephalitis—measles virus.
(E) progressive multifocal leukoencephalopathy—leukemia or lymphoma.

7. All of the following are associated with multiple sclerosis EXCEPT

(A) increased incidence in association with certain HLA haplotypes.
(B) irregularly scattered focal areas of demyelination in the brain and spinal cord.
(C) optic nerve, brain stem, and paraventricular areas favored sites.
(D) progressive, highly variable course, characterized by exacerbations with long asymptomatic remissions.
(E) widespread demyelination following a viral illness, such as measles, mumps, rubella, or chicken pox.

8. All of the following are characteristics of amyotrophic lateral sclerosis EXCEPT

(A) association with a papovavirus.
(B) involvement of anterior motor neurons.
(C) involvement of lateral corticospinal tracts.
(D) symmetric hyperreflexia and spasticity.
(E) symmetric muscle atrophy and fasciculation.

9. All of the following disorders are correctly matched with the appropriate association or characteristic EXCEPT

(A) Guillain-Barré syndrome—albumino-cytologic dissociation.
(B) Alzheimer's disease—focal spherical collections of swollen nerve cell processes with a central amyloid core.
(C) Huntington's disease—hereditary disorder with delay of clinical onset until age 30 to 40.
(D) Pick's disease—Lewy bodies.
(E) Parkinson's disease—depigmentation of cells of substantia nigra.

10. Which of the following characteristics is associated with meningioma?

(A) Amenability to surgical cure
(B) "Fried egg" appearance of tumor cells
(C) Multiple areas of necrosis and hemorrhage within the tumor
(D) Peak incidence in early childhood
(E) Tumor cells arranged in a rosette pattern

11. A lesion similar to that shown in the illustrations below was found at autopsy in a 55-year-old woman. This is an example of

(A) glioblastoma multiforme.
(B) meningioma.
(C) oligodendroglioma.
(D) medulloblastoma.
(E) ependymoma.

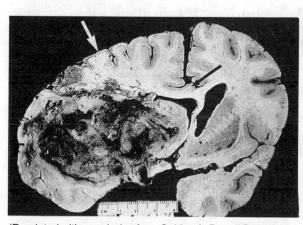
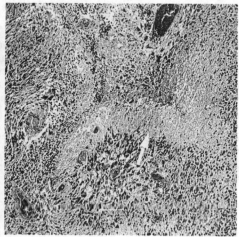

(Reprinted with permission from Golden A, Powell D, and Jennings C: *Pathology: Understanding Human Disease,* 2nd ed. Baltimore, Williams & Wilkins, 1985, p 266, p 267.)

Answers and Explanations

1–A. Embolic obstruction of cerebral vessels with resultant infarction is less frequent than local thrombotic occlusion associated with atherosclerotic disease. However, in patients such as those with chronic atrial fibrillation, the development of atrial mural thrombi and subsequent cerebral embolization is a threat. Cerebral hemorrhage is often associated with hypertension; when hemorrhage is subarachnoid in distribution, rupture of a berry aneurysm of the circle of Willis is a frequent finding.

2–C. Subdural hematoma is characteristically caused by venous bleeding, most often from veins that join the cerebrum to venous sinuses within the dura. The venous hemorrhage typically arrests early, but the volume of the hematoma gradually increases because of osmotic imbibement of water. This results in a slowly enlarging tumor-like mass characterized clinically by gradual signs of cerebral compression occurring hours to days or even weeks after head injury.

3–B. Pyogenic meningitis in older infants and young children is most frequently caused by *H. influenzae*. In newborns, the most likely agent is *E. coli;* in young adults, the most frequent agent is *N. meningitidis*. In older adults, especially those with impaired resistance to infection, the most common etiologic agent is *S. pneumoniae*.

4–D. In the infantile form of toxoplasmosis, *Toxoplasma gondii* is characteristically transmitted transplacentally from an infected mother and not by ingestion of foods contaminated by animal urine or feces, as occurs in older children.

5–B. Herpes simplex encephalitis is an uncommon complication of HSV infection but is, nonetheless, the most common form of severe viral encephalitis.

6–A. Cells of monocyte–macrophage origin are considered to be the probable vehicle by which HIV infection enters the CNS, and these cells most likely function as a viral reservoir.

7–E. Demyelination following an acute viral illness is characteristic of acute disseminated encephalomyelitis (postinfectious encephalitis), not multiple sclerosis. The incidence of multiple sclerosis is increased in association with HLA haplotypes A3, B7, DR2, and DW2, suggesting that immune factors may play a role. The disease is associated with plaques scattered irregularly throughout the CNS or the peripheral nervous system. Common sites are the optic nerve, brain stem, and paraventricular areas. Although characterized by exacerbations and remissions, the course is progressive, leading to increasing disability.

8–A. The JC polyoma papovavirus is associated with progressive multifocal leukoencephalopathy. The cause of amyotrophic lateral sclerosis (Lou Gehrig's disease) remains unknown.

9–D. Lewy bodies are characteristic eosinophilic intracytoplasmic inclusions observed in idiopathic Parkinson's disease, not Pick's disease, and are noted within the depigmented cells of the substantia nigra, which are also characteristic of this disorder.

10–A. Meningioma is a benign, slowly growing tumor located external to the brain and is often amenable to surgical resection. The tumor occurs most often in women older than age 40.

11–A. The lesion shown in the illustrations is a glioblastoma multiforme, the most frequently occurring neoplasm of the CNS. Characteristic features include the intracerebral location, prominent hemorrhage and necrosis, and the pseudopalisading appearance of the pleomorphic tumor cells.

Comprehensive Examination

Directions: Each of the numbered items or incomplete statements in this section is followed by answers or by completions of the statement. Select the **one** lettered answer or completion that is **best** in each case.

1. Increased free radical formation is implicated in the pathogenesis of injury caused by all of the following EXCEPT

(A) ingestion of carbon tetrachloride (CCl_4).
(B) ionizing radiation.
(C) metastatic calcification.
(D) oxygen toxicity.
(E) reperfusion after ischemia.

2. All of the following cellular changes are reversible EXCEPT

(A) fatty change.
(B) formation of cell blebs.
(C) formation of myelin figures.
(D) nuclear pyknosis.
(E) swelling of organelles.

3. A 65-year-old woman fell and sustained a pelvic fracture. The woman died after a short period of rapidly progressive mental confusion and respiratory insufficiency. Numerous conjunctival petechiae were noted. These abnormalities were most likely due to which one of the following conditions?

(A) Epidural hematoma
(B) Aspiration pneumonia
(C) Fat embolization
(D) Acute tubular necrosis
(E) Saddle embolus occluding bifurcation of pulmonary arteries

4. All of the following clinical disorders are appropriately matched with effector substances or cells EXCEPT

(A) erythroblastosis fetalis—C5b-9.
(B) Graves' disease—anti-receptor antibody.
(C) poison ivy—CD4 + T cells.
(D) polyarteritis nodosa—immune complexes.
(E) serum sickness—mast cells

5. Which one of the following viruses is associated with nasopharyngeal carcinoma?

(A) Cytomegalovirus
(B) Epstein-Barr virus (EBV)
(C) Measles virus
(D) Papillomavirus
(E) Parvovirus

6. Which of the following characteristics of neoplastic cells is the most reliable indicator of malignancy?

(A) Appearance of oncofetal antigens
(B) Chromosomal aneuploidy
(C) Loss of contact inhibition in tissue culture
(D) Spread to distal sites
(E) Ultrastructural alterations

7. The combination of pulmonary emphysema and cirrhosis of the liver may be caused by deficiency of

(A) α-1-antitrypsin.
(B) galactokinase.
(C) glucose-6-phosphatase.
(D) glucocerebrosidase.
(E) phenylalanine hydroxylase.

8. Which of the following gastrointestinal lesions most frequently leads to adenocarcinoma?

(A) Colorectal villous adenoma
(B) Crohn's disease
(C) Duodenal peptic ulcer
(D) Familial multiple polyposis
(E) Ulcerative colitis

9. Which one of the following tumors is associated with Paget's disease of bone?

(A) Ewing's sarcoma
(B) Giant cell tumor
(C) Metastatic duct carcinoma of the breast
(D) Multiple enchondromas
(E) Osteosarcoma

10. Increased serum human chorionic gonado-tropin (HCG) may be observed in all of the following conditions EXCEPT

(A) choriocarcinoma.
(B) hydatidiform mole.
(C) normal pregnancy.
(D) ovarian granulosa cell tumor.
(E) testicular mixed germ cell tumor.

11. A 21-year-old basketball player died suddenly during a game. Autopsy revealed hypertrophy of the left ventricular wall, especially of the ventricular septum. Histologically, the myocardial fibers were arranged in a disorganized pattern. Which of the following best characterizes this disorder?

(A) Can be a manifestation of primary amyloidosis
(B) Can be a result of myocarditis
(C) Is often associated with alcohol abuse
(D) Is often associated with coronary artery disease
(E) Often demonstrates autosomal dominant inheritance

12. Which finding would be least expected in disseminated intravascular coagulation (DIC)?

(A) Increased fibrin degradation products
(B) Prolonged activated partial thromboplastin time
(C) Prolonged prothrombin time
(D) Prolonged thrombin time
(E) Thrombocytosis

Questions 13 and 14

13. Which one of the following findings is most likely in the cerebrospinal fluid (CSF) of a 10-day-old infant with high fever and nuchal rigidity?

(A) Decreased protein, decreased glucose
(B) Decreased protein, increased glucose
(C) Increased protein, decreased glucose
(D) Increased protein, increased glucose
(E) Normal protein, decreased glucose

14. CSF culture from this patient is most likely to yield

(A) *Escherichia coli*.
(B) *Haemophilus influenzae*.
(C) *Neisseria meningitidis*.
(D) *Streptococcus pneumoniae*.
(E) none of the above.

15. Mutations of the *ras* oncogene result in a protein product that has

(A) decreased GTPase activity.
(B) decreased reverse transcriptase activity.
(C) increased protein phosphatase activity.
(D) increased responsiveness to growth factors.
(E) increased tyrosine kinase activity.

16. A 68-year-old woman presents with fever, chills, and cough productive of blood-tinged sputum. Fluid aspirated from the right pleural space would most likely

(A) be clear and straw-colored in appearance.
(B) contain large numbers of neutrophils.
(C) have a glucose content somewhat higher than the serum glucose.
(D) have a protein content of less than 1 g/dl.
(E) have a specific gravity of 1.012.

17. Microcephaly apparent at birth can be caused by any of the following EXCEPT

(A) cytomegalovirus.
(B) herpes simplex virus.
(C) homozygous deficiency of phenylalanine hydroxylase.
(D) maternal alcohol abuse.
(E) rubella virus.

18. An adult patient is evaluated for anemia and splenomegaly. Which one of the following sets of associated findings would be least likely?

(A) Atypical lymphocytes and sheep cell agglutinins
(B) Positive sickle cell preparation
(C) Marked leukocytosis, many immature granulocytes, and increased number of basophils
(D) Spherocytosis and acholuric jaundice
(E) Teardrop-shaped red cells, small numbers of nucleated red cells, and immature granulocytes

19. All of the following are associated with carcinoma of the urinary bladder EXCEPT

(A) early hematogenous metastasis.
(B) hematuria.
(C) high recurrence rate.
(D) increased incidence in aniline dye workers.
(E) transitional cell morphology.

20. Which of the following parathyroid disorders is characterized by renal end-organ unresponsiveness?

(A) Primary hyperparathyroidism
(B) Secondary hyperparathyroidism
(C) Tertiary hyperparathyroidism
(D) Hypoparathyroidism
(E) Pseudohypoparathyroidism

21. Diffuse demineralization of bone associated with hypercalcemia, anemia, hypergammaglobulinemia, proteinuria, and normal serum alkaline phosphatase is most suggestive of

(A) Ewing's sarcoma.
(B) hyperparathyroidism.
(C) multiple myeloma.
(D) osteomalacia.
(E) Paget's disease of bone.

22. Which one of the following thyroid tumors is associated with amyloid stroma?

(A) Epidermoid carcinoma
(B) Follicular carcinoma
(C) Medullary carcinoma
(D) Papillary carcinoma
(E) Undifferentiated carcinoma

23. Which one of the following myocardial changes is the most frequent cause of cardiac rupture?

(A) Abscess formation and tissue destruction due to infective endocarditis
(B) Fatty change due to interaction of diphtheria exotoxin and carnitine
(C) Inflammation associated with Aschoff bodies
(D) Inflammation due to coxsackie B infection
(E) Necrosis due to coronary artery obstruction

24. Hypersensitivity (leukocytoclastic) vasculitis is characterized by

(A) a heterogeneous mix of newly formed and older lesions.
(B) delayed (cell-mediated) hypersensitivity.
(C) palpable purpura in the skin.
(D) a predilection for medium- to large-sized vessels.
(E) sparing of glomeruli.

25. Which pattern of serum iron and total iron binding capacity (TIBC) is characteristic of long-standing idiopathic hemochromatosis?

(A) Serum iron increased, TIBC increased
(B) Serum iron increased, TIBC decreased
(C) Serum iron normal, TIBC increased
(D) Serum iron decreased, TIBC increased
(E) Serum iron decreased, TIBC decreased

26. Alveolar hyaline membrane formation is associated with all of the following causative factors EXCEPT

(A) high-concentration oxygen therapy.
(B) infection with *Mycoplasma pneumoniae*.
(C) long-standing pulmonary emphysema.
(D) shock.
(E) uremia.

27. Characteristics of neuroblastoma include all of the following EXCEPT

(A) catecholamine production.
(B) differentiation to more mature form.
(C) oncogene amplification.
(D) peak incidence in infancy and childhood.
(E) posterior cranial fossa most frequent site of origin.

28. The microscopic appearance of the organisms in disseminated histoplasmosis is best described as

(A) budding yeast forms surrounded by empty haloes.
(B) cup-shaped forms demonstrable by silver stain within a foamy amorphous intra-alveolar exudate.
(C) intracavitary mycelial forms.
(D) minute fungal yeast forms within phagocytes.
(E) thick-walled spherules filled with endospores.

29. A linear pattern of glomerular immunofluorescence for IgG is observed in a renal biopsy. The most likely associated laboratory finding is a positive antibody test for

(A) antistreptolysin O.
(B) C3 convertase.
(C) glomerular and alveolar basement membranes.
(D) hepatitis B virus.
(E) Sm (Smith) nuclear antigen.

30. After being picked up by the police, a runaway adolescent girl became increasingly somnolent, lapsing into a deep coma 72 hours later. Her respirations were rapid and deep, and she appeared to be severely dehydrated. Laboratory studies revealed a marked reduction in serum bicarbonate and a significant anion gap, as well as neutrophilic leukocytosis. The most likely additional laboratory abnormality is

(A) a BUN:creatinine ratio of less than 1:10.
(B) decreased serum cortisol.
(C) decreased serum thyroxine (T_4).
(D) increased CSF protein with no parallel increase in cell count.
(E) increased serum glucose.

31. All of the following item pairs are correct effects or associations EXCEPT

(A) Duffy blood group antigen—susceptibility to malaria.
(B) folate deficiency—hypochromic erythrocytes.
(C) hereditary spherocytosis—increased mean corpuscular hemoglobin concentration (MCHC).
(D) increased plasma volume—decreased hematocrit in pregnancy.
(E) suppressed β chain synthesis—thalassemia.

32. A 56-year-old man collapsed at work and died 20 minutes later in the emergency room while blood was being drawn. The patient's history revealed an episode of prolonged chest discomfort 3 months earlier. Which of the following is least likely?

(A) Death from arrhythmia
(B) Fibrotic scar in the ventricular septum
(C) Loss of myocardial striations and beginning infiltration with neutrophils
(D) Normal values for serum creatine phosphokinase (CPK), aspartate aminotransferase (AST), and lactate dehydrogenase (LDH)
(E) Severe atherosclerotic narrowing of the anterior descending branch of the left coronary artery with overlying thrombus formation

33. Which structure is most resistant to infection with *Neisseria gonorrhoeae*?

(A) Urethra
(B) Prostate
(C) Seminal vesicles
(D) Epididymis
(E) Testes

34. Bacillary forms demonstrable by electron microscopy within PAS-positive macrophages are characteristic of

(A) celiac disease.
(B) Crohn's disease.
(C) disaccharidase deficiency.
(D) tropical sprue.
(E) Whipple's disease.

35. A prolonged bleeding time and a prolonged activated partial thromboplastin time, when associated with a normal platelet count, suggest

(A) Christmas disease.
(B) classic hemophilia.
(C) congenital afibrinogenemia.
(D) Glanzmann's thrombasthenia.
(E) von Willebrand's disease.

36. All of the following pairs of environmental exposures and associated malignant tumors are correct EXCEPT

(A) aflatoxin B—hepatocellular carcinoma.
(B) arsenic—mesothelioma.
(C) β-naphthylamine —transitional cell carcinoma of the bladder.
(D) diethylstilbestrol—clear cell adenocarcinoma of the vagina.
(E) ionizing radiation—carcinoma of the thyroid.

37. The pathogenesis of carcinoma of the endometrium is associated with all of the following EXCEPT

(A) adenomatous hyperplasia of the endometrium.
(B) coexisting granulosa cell tumor of the ovary.
(C) diabetes mellitus.
(D) endometriosis.
(E) obesity.

38. Which of the following cells reaches the site of an acute inflammatory reaction first?

(A) Basophils
(B) Lymphocytes
(C) Monocytes–macrophages
(D) Neutrophils
(E) Plasma cells

39. Acute leukemia occurs with increased frequency in which one of the following syndromes?

(A) Cri du chat syndrome
(B) Down's syndrome
(C) Fragile X syndrome
(D) Klinefelter's syndrome
(E) Turner's syndrome

40. Repeated intravenous injections of foreign protein result in a characteristic glomerular lesion in experimental animals. The pathogenesis of this lesion is similar to that of each of the following human disorders EXCEPT

(A) lipoid nephrosis.
(B) lupus nephropathy.
(C) membranous glomerulonephritis.
(D) polyarteritis nodosa.
(E) poststreptococcal glomerulonephritis.

41. A tumor secreting which one of the following hormones is likely to be a cause of hyperglycemia?

(A) Catecholamines
(B) Cortisol
(C) Growth hormone
(D) Thyroxine
(E) All of the above

42. Likely urinary findings in acute pyelonephritis include all of the following EXCEPT

(A) positive test for protein.
(B) red blood cells.
(C) red blood cell casts.
(D) white blood cells.
(E) white blood cell casts.

43. A 10-day-old boy with projectile vomiting and a palpable midepigastric mass most likely has

(A) congenital pyloric stenosis.
(B) infantile polycystic kidney.
(C) intussusception.
(D) tracheoesophageal fistula.
(E) Wilms' tumor.

44. All of the following are likely complications of atherosclerosis EXCEPT

(A) aneurysm of ascending aorta.
(B) cerebral infarct.
(C) gangrene of small bowel.
(D) mural thrombosis.
(E) myocardial infarct.

45. All of the following procedures are useful in distinguishing iron deficiency anemia from β-thalassemia minor EXCEPT

(A) bone marrow Prussian blue stain.
(B) hematocrit.
(C) serum ferritin.
(D) serum iron.
(E) total iron binding capacity (TIBC).

46. Which form of Hodgkin's disease has the poorest prognosis?

(A) Lymphocytic predominance
(B) Mixed cellularity
(C) Lymphocytic depletion
(D) Nodular sclerosis

47. All of the following findings are expected in hemolytic anemia EXCEPT

(A) decreased haptoglobin.
(B) increased urinary bilirubin.
(C) increased reticulocyte count.
(D) jaundice.
(E) normoblastic erythroid hyperplasia.

48. All of the following lesions are associations or precursors of malignancy EXCEPT

(A) acanthosis nigricans.
(B) actinic keratosis.
(C) dysplastic nevus.
(D) juvenile melanoma.
(E) xeroderma pigmentosum.

49. Histologic features of alcoholic hepatitis include all of the following EXCEPT

(A) fatty change.
(B) focal liver cell necrosis.
(C) giant cells.
(D) infiltrates of neutrophils.
(E) Mallory bodies.

50. Which one of the following disorders is often caused by T-cell mediated hypersensitivity?

(A) Contact dermatitis
(B) Graves' disease
(C) Hemolytic disease of the newborn
(D) Polyarteritis nodosa
(E) Urticaria

51. All of the following are characteristics or associations of sarcoidosis EXCEPT

(A) anergy to tuberculin.
(B) caseating granulomas.
(C) hilar lymphadenopathy.
(D) hypercalcemia.
(E) increased serum angiotensin-converting enzyme.

52. The following items pair predisposing risk factors for cancer with the appropriate site of involvement. Which pair is incorrect?

(A) Aflatoxin B ingestion—oral mucosa and tongue
(B) Cirrhosis and hepatitis B virus infection—liver
(C) Diet low in fiber and high in animal fat—colon
(D) *Helicobacter pylori* infection and diet high in salt—stomach
(E) Tobacco and alcohol abuse—esophagus

53. Characteristics or associations of small cell carcinoma of the lung include all of the following EXCEPT

(A) frequently centrally located.
(B) clear association with cigarette smoking.
(C) ectodermal origin.
(D) inappropriate ADH or ACTH secretion.
(E) intracytoplasmic neurosecretory granules.

54. All of the following complement components are correctly paired with the appropriate effect EXCEPT

(A) C3a and C5a—degranulation of mast cells.
(B) C3b—phagocytosis.
(C) C4a—release of interleukin-1.
(D) C5a—chemotaxis.
(E) C5b-9—cytolysis.

55. The most frequent cause of coagulation necrosis is

(A) autolytic digestion by intracellular enzymes.
(B) deposition of protein into arteriolar walls.
(C) granulomatous inflammation.
(D) heterolytic digestion by invading bacteria.
(E) ischemia caused by interruption of blood supply.

56. All of the following are characteristic of pseudomembranous colitis EXCEPT

(A) associated with broad-spectrum antibiotic therapy.
(B) caused by overgrowth of commensal microorganisms indigenous to the bowel.
(C) characterized clinically by fever, toxicity, and diarrhea.
(D) marked morphologically by superficial mucosal erosions with overlying necrotic, loosely adherent mucosal debris.
(E) often complicated by widespread dissemination of causative microorganisms.

57. All of the following conditions may be complications of infective endocarditis EXCEPT

(A) cerebral abscess.
(B) dissecting aortic aneurysm.
(C) focal glomerulonephritis.
(D) perforation of valve leaflets.
(E) renal infarction.

58. Multiple cutaneous punctate hemorrhages are characteristic of all of the following conditions EXCEPT

(A) ascorbic acid deficiency.
(B) Christmas disease.
(C) disseminated intravascular coagulation.
(D) Rocky Mountain spotted fever.
(E) thrombocytopenia.

59. All of the following characteristics of Hashimoto's thyroiditis are suggestive of an autoimmune etiology EXCEPT

(A) anti-thyroglobulin and antimicrosomal antibodies.
(B) association with other autoimmune disorders.
(C) atrophy of thyroid follicles.
(D) increased incidence in HLA-DR5 and HLA-B5 positive persons.
(E) presence of lymphoid follicles within the thyroid gland.

60. An autopsy is performed on a 60-year-old man with a history of sustained ethanol abuse. There had been a history of progressive dementia with marked memory loss manifest by a tendency to fabricate false accounts of recent events. Additionally, confusion, ataxic gait, and paralysis of eye movements had been noted. The most likely findings in the brain are

(A) amyloid-containing neuritic plaques within cerebral cortex, amygdala, and hippocampus.
(B) degeneration of mamillary bodies and paramedian masses of gray matter.
(C) depigmentation of substantia nigra and locus ceruleus.
(D) diffuse cortical atrophy with hydrocephalus ex vacuo.
(E) multiple lacunar infarcts and progressive subcortical demyelination.

61. All of the following statements about endocarditis are true EXCEPT

(A) Libman-Sacks endocarditis is characterized by small vegetations on either or both surfaces of valve leaflets.
(B) marantic endocarditis is a frequent feature of systemic lupus erythematosus (SLE).
(C) the vegetations of acute rheumatic endocarditis are characteristically localized to the lines of closure of the valve leaflet on the surface exposed to the flow of blood.
(D) the vegetations of infective endocarditis are much more likely to result in embolism than those of rheumatic endocarditis.
(E) mitral prolapse is a predisposing lesion to infective endocarditis.

62. Which of the following viruses is the most common cause of transfusion-mediated hepatitis?

(A) Hepatitis A
(B) Hepatitis B
(C) Hepatitis C
(D) Hepatitis D
(E) Hepatitis E

63. Agnogenic myeloid metaplasia is characterized by all of the following features EXCEPT

(A) depletion of bone marrow megakaryocytes.
(B) hepatosplenomegaly.
(C) myelofibrosis.
(D) nucleated red cells in peripheral blood smear.
(E) teardrop-shaped erythrocytes.

64. An autopsy is performed on a 35-year-old black man who died after a brief illness characterized by papilledema, severe hypertension, left ventricular hypertrophy and failure, and renal dysfunction. The most likely findings in the kidney are

(A) finely granular renal surface and hyaline arteriolosclerosis of afferent arterioles.
(B) swollen, hypercellular, "bloodless" glomeruli.
(C) nodular mesangial accumulations of basement membrane-like material and hyaline arteriolosclerosis of afferent and efferent arterioles.
(D) surface covered with multiple petechial hemorrhages, hyperplastic arteriolosclerosis, and necrotizing glomerulitis.
(E) swollen, pale kidneys and marked accumulation of lipid in convoluted tubules.

65. The most likely diagnosis in a 24-year-old woman with the nephrotic syndrome, progressive azotemia, and thickening of glomerular capillary loops apparent on light microscopy is

(A) Alport's syndrome (IgA nephropathy).
(B) diabetic nephropathy.
(C) focal and segmental glomerulosclerosis.
(D) lipoid nephrosis.
(E) membranous glomerulonephritis.

66. All of the following statements are true of maternal-fetal rubella infection EXCEPT

(A) associated fetal defects are not limited to the cardiovascular system.
(B) the fetus is most vulnerable during the first trimester of pregnancy.
(C) the majority of cases of congenital heart disease are caused by rubella or other intrauterine infections.
(D) patent ductus arteriosus and septal defects are the most frequent congenital cardiac abnormalities associated with rubella infection.
(E) a predominant IgM antibody response indicates recent primary infection.

67. A bone marrow aspiration from a 65-year-old man with long-standing profound anemia shows megaloblastic erythroid hyperplasia. Which of the following is the most likely diagnosis?

(A) Anemia of chronic disease
(B) Pelger-Huet anomaly
(C) Pernicious anemia
(D) Homozygous hemoglobin E
(E) Thalassemia

68. A 65-year-old man is evaluated for abdominal pain radiating through to the back, jaundice, anorexia, and recent weight loss. An additional likely finding is

(A) history of thorium dioxide (Thorotrast) exposure.
(B) increased alpha-fetoprotein.
(C) migratory venous thrombosis.
(D) pancreatic calcification and pseudocyst formation.
(E) urine test negative for bilirubin.

69. Which pigmented neoplasm is most likely to metastasize early?

(A) Dysplastic nevus
(B) Nodular melanoma
(C) Pigmented nevus
(D) Spitz nevus
(E) Superficial spreading melanoma

70. All of the following are well-known causes of megaloblastic anemia EXCEPT

(A) hookworm infestation.
(B) intestinal blind loops.
(C) pregnancy.
(D) severe malnutrition.
(E) strict vegetarian diet.

71. A 10-month-old girl presents with recurrent pulmonary infections, steatorrhea, and failure to thrive. Measurement of which substance is the most appropriate procedure in this patient?

(A) Erythrocyte glucose-6-phosphate dehydrogenase
(B) Serum ceruloplasmin
(C) Serum β-lipoprotein
(D) Serum phenylalanine
(E) Sweat chloride

72. Granulation tissue formation is associated with

(A) cat-scratch disease.
(B) foreign body reaction.
(C) histoplasmosis.
(D) tuberculosis.
(E) wound healing.

73. A tumor-like scar that developed following piercing of the ears in a young black woman is most likely a

(A) benign fibrous histiocytoma.
(B) dermatofibrosarcoma protuberans.
(C) fibroepithelial polyp.
(D) keloid.
(E) xanthoma.

74. Localized or systemic deposition of amyloid is associated with all of the following EXCEPT

(A) Alzheimer's disease.
(B) exocrine deficiency of the pancreas.
(C) medullary carcinoma of the thyroid.
(D) multiple myeloma.
(E) rheumatoid arthritis.

75. While being investigated for long-standing hypertension, a 55-year-old woman is found to have the following serum laboratory test values: normal creatinine, total protein, albumin, and globulin; increased calcium and alkaline phosphatase; and decreased phosphorus. These findings suggest the presence of

(A) carcinoma metastatic to bone.
(B) excessive dietary calcium intake.
(C) multiple myeloma.
(D) parathyroid adenoma.
(E) sarcoidosis.

76. Which one of the following disorders is characterized by multiple angiomas along with liver, kidney, and pancreas cysts?

(A) Von Hippel-Lindau disease
(B) Von Recklinghausen's disease
(C) Marfan's syndrome
(D) Familial hypercholesterolemia
(E) Tuberous sclerosis

77. Necrosis in which one of the following sites is caused by phenacetin abuse?

(A) Basal ganglia
(B) Epithelioid granulomas
(C) Myocardium
(D) Renal papillae
(E) Splenic arterioles

78. Which of the following is characteristic of true hermaphroditism?

(A) Barr body absent
(B) Both testicular and ovarian tissue present
(C) Cellular resistance to male hormones
(D) Clinical manifestations delayed until puberty

79. A 62-year-old man is seen because of a change in bowel habits. A lesion similar to that illustrated below is resected from the sigmoid colon. The diagnosis is

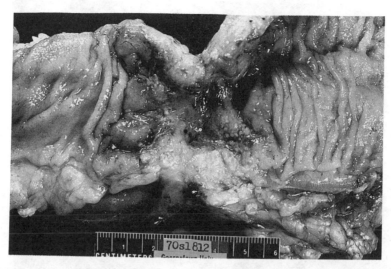

(Reprinted with permission from Golden A, Powell D, and Jennings C: *Pathology: Understanding Human Disease,* 2nd ed. Baltimore, Williams & Wilkins, 1985, p 144.)

(A) adenocarcinoma.
(B) Crohn's disease.
(C) lymphoma.
(D) pseudomembranous colitis.
(E) tubular adenoma.

80. Which one of the following metabolic processes is catalyzed by phospholipase A_2?

(A) Cyclooxygenase pathway
(B) Liberation of arachidonic acid from membrane phospholipids
(C) Lipoxygenase pathway
(D) Synthesis of prostacyclin (PGI_2)
(E) Synthesis of thromboxane A_2 (TxA_2)

81. Which one of the following processes causes increased bulk of skeletal muscle after exercise?

(A) Hypertrophy
(B) Hyperplasia
(C) Both hypertrophy and hyperplasia
(D) Neither hypertrophy nor hyperplasia

82. Which one of the following disorders is thought to be associated with measles virus?

(A) Creutzfeldt-Jakob disease
(B) Guillain-Barré syndrome
(C) Kuru
(D) Progressive multifocal leukoencephalopathy
(E) Subacute sclerosing panencephalitis

83. A 20-year-old man is hospitalized with fever, shaking chills, and widespread cutaneous hemorrhages. He complains of severe headache, and nuchal rigidity is noted on physical examination. Examination of the peripheral blood and CSF reveals gram-negative diplococci within neutrophils. A well-known complication of this disorder is hemorrhage into the

(A) adrenal cortex.
(B) anterior pituitary.
(C) brain stem.
(D) pancreas.
(E) subarachnoid space.

84. Which of the following is an example of metastatic calcification?

(A) Calcification of atheromatous plaques in coronary arteries
(B) Calcification of caseating granulomas in Ghon complex
(C) Calcification in healed rheumatic mitral valvulitis
(D) Cerebral calcifications in congenital toxoplasmosis
(E) Nephrocalcinosis in the milk-alkali syndrome

85. The diagnosis suggested by the illustrated glomerular change is supported by prolongation of or increase in all of the following indices EXCEPT

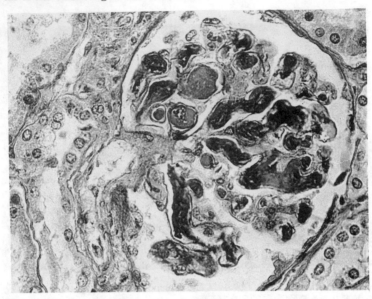

(Reprinted with permission from Golden A, Powell D, and Jennings C: *Pathology: Understanding Human Disease,* 2nd ed. Baltimore, Williams & Wilkins, 1985, p 83.)

(A) activated partial thromboplastin time.
(B) fibrin and fibrinogen degradation products.
(C) platelet count.
(D) prothrombin time.
(E) thrombin time.

86. A 28-year-old man was evaluated for progressive weakness, weight loss, and anorexia. He was found to be hypotensive, and generalized hyperpigmentation involving exposed surfaces of the skin, lips, and buccal mucosa was noted. All of the following laboratory findings are expected in this patient EXCEPT

(A) decreased serum sodium.
(B) increased serum potassium.
(C) decreased serum glucose.
(D) decreased plasma cortisol corrected by administration of ACTH.
(E) decreased urinary 17-ketosteroids.

87. Which one of the following autosomal disorders remains clinically silent until adulthood?

(A) Huntington's disease
(B) Osteogenesis imperfecta
(C) Phenylketonuria
(D) Sickle cell anemia
(E) Tuberous sclerosis

88. Membranous glomerulonephritis is found at autopsy in a 25-year-old woman who died in renal failure. Other autopsy findings include pleuritis, diffuse interstitial fibrosis of the lungs, concentric rings of collagen surrounding splenic arterioles, and warty vegetations of the mitral and tricuspid valves affecting the surfaces behind the cusps as well as the surfaces exposed to the forward flow of blood. Which of the following is an expected laboratory finding?

(A) Increased titer of antistreptolysin O (ASO)
(B) Lymphocytosis
(C) Peripheral rim pattern of antinuclear antibody fluorescence
(D) Positive blood cultures for *Streptococcus viridans*
(E) Serum antibodies reactive with glomerular and pulmonary alveolar basement membranes

89. A single nodule was resected from the peripheral portion of the right lower lobe of the lung of a 45-year-old woman. The microscopic findings were similar to those shown in the illustration. The diagnosis is

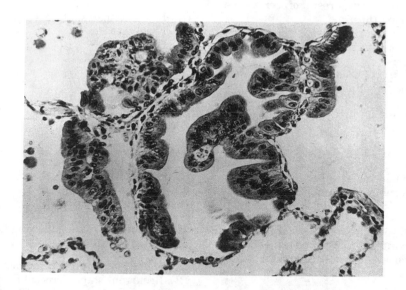

(Reprinted with permission from Rosai J: *Ackerman's Surgical Pathology,* 7th ed. St. Louis, CV Mosby, 1989, p 301.)

(A) bronchioloalveolar carcinoma.
(B) carcinoid.
(C) mesothelioma.
(D) small cell carcinoma.
(E) squamous cell carcinoma.

90. Recurrent intractable peptic ulcer disease suggests an underlying

(A) adenocarcinoma of the pancreas.
(B) adenoma of the adrenal medulla.
(C) carcinoid of the jejunum.
(D) islet cell tumor of the pancreas.
(E) pheochromocytoma.

91. Conjugated hyperbilirubinemia, positive urine tests for bilirubin and total absence of urobilinogen in the urine and stools suggest

(A) adenocarcinoma of the pancreas.
(B) amebic abscess of the liver.
(C) hepatic vein thrombosis.
(D) hepatitis A infection.
(E) hereditary spherocytosis.

92. Pheochromocytoma results in increased urinary excretion of all of the following EXCEPT

(A) epinephrine.
(B) metanephrine.
(C) norepinephrine.
(D) serotonin.
(E) vanillylmandelic acid.

93. Autophagic granules are characteristic findings in

(A) erythrocytic precursor cells after acute blood loss.
(B) gonadal structures in Turner's syndrome.
(C) myocardial cells in hypertensive cardiovascular disease.
(D) myometrial cells during pregnancy.
(E) skeletal muscle cells after prolonged immobilization.

94. All of the following are true of fatty change EXCEPT

(A) it is observed most frequently in the liver.
(B) it often occurs as a result of decreased apoprotein synthesis.
(C) it can be associated with starvation.
(D) it can result from increased triglyceride synthesis.
(E) it is characterized by triglyceride deposition within adipocytes.

95. The most frequently occurring salivary gland tumor is

(A) acinic cell tumor.
(B) adenoid cystic carcinoma.
(C) mucoepidermoid tumor.
(D) pleomorphic adenoma.
(E) Warthin's tumor.

96. A 2-year-old girl with a history of repeated pulmonary infections is found to have elevated chloride in a sweat test. An additional expected finding is

(A) hypercalcemia.
(B) hypotension.
(C) increased metabolism.
(D) renal failure.
(E) steatorrhea.

97. Which of the following is not a characteristic of berry aneurysms?

(A) Localized to sites of arterial bifurcation
(B) Frequent cause of subarachnoid hemorrhage
(C) Most frequently located in or near the circle of Willis
(D) Most often due to severe atherosclerosis
(E) Are often associated with polycystic kidney

98. Which of the following intracellular changes is characteristic of severe ischemic cell injury?

(A) Decreased calcium
(B) Decreased pH
(C) Decreased sodium
(D) Increased activity of Na^+K^+ pump
(E) Increased ATP

99. Which one of the following clinical manifestations or complications is least likely in a patient with pneumonia caused by *Streptococcus pneumoniae*?

(A) Blood-stained sputum
(B) Empyema
(C) Hypoxia
(D) Leukocytosis
(E) Pneumothorax

100. The epithelioid cells and multinucleated giant cells of granulomatous inflammation are derived from

(A) basophils.
(B) CD4+ lymphocytes.
(C) eosinophils.
(D) monocytes–macrophages.
(E) plasma cells.

101. Which one of the following is most likely associated with T-cell deficiency?

(A) *Haemophilus influenzae* meningitis
(B) Recurrent staphylococcal furunculosis
(C) Absence of germinal centers in spleen and lymph nodes
(D) *Pneumocystis carinii* pneumonia
(E) Severe anaphylactic reaction to IgA in transfused blood

102. Vasospasm of the arterioles and small arteries of the fingers is most characteristic of

(A) Buerger's disease (thromboangiitis obliterans).
(B) Raynaud's disease.
(C) Wegener's granulomatosis.
(D) Kawasaki disease.
(E) Takayasu's arteritis.

103. Characteristics of vitamin C deficiency include all of the following EXCEPT

(A) abnormal bleeding.
(B) defective collagen formation.
(C) defective osteoid matrix formation.
(D) impaired wound healing.
(E) increased intestinal absorption of iron.

104. Grading of a malignant tumor is based on all of the following characteristics EXCEPT

(A) the cell of origin.
(B) the degree of anaplasia.
(C) the degree of differentiation of tumor cells.
(D) the distribution and extent of the disease.
(E) the number of mitotic figures.

105. Which one of the following conditions is suggestive of an underlying malignancy?

(A) Acanthosis nigricans
(B) Clubbing of the fingers
(C) Marantic endocarditis
(D) Venous thrombosis
(E) All of the above

106. All of the following are characteristics of leiomyoma of the uterus EXCEPT

(A) frequent cause of menometrorrhagia.
(B) high incidence of malignant transformation.
(C) higher incidence in black women.
(D) often multifocal in location.
(E) regression after menopause.

107. All of the following are associated with lead poisoning EXCEPT

(A) dark precipitate along gingival margins.
(B) degeneration of the optic nerve.
(C) punctate basophilic stippling of erythrocytes.
(D) radiopaque deposits in epiphyses.
(E) urinary excretion of delta-aminolevulinic acid.

108. All of the following conditions are associated with increased HCG EXCEPT

(A) gestational carcinomas.
(B) granulosa cell tumor.
(C) hydatidiform mole.
(D) pregnancy.
(E) seminoma.

109. Which one of the following tumors is the most frequently occurring primary neoplasm of bone?

(A) Osteochondroma
(B) Osteosarcoma
(C) Giant cell tumor
(D) Ewing's sarcoma
(E) Chondrosarcoma

110. The degree of amplification of the HER-2/*neu* oncogene is a negative prognostic indicator in carcinoma of the

(A) adrenal.
(B) breast.
(C) kidney.
(D) stomach.
(E) thyroid.

111. All of the following features are associated with carcinoma of the cervix EXCEPT

(A) early sexual activity.
(B) frequent origin at the squamocolumnar junction.
(C) a history of estrogen therapy.
(D) infection with human papillomavirus.
(E) squamous cell morphology.

Questions 112 and 113

112. A male infant was seen for recurrent bacterial infections beginning at age 6 months. Immunoglobulin assay reveals absent IgG. An additional expected finding is

(A) absence of germinal centers in the lymph nodes.
(B) autosomal recessive inheritance.
(C) decreased CD4 + :CD8 + T-lymphocyte ratio.
(D) defective leukocytic bacterial killing.
(E) impaired phagocytosis.

113. In this infant, the period of well-being for the first 6 months of life is best explained by

(A) antibacterial substances supplied by breast-feeding.
(B) deficient opsonization due to immaturity of complement synthesis.
(C) delayed responsiveness of lymphocytes to mitogenic stimuli.
(D) protection by maternal antibodies.
(E) need for a viral infection to trigger immune destruction of thymic tissue.

114. Which of the following is not a feature of acute hematogenous osteomyelitis?

(A) Surgical drainage almost always required
(B) More common in males
(C) Most commonly affects the metaphyseal ends of long bones
(D) Most commonly is caused by *Staphylococcus aureus*
(E) Occurs with peak incidence in children

115. All of the following toxic agents are correctly paired with the appropriate disease process EXCEPT

(A) carbon tetrachloride (CCl_4)—hepatic centrilobular fatty change and necrosis.
(B) carbon monoxide (CO)—neuronal loss in the basal ganglia.
(C) ethanol—coronary artery disease.
(D) phenacetin—renal papillary necrosis.
(E) polychlorinated biphenyls (PCBs)—chloracne.

116. A 68-year-old woman has fever, generalized lower abdominal pain, and bright red blood in the stools. The white blood cell count is 15,000/μl, with 85% segmented neutrophils. The most likely diagnosis is

(A) acute appendicitis.
(B) carcinoma of the rectum.
(C) Crohn's disease.
(D) diverticulitis.
(E) tubular adenoma in sigmoid colon.

117. Which of the following is a predisposing factor in the pathogenesis of clear cell adenocarcinoma of the vagina?

(A) Excess estrogen stimulation
(B) Herpes simplex virus infection
(C) Human papillomavirus infection
(D) In utero exposure to diethylstilbestrol (DES)
(E) Oral contraceptive therapy

118. Disordered metabolism of bone is associated with deficiency of

(A) vitamin C.
(B) vitamin D.
(C) both vitamin C and vitamin D.
(D) neither vitamin C nor vitamin D.

119. All of the following statements concerning benign nodular hyperplasia and adenocarcinoma of the prostate are true EXCEPT

(A) adenocarcinoma is often responsive to orchiectomy or endocrine therapy.
(B) adenocarcinoma tends to arise in the peripheral group of prostatic glands.
(C) both benign nodular hyperplasia and adenocarcinoma have a peak incidence in elderly men.
(D) an increase in serum acid phosphatase is useful in the detection of early adenocarcinoma.
(E) an increase in serum prostate-specific antigen may occur with both benign nodular hyperplasia and adenocarcinoma.

120. All of the following factors contribute to the production of ascites in cirrhosis of the liver EXCEPT

(A) hypoalbuminemia.
(B) increased hepatic lymph formation.
(C) increased portal venous pressure.
(D) portal-systemic venous shunting.
(E) renal retention of sodium and water.

121. After localized injury and cell death, which of the following cell types is least likely to undergo regeneration with restoration of normal structure?

(A) Bronchial epithelial cells
(B) Gastric mucosal cells
(C) Hepatocytes
(D) Hippocampal neurons
(E) Renal tubular cells

122. Exposure to asbestos is most closely linked to

(A) basal cell carcinoma.
(B) hepatocellular carcinoma.
(C) mesothelioma.
(D) nasopharyngeal carcinoma.
(E) pheochromocytoma.

123. Which of the following is not a characteristic of multiple sclerosis?

(A) Association with certain HLA haplotypes
(B) Axonal degeneration
(C) Differing incidence according to geographic location
(D) Multiple cerebrospinal fluid oligoclonal immunoglobulin bands
(E) Optic nerve, brain stem, and paraventricular areas are favored sites

124. Which one of the following aneurysms is frequently associated with adult polycystic kidney?

(A) Berry aneurysm of the circle of Willis
(B) Dissecting aneurysm
(C) Fusiform aneurysm of the abdominal aorta
(D) Saccular aneurysm of the thoracic aorta

Directions: Each group of items in this section consists of lettered options followed by a set of numbered items. For each item, select the **one** lettered option that is most closely associated with it. Each lettered option may be selected once, more than once, or not at all.

Questions 125–127

Match the vascular source of bleeding with the site of intracranial hemorrhage.

(A) Brain substance of cerebral hemisphere
(B) Cerebral ventricles
(C) Epidural space
(D) Subarachnoid space
(E) Subdural space

125. Bridging cerebral veins

126. Middle meningeal artery

127. Berry aneurysm of the circle of Willis

Questions 128 and 129

Match the characteristic below with the appropriate intracranial neoplasm.

(A) Glioblastoma multiforme
(B) Medulloblastoma
(C) Meningioma
(D) Neurilemmoma
(E) Oligodendroglioma

128. Peak incidence in young children

129. Posterior cranial fossa most frequent site

Questions 130–132

Match the characteristic below with the appropriate disorder.

(A) Alzheimer's disease
(B) Huntington's disease
(C) Idiopathic Parkinson's disease
(D) Myasthenia gravis
(E) Wernicke-Korsakoff syndrome

130. Depigmentation of the substantia nigra and locus ceruleus

131. Autoantibodies to acetylcholine receptors

132. Atrophy of the caudate nucleus

Questions 133 and 134

Match the characteristic below with the appropriate disorder.

(A) Ankylosing spondylitis
(B) Hypertrophic osteoarthropathy
(C) Osteoarthritis
(D) Rheumatoid arthritis
(E) Felty's syndrome

133. Typically secondary to lung disease

134. Splenomegaly and neutropenia

Questions 135 and 136

Match the characteristic below with the testicular tumor associated with it.

(A) Androblastoma
(B) Endodermal sinus tumor
(C) Mature teratoma
(D) Mixed germ cell tumor
(E) Seminoma

135. Usually benign

136. Analogous to dysgerminoma

Questions 137 and 138

Match the clinical finding below with the associated disorder.

(A) Renal amyloidosis
(B) Diabetic nephropathy
(C) Focal and segmental glomerulosclerosis
(D) Membranous glomerulonephritis
(E) Minimal change disease
(F) Poststreptococcal glomerulonephritis

137. Nephritic syndrome

138. Impetigo

Questions 139 and 140

Match the characteristic below with the congenital infection associated with it.

(A) Cytomegalovirus
(B) Toxoplasma
(C) Both cytomegalovirus and Toxoplasma
(D) Neither cytomegalovirus nor Toxoplasma

139. Intracranial calcifications

140. Multisystem involvement

Answers and Explanations

1–C. Metastatic calcification is the deposition of calcium in organs and tissues and is associated with hypercalcemia. CCl_4 injury is the classic model of membrane injury by free radical formation. In this instance, CCl_4 is converted to the active free radical $CCl_3\cdot$ in the smooth endoplasmic reticulum by the P-450 system of mixed function oxidases. Injury from ionizing radiation, oxygen toxicity, and injury from reperfusion after ischemia are examples of free radical-mediated injury.

2–D. Nuclear pyknosis, along with karyorrhexis and karyolysis, is a sign of necrosis and is of course irreversible. Fatty change, formation of cell blebs or myelin figures, and swelling of the cell or of organelles are all reversible changes.

3–C. The fat embolism syndrome occurs 2 to 3 days after severe fracture injury and includes progressive CNS dysfunction and severe respiratory insufficiency. Thrombocytopenia with petechial bleeding is common, and petechial hemorrhages can result from obstruction of the microvasculature by embolic fat droplets. Respiratory insufficiency may be due to injury to pulmonary microvessels with leakage of fluid into the alveoli, resulting in adult respiratory distress syndrome (ARDS).

4–E. Serum sickness is the classic example of systemic immune complex disease and is unrelated to tissue mast cells.

5–B. EBV is associated with nasopharyngeal carcinoma. It also is associated with Burkitt's lymphoma and with infectious mononucleosis, a benign, self-limited lymphoproliferative disorder.

6–D. The clinical behavior of neoplasms is the underlying basis for all other indicators that distinguish malignant from benign lesions. For example, some extremely well-differentiated, otherwise benign-appearing lesions are known to metastasize and thus are classified as malignant.

7–A. Homozygous α-1-antitrypsin deficiency is associated with the combination of panacinar emphysema and hepatic cirrhosis.

8–D. The risk of malignant transformation in familial multiple polyposis approaches 100%. Colorectal villous adenomas undergo malignant change in about 30% of cases. There is a markedly increased incidence of colon cancer in long-standing cases of ulcerative colitis. The incidence of colon cancer is also increased in Crohn's disease but to a lesser degree than in ulcerative colitis. Peptic ulcer of the duodenum is not a precursor lesion to carcinoma.

9–E. Paget's disease of bone may lead to osteosarcoma. It should not be confused with Paget's disease of the breast, which is closely associated with an underlying duct carcinoma.

10–D. Granulosa cell tumors of the ovary characteristically produce estrogen, not HCG.

11–E. Hypertrophic cardiomyopathy, a condition that is usually inherited as an autosomal dominant disorder, is often associated with sudden death in young athletes. The ventricular septum is especially involved, with protrusion into the left ventricular cavity (asymmetric septal hypertrophy), sometimes leading to left ventricular outflow tract obstruction.

12–E. DIC is characterized by widespread clotting with consumption of platelets. Thus thrombocytopenia, not thrombocytosis, is an expected finding. The consumption of coagulation factors results in prolongation of the prothrombin time (a measure of the extrinsic pathway of coagulation), activated partial thromboplastin time (a measure of the intrinsic pathway of coagulation), and thrombin time (a measure of the fibrinogen concentration). Widespread thrombosis activates the fibrinolytic system, with degradation of both fibrin and fibrinogen, and is therefore marked by increased fibrin and fibrinogen degradation products.

13–C. The most common form of meningitis in the newborn is pyogenic meningitis. CSF findings include numerous neutrophils, increased protein, and decreased glucose.

14–A. Pyogenic meningitis in newborns is most frequently caused by *E. coli;* in older infants and young children, by *H. influenzae;* in young adults, by *N. meningitidis;* and in older persons, by *S. pneumoniae.*

15–A. GTPase activity, which is required for inactivation, is decreased in mutant Ras (p21) proteins. This change is mediated by reduced responsiveness to GTPase-activating protein.

16–B. The clinical history is strongly suggestive of bacterial pneumonia. Pleural fluid from this patient would typically be an exudate rather than a transudate, and would be expected to be cloudy and contain many neutrophils. The fluid would also demonstrate reduced glucose, increased protein, and increased specific gravity.

17–C. Brain damage in phenylketonuria (caused by homozygous deficiency of phenylalanine hydroxylase) is delayed until the postnatal period since phenylalanine can be metabolized by maternal mechanisms prior to birth. Fetal alcohol syndrome is an important cause of congenital microcephaly. Microcephaly can also be part of the TORCH complex, a group of congenital manifestations caused by infection with *T*oxoplasma, *O*ther viral etiologies, *R*ubella virus, *C*ytomegalovirus, or *H*erpes simplex virus.

18–B. The sickle cell preparation is positive in sickle cell anemia and other hemoglobin S disorders. Splenomegaly occurs in children with sickle cell anemia, but repeated bouts of splenic infarction and fibrosis reduce the spleen to a fibrous remnant in adults (autosplenectomy).

19–A. Carcinoma of the urinary bladder, almost always transitional cell carcinoma, most often spreads by local extension to surrounding tissues. Hematogenous dissemination is a late finding.

20–E. Pseudohypoparathyroidism is characterized by chemical indicators of hypoparathyroidism. However, parathyroid hormone activity is normal or even increased. The disorder is thought to be caused by renal end-organ unresponsiveness to parathyroid hormone.

21–C. Multiple myeloma often presents with diffuse demineralization of bone, even though punched-out lesions are more characteristic. Findings that distinguish multiple myeloma from other conditions also characterized by bony demineralization include anemia, hypergammaglobulinemia, proteinuria, and normal (rather than increased) serum alkaline phosphatase.

22–C. Medullary carcinoma is characterized histologically by sheets of tumor cells in an amyloid-containing stroma. This neoplasm is a calcitonin-producing tumor derived from C cells of the thyroid. Medullary carcinoma can occur as a component of multiple endocrine neoplasia (MEN) syndromes types IIa and IIb.

23–E. The most frequent cause of cardiac rupture is myocardial infarction. This complication, which often results in hemopericardium and cardiac tamponade, occurs with peak incidence within 4 to 10 days after infarction.

24–C. Hypersensitivity (leukocytoclastic) vasculitis is an immune complex disease characterized by involvement of small vessels (venules, capillaries, arterioles) and by multiple lesions, all about the same age. The disorder may involve only the skin, presenting as palpable purpura, or it may involve a variety of other sites, including the glomeruli, gastrointestinal tract, lungs, or brain.

25–B. In long-standing idiopathic hemochromatosis, serum iron is markedly increased and TIBC is moderately reduced. This combination often results in almost 100% saturation of iron binding capacity.

26–C. Emphysema has no association with hyaline membrane formation. Alveolar hyaline membrane formation is a characteristic finding in both the neonatal and adult respiratory distress syndromes. The common factor is diffuse alveolar damage induced by a number of agents or conditions.

27–E. Most neuroblastomas are peripheral, and the most frequent site of origin is the adrenal medulla or adjacent tissues. CNS neuroblastomas are less common, and most often involve the cerebral hemispheres. Origin in the posterior cranial fossa is rare. Amplification of *N-myc* is characteristic, and the degree of amplification is a negative prognostic indicator. The tumor may occasionally undergo differentiation to a benign ganglioneuroma. Neuroblastoma is one of the most common malignancies of childhood.

28–D. Disseminated histoplasmosis is characterized by widespread dissemination of macrophages filled with fungal yeast forms.

29–C. A linear pattern of glomerular immunofluorescence for IgG is found in Goodpasture's syndrome, which is caused by antibodies that react with both glomerular and alveolar basement membranes.

30–E. Progressive somnolence leading to metabolic acidosis (low bicarbonate with significant anion gap), coma, and severe dehydration, often with prerenal azotemia, are all strongly suggestive of diabetic ketoacidosis. Expected findings in this condition include increased serum and urine glucose and ketones.

31–B. Folate deficiency leads to megaloblastic anemia. The red cells are macrocytic and normochromic. Since the thickened red cells appear more dense on peripheral blood smears, these cells are often erroneously thought to be hyperchromic; however, the MCHC is normal.

32–C. In the first several hours after myocardial infarction, the most common cause of death is arrhythmia. Although evidence of acute coronary artery obstruction may be found, morphologic myocardial changes and serum enzyme elevations are most often delayed for several hours. A myocardial fibrotic scar is evidence of old prior myocardial infarction.

33–E. Gonorrhea is most often manifest in men as acute purulent urethritis; without treatment, it can extend to the prostate and seminal vesicles and sometimes to the epididymis. The testes are rarely involved.

34–E. Whipple's disease, a systemic illness invariably involving the small intestine, is characterized morphologically by distinctive PAS-positive macrophages within affected organs. On electron microscopy, the macrophages contain numerous bacillary forms suggestive of microorganisms. The disorder responds to antibacterial therapy.

35–E. Von Willebrand's disease (congenital deficiency of von Willebrand's factor) is characterized by defective platelet adhesion, resulting in a prolonged bleeding time even though the platelets are qualitatively and quantitatively normal. The activated thromboplastin time is also prolonged because of a secondary deficiency of factor VIII. Factor VIII normally circulates in a complex with von Willebrand's factor and is unstable when von Willebrand's factor is deficient.

36–B. Pleural and peritoneal mesotheliomas are associated with exposure to asbestos, not arsenic.

37–D. Endometriosis is not a neoplasm and has no relation to malignancy. The most important factor in the pathogenesis of endometrial carcinoma appears to be prolonged estrogen stimulation such as that associated with estrogen therapy or with estrogen-secreting tumors. Adenomatous hyperplasia, itself a result of estrogen stimulation, is a frequent precursor to endometrial carcinoma. Obesity and conditions associated with it, such as diabetes mellitus or hypertension, may contribute to hyperestrinism because estrone can be synthesized in peripheral fat cells.

38–D. During the first several hours of an inflammatory process, the predominant inflammatory cells are neutrophils. After 1 or 2 days, neutrophils are largely replaced by longer-lived monocytes–macrophages.

39–B. Down's syndrome is associated with a markedly increased incidence of acute leukemia.

40–A. Except for lipoid nephrosis (minimal change disease), all of the listed entities are examples of immune complex disease, as is experimental serum sickness.

41–E. Endocrine disorders associated with hyperglycemia include pheochromocytoma, with hypersecretion of catecholamines; Cushing's syndrome, either pituitary or adrenal, with hypersecretion of corticotropin or cortisol; acromegaly, with hypersecretion of growth hormone; and hyperthyroidism, with hypersecretion of thyroxine.

42–C. Red blood cell casts are a specific indicator of glomerular inflammation. Although microscopic hematuria is a frequent finding in acute pyelonephritis and other urinary tract infections, red cell casts are not seen since the glomeruli tend to be spared in renal infection.

43–A. Congenital pyloric stenosis is an obstruction of the gastric outlet caused by hypertrophy of the pyloric muscularis. The hypertrophic muscle is often perceived as a palpable mass. The principal manifestation of this condition, more common in boys, is projectile vomiting, most often occurring in the first 2 weeks of life.

44–A. Although atherosclerosis can affect all portions of the aorta, aneurysm of the thoracic aorta, especially the ascending portion, is unusual. Most atherosclerotic aortic aneurysms involve the abdominal aorta.

45–B. The hematocrit (as well as the hemoglobin and red cell count) does not distinguish one form of anemia from another. In iron deficiency anemia, serum iron is decreased, TIBC is increased, and storage iron is depleted, as indicated by decreased serum ferritin and absent bone marrow hemosiderin on Prussian blue stain.

46–C. Among the variants of Hodgkin's disease, lymphocytic depletion has the poorest prognosis. This form of Hodgkin's disease is characterized by lymphocytic depletion and the presence of numerous Reed-Sternberg cells, both of which are indicators of poor prognosis.

47–B. The jaundice of hemolytic anemia is due to increased unconjugated bilirubin. Since unconjugated bilirubin is not excreted into the urine, the type of jaundice is acholuric, jaundice without bilirubin pigment in the urine.

48–D. Juvenile melanoma, or Spitz nevus, is a benign lesion that can be confused with malignant melanoma. Acanthosis nigricans is sometimes an indicator of visceral malignancy. Actinic keratosis is a premalignant epidermal lesion. Dysplastic nevus may transform into malignant melanoma. Xeroderma pigmentosum is associated with a markedly increased incidence of skin cancer caused by failure of DNA repair.

49–C. Giant cells are not a feature of alcoholic hepatitis, which is characterized by fatty change, focal liver cell necrosis, infiltrates of neutrophils, and intracytoplasmic hyaline inclusions referred to as Mallory bodies.

50–A. Contact dermatitis can be caused by T-cell mediated (type IV) hypersensitivity or by direct chemical injury to the skin. Graves' disease, hemolytic disease of the newborn, polyarteritis nodosa, and urticaria are all antibody-mediated disorders.

51–B. The granulomas of sarcoidosis are characteristically noncaseating.

52–A. Aflatoxin B is associated with hepatocellular carcinoma, not cancer of the mouth and tongue. Oral cancers, like cancer of the esophagus, have a marked association with the combined abuse of tobacco and alcohol.

53–C. In spite of morphologic differences, the bronchogenic carcinomas, including small cell carcinoma, all share a common endodermal origin.

54–C. C4a has no association with the release of interleukin-1. C3a and C5a (anaphylatoxins) mediate degranulation of basophils and mast cells. In addition, C5a is a potent chemotactic agent for neutrophils. C3b is an important opsonin. C5b-9 is the membrane attack complex that mediates complement-induced cell lysis.

55–E. Coagulation necrosis is marked by initial preservation of tissue architecture and is most often caused by interruption of the blood supply to the affected tissue.

56–E. Pseudomombranous colitis is caused by intraluminal proliferation of *Clostridium difficile,* a normally occurring commensal organism. The clostridia remain intraluminal but secrete an enterotoxin that is responsible for the clinical and pathologic manifestations of the disorder.

57–B. Septic cerebrovascular emboli from the bacteria-laden vegetations of infective endocarditis can result in cerebral abscess formation. Renal complications of infective endocarditis include embolization with renal infarction of focal glomerulonephritis (either septic or immune complex in type). Local effects in the heart include abscess formation and local tissue destruction, resulting in complications such as ruptured chordae tendineae, perforation of valve leaflets, and even perforation of the interventricular septum. Dissecting aortic aneurysm is predisposed by cystic medial necrosis and hypertension, and is unrelated to infective endocarditis.

58–B. Punctate cutaneous bleeding is an indicator of primary hemostatic bleeding, as seen in defects involving the microvasculature (scurvy, rickettsial infections) or the platelets. Platelet disorders include thrombocytopenia, which may be either primary (as in idiopathic thrombocytopenic purpura) or secondary (as in disseminated intravascular coagulation). Christmas disease (factor IX deficiency), a disorder of the intrinsic pathway of coagulation clinically indistinguishable from classic hemophilia, is characterized by secondary hemostatic bleeding.

59–C. Autoantibodies, association with certain HLA types, and increased incidence in persons with other autoimmune disorders are frequent occurrences in autoimmune disorders. In addition, Hashimoto's thyroiditis is characterized by dense lymphocytic infiltrates with germinal center formation, striking morphologic evidence of immune cell (B lymphocyte) participation.

60–B. Sustained ethanol abuse and progressive dementia are strongly suggestive of the Wernicke-Korsakoff syndrome, which is due to thiamine deficiency, most often in association with chronic alcoholism. Clinical characteristics include Wernicke's triad (confusion, ataxia, and ophthalmoplegia) and often Korsakoff's psychosis, characterized by memory loss and confabulation (making up stories in an attempt to hide the inability to remember).

61–B. Marantic endocarditis is associated with a variety of wasting diseases, such as end-stage widely disseminated cancer, and has no association with SLE.

62–C. The most frequent cause of transfusion-related hepatitis is hepatitis C virus infection. Hepatitis C virus is the most frequent cause of what was formerly termed non-A, non-B hepatitis.

63–A. Agnogenic (idiopathic) myeloid metaplasia is characterized by extensive myelofibrosis and extramedullary hematopoiesis resulting in hepatosplenomegaly. Myeloid (granulocytic) and erythroid precursor cells are depleted. Megakaryocytes are not only spared but are most often increased in number.

64–D. A rapidly fatal course with severe hypertension, left ventricular hypertrophy and failure, papilledema, and renal dysfunction is characteristic of malignant hypertension. This syndrome is most frequently seen in relatively young black men. The defining renal arteriolar lesion, malignant nephrosclerosis (hyperplastic arteriolosclerosis, fibrinoid necrosis, necrotizing arteriolitis), and the associated necrotizing glomerular lesion result in capillary rupture and the consequent "flea-bitten" kidney appearance due to petechial hemorrhages covering the surfaces of the kidneys.

65–E. The observation of thickened glomerular capillary loops apparent on light microscopy permits the diagnosis of membranous glomerulonephritis. This condition is most frequent in young women and is characterized clinically by the nephrotic syndrome and progressive azotemia.

66–C. The cause of congenital heart disease is most often unknown. Only a small minority of cases are clearly associated with maternal-fetal infections.

67–C. The hallmark of the megaloblastic anemias is the finding of megaloblastic erythroid hyperplasia in the bone marrow; pernicious anemia is a megaloblastic anemia.

68–C. Carcinoma of the pancreas with common bile duct obstruction is strongly suggested by the clinical findings. Trousseau's sign, spontaneous migratory venous thrombosis with visceral neoplasms, was first described as an association of adenocarcinoma of the pancreas.

69–B. Nodular melanoma tends to expand vertically rather than horizontally, a phenomenon associated with a more aggressive course and a greater likelihood of metastasis. Among the malignant melanomas, nodular melanoma has the poorest prognosis.

70–A. Hookworm infestation causes chronic blood loss with resultant iron deficiency anemia and should not be confused with fish tapeworm infestation, which causes megaloblastic anemia. Folate deficiency with megaloblastic anemia can occur in severely malnourished persons (often alcoholics) and in association with increased demand for folate in pregnancy. Cobalamin (vitamin B_{12}) deficiency megaloblastic anemia can occur in strict vegetarians (vitamin B_{12} is found in foods of animal origin only) and is associated with surgically induced intestinal blind loops overgrown with microorganisms with high avidity for cobalamin.

71–E. In a pediatric patient, the combination of recurrent pulmonary infections and steatorrhea (presumably due to pancreatic insufficiency) is strongly suggestive of cystic fibrosis. This disorder is characterized by a generalized defect in the reabsorption of anions, leading to increased sweat chloride concentration, an important diagnostic indicator.

72–E. Granulation tissue is formed in healing wounds and consists of young fibroblasts and newly formed capillaries. Cat-scratch disease, foreign body reaction, histoplasmosis, and tuberculosis are all well-known causes of granulomatous inflammation and have nothing to do with granulation tissue.

73–D. A keloid is a result of excessive production of collagenous fibrous tissue and is characterized by a tumor-like scar consisting of dense bundles of structurally abnormal collagen. Keloids have a marked tendency to recur after resection. Propensity to keloid formation is markedly increased in blacks.

74–B. Multiple myeloma is frequently complicated by systemic accumulations of amyloid derived from immunoglobulin light chains. Secondary systemic (reactive) amyloidosis is associated with chronic inflammation, most frequently rheumatoid arthritis. Localized accumulations of amyloid within neuritic plaques may play a pathogenetic role in Alzheimer's disease. Amyloid stroma is a characteristic feature of medullary carcinoma of the thyroid.

75–D. The combination of increased serum calcium and alkaline phosphatase along with decreased serum phosphorus is most consistent with primary hyperparathyroidism. The most frequent cause of this endocrine abnormality is a parathyroid adenoma. Decreased phosphorus would not be an expected finding in metastatic carcinoma. The normal serum proteins mitigate against multiple myeloma and sarcoidosis. Additionally, the alkaline phosphatase is usually normal in multiple myeloma. Hypercalcemia from increased intake (as in the milk-alkali syndrome) is usually unaccompanied by significant changes in phosphorus or alkaline phosphatase.

76–A. Von Hippel-Lindau disease is an autosomal dominant disorder characterized by multiple vascular tumors and cysts of the liver, kidney, and pancreas.

77–D. Renal papillary necrosis is a frequent complication of chronic analgesic nephritis, which is caused by long-term abuse of phenacetin or its metabolite, acetaminophen, most often in combination with aspirin or another nonsteroidal anti-inflammatory drug. Another major cause of renal papillary necrosis is diabetes mellitus. Phenacetin abuse is also associated with a markedly increased incidence of transitional cell carcinoma of the renal pelvis.

78–B. True hermaphroditism requires the presence of both ovarian and testicular tissue. The karyotype is either XX (with translocation of at least part of the Y chromosome to an X chromosome or to an autosome) or a mosaicism such as XX/XXY. A Barr body is present.

79–A. The illustration demonstrates an adenocarcinoma diffusely infiltrating the wall of the colon, with marked constriction of the lumen and ulceration of the mucosa.

80–B. Phospholipase A_2 catalyzes the release of arachidonic acid from membrane phospholipids. Arachidonic acid metabolism then proceeds through two major pathways, the lipoxygenase and cyclooxygenase pathways. The lipoxygenase pathway yields HETE and leukotrienes. The cyclooxygenase pathway yields thromboxanes and prostaglandins. PGI_2 is synthesized in endothelial cells, and TxA_2 is synthesized in platelets.

81–A. The increase in size of skeletal muscle after exercise is the classic example of hypertrophy, an increase in organ size due to an increase in the size of cells. Striated muscle cells are unable to proliferate in number in adults.

82–E. Subacute sclerosing panencephalitis, one of the slow virus infections, is thought to be caused by persistent infection with a defective measles virus. The virus lacks the M component, a protein required for extracellular spread of the virus. This deficiency is thought to explain the slow nature of the infection.

83–A. The findings are characteristic of meningococcemia with meningococcal meningitis. A well-recognized complication of meningococcemia is the Waterhouse-Friderichsen syndrome, which is catastrophic adrenal insufficiency and vascular collapse caused by hemorrhagic necrosis of the adrenal cortex, often with associated disseminated intravascular coagulation.

84–E. Metastatic calcification refers to deposition of calcium caused by hypercalcemia. The milk-alkali syndrome is hypercalcemia caused by increased calcium intake in the form of milk and antacid (often calcium-containing) therapy. Calcification of previously damaged tissue is termed dystrophic calcification.

85–C. The illustration demonstrates thrombotic obliteration of glomerular capillary loops and is typical of disseminated intravascular coagulation (DIC). In this disorder, sometimes termed consumption coagulopathy, coagulation factors, fibrinogen, and platelets are depleted by the widespread thrombotic process. Thus the coagulation assays are prolonged and the platelet count is decreased. Increased fibrin and fibrinogen degradation products are sensitive indicators of DIC.

86–D. Progressive weakness, hypotension, and hyperpigmentation are strongly suggestive of adrenocortical deficiency. Primary adrenocortical deficiency (Addison's disease), as distinguished from adrenal cortical insufficiency secondary to pituitary hypofunction, is indicated by the presence of pigmentation. Decreased plasma cortisol in Addison's disease is unresponsive to ACTH administration.

87–A. Clinical manifestations of Huntington's disease, an autosomal dominant disorder, are characteristically delayed until age 30 to 40. Persons at risk can be identified by restrictive fragment length polymorphism (RFLP) analysis.

88–C. The combination of membranous glomerulonephritis, pleuritis, and Libman-Sacks endocarditis (vegetations on both surfaces of the mitral or tricuspid valves) as well as proliferative splenic arteriolitis is characteristic of systemic lupus erythematosus (SLE). Diffuse interstitial pulmonary fibrosis also occurs in SLE. A variety of antinuclear antibodies (ANAs) are found; the most specific are antibodies to the Sm (Smith) antigen, antibodies to double-stranded DNA, and antibodies that result in a peripheral rim pattern of nuclear immunofluorescence.

89–A. In a typical well-differentiated bronchioloalveolar carcinoma, tumor cells line the walls of terminal air spaces, as shown in the illustration. When the tumor is localized to a single nodule, it is potentially curable by surgical resection.

90–D. The Zollinger-Ellison syndrome, characterized by markedly increased gastric acid production and intractable peptic ulcer, is caused by hypersecretion of a gastrin-producing islet cell tumor (gastrinoma).

91–A. Conjugated hyperbilirubinemia and positive urine tests for bilirubin are indicative of obstructive jaundice. The complete absence of urine and stool urobilinogen further indicates total common bile duct obstruction and strongly suggests that the etiology is a malignant tumor such as adenocarcinoma of the pancreas.

92–D. Pheochromocytoma of the adrenal medulla (and its extra-adrenal counterpart paraganglioma) secretes the catecholamines epinephrine and norepinephrine. Increased urinary excretion of catecholamines or their metabolites metanephrine and vanillylmandelic acid is a clinical indicator of this tumor. Increased urinary excretion of serotonin is an indicator of a carcinoid tumor, not pheochromocytoma.

93–E. Autophagic granules are intracytoplasmic vacuoles containing debris from degraded organelles such as mitochondria. They are especially prominent in cells that have become atrophic, such as skeletal muscle cells after prolonged immobilization.

94–E. Fatty change is defined as deposition of triglycerides within parenchymal cells. The liver is most often affected, but it also can occur in myocardial and renal tubular cells.

95–D. The majority of salivary gland tumors occur in the parotid, and most are pleomorphic adenomas. These tumors most often present as a painless mass just anterior to the ear.

96–E. Repeated pulmonary infections and a positive sweat test are characteristic of cystic fibrosis. In this condition, viscid secretions cause defective exocrine gland function. The lungs and pancreas are the most significant sites of involvement, and the disorder is marked by repeated bouts of pneumonia and by pancreatic failure with wasting and steatorrhea.

97–D. Berry aneurysms occur at sites of discontinuity of the arterial media, most frequently at bifurcations of vessels of the circle of Willis. The most common locations are the junction of the anterior cerebral and anterior communicating arteries, the bifurcation of the middle cerebral artery, the junction of the internal carotid and posterior communicating arteries, and the junction of the basilar and posterior cerebral arteries. Berry aneurysms are the most frequent cause of subarachnoid hemorrhage. An increased incidence is associated with adult polycystic kidney. There is no association with atherosclerosis.

98–B. Intracellular pH is decreased in severe ischemic cell injury. This change is caused by mitochondrial damage, which in turn results in decreased oxidative phosphorylation and diminished ATP synthesis. Decreased ATP stimulates glycolysis, with lactate formation, thus resulting in decreased intracellular pH. Decreased ATP also diminishes the activity of the membrane-associated Na^+K^+ pump, allowing an influx of sodium and water. The final steps leading to cell death in severe ischemic injury are associated with massive influx of extracellular calcium.

99–E. Although a lung abscess may lead to spontaneous pneumothorax, abscess formation is unusual in *S. pneumoniae* infection. The most common cause of spontaneous pneumothorax is emphysema.

100–D. Both epithelioid cells and multinucleated giant cells are modified macrophages.

101–D. Opportunistic infection with *P. carinii* affects approximately half of the patients with AIDS, which is the classic example of T-cell immunodeficiency. In T-cell dysfunction or deficiency, resistance to bacterial infection is largely unimpaired. Absence of lymphoid germinal centers suggests B-cell rather than T-cell dysfunction. Anaphylactic reactions depend on preformed IgE antibody synthesized by plasma cells (derived from B cells).

102–B. Raynaud's disease is cold-induced vasospasm of arterioles and small arteries, most often involving the fingers and sometimes the hands or feet. Young, otherwise healthy women are most often affected.

103–E. Vitamin C is required for a variety of hydroxylations, especially of proline and lysine, both of which are required steps in collagen and osteoid matrix synthesis. Poor collagen formation contributes to impaired wound healing as well as to fragility of capillary walls, which in turn leads to abnormal bleeding. Vitamin C also maintains the reduced state of metabolically active agents, such as iron and tetrahydrofolate. The maintenance of iron in its divalent ferrous form is required for intestinal iron absorption. Thus iron absorption is decreased rather than increased in vitamin C deficiency.

104–D. Grading is based on histopathologic evaluation of a malignant neoplasm and is contrasted with staging, which is based on clinical evaluation of the distribution and extent of the disease process.

105–E. Acanthosis nigricans is associated with an increased incidence of visceral malignancy, as is venous thrombosis. Clubbing of the fingers may be associated with a number of disorders, including carcinoma of the lung. Marantic endocarditis is associated with wasting diseases such as cancer.

106–B. Leiomyoma of the uterus, the most frequently occurring neoplasm of women, is benign. Malignant transformation is extremely rare. Most leiomyosarcomas are thought to arise de novo.

107–B. Classic features of lead poisoning include a gingival lead line consisting of precipitated lead sulfide, basophilic stippling of erythrocytes, radiopaque deposits in epiphyses, and increased urinary delta-aminolevulinic acid. Although lead poisoning is associated with peripheral neuropathy and a variety of CNS changes, degeneration of the optic nerve is not observed.

108–B. Granulosa cell tumors typically secrete estrogen and are independent of HCG stimulation.

109–B. The most frequently occurring primary tumor of bone is osteosarcoma.

110–B. Amplification of the HER-2/*neu* oncogene is frequently observed in breast cancer, and the degree of amplification is thought to be a negative prognostic indicator.

111–C. Hyperestrinism from estrogen therapy or other causes is associated with endometrial carcinoma, not carcinoma of the cervix.

112–A. The findings described are characteristic of congenital agammaglobulinemia of Bruton, an X-linked disorder characterized morphologically by agammaglobulinemia, absence of plasma cells, and absent or poorly defined germinal centers in the lymph nodes. Leukocyte functions, such as phagocytosis and bacterial killing, are unimpaired. T lymphocytes are unaffected.

113–D. Maternal antibodies provide passive immunization and protection from bacterial infection during the first months of life in children with congenital agammaglobulinemia.

114–A. In the acute stage, pyogenic osteomyelitis often resolves with antibiotic therapy. If the disorder is allowed to progress to necrosis and sequestrum formation, surgical intervention is usually required.

115–C. Ethanol intake is unrelated to coronary artery disease. Moderate ethanol intake may induce a beneficial rise in HDL cholesterol. CCl_4 poisoning leads to centrilobular fatty change in the liver and sometimes to liver cell necrosis. CO interferes with oxygen transport by hemoglobin, leading to systemic hypoxia. Neurons, particularly those of the basal ganglia and lenticular nuclei, are especially susceptible to CO-mediated hypoxic damage. The therapeutic use of phenacetin has been largely discontinued because of its nephrotoxicity, which is manifest by renal papillary necrosis and chronic tubulointerstitial nephritis. Indestructible PCBs have been banned from manufacturing because of their association with chloracne, impaired vision, and impotence.

116–D. Generalized lower abdominal pain, bloody stools, and signs of acute inflammation in an older patient are classic findings in diverticulitis. Appendicitis and Crohn's disease occur more often in younger persons, and bloody stools would not be expected. Signs of acute inflammation would not be expected in carcinoma of the rectum or in tubular adenoma.

117–D. Clear cell adenocarcinoma of the vagina is a rare malignant tumor that is markedly increased in incidence in daughters of women who received DES therapy during pregnancy.

118–C. Vitamin C deficiency results in defective osteoid matrix formation caused by impaired synthesis of hydroxyproline and hydroxylysine. Vitamin D deficiency causes deficient calcification of osteoid matrix and is clinically manifest as rickets in children and osteomalacia in adults.

119–D. Serum acid phosphatase remains normal in adenocarcinoma of the prostate until the tumor has penetrated the capsule into the adjacent tissues. The most useful measure for early diagnosis is digital rectal examination along with measurement of prostate-specific antigen.

120–D. Portal-systemic venous shunting leads to esophageal varices, rectal hemorrhoids, and distention of periumbilical venous collaterals; it can also lead to encephalopathy but does not contribute to ascites.

121–D. Neurons are permanent cells that do not proliferate during adult life. Bronchial epithelial cells, gastric mucosal cells, and renal tubular cells are labile cells, and hepatocytes are stable cells. Both labile and stable cells are fully capable of proliferation and regeneration.

122–C. Exposure to asbestos markedly predisposes to mesothelioma of the pleura or peritoneum and is also closely linked to bronchogenic carcinoma.

123–B. Multiple sclerosis is the most common of the demyelinating diseases, a group of disorders characterized by destruction of myelin with preservation of axons.

124–A. Adult polycystic kidney is frequently associated with berry aneurysm of the circle of Willis, often in association with cysts in the liver or pancreas.

125–E. Subdural hematoma is caused by venous bleeding, most often from bridging veins joining the cerebral vessels to venous sinuses within the dura.

126–C. Epidural hematoma is most often caused by skull fracture with laceration of branches of the middle meningeal artery.

127–D. Subarachnoid hemorrhage is often caused by rupture of a berry aneurysm of the circle of Willis.

128–B. Medulloblastoma, a highly malignant tumor of the cerebellum, is one of the most frequently occurring malignancies of early childhood (along with acute leukemia, Wilms' tumor, and adrenal neuroblastoma).

129–B. Medulloblastoma, a cerebellar tumor, is sited in the posterior cranial fossa.

130–C. Idiopathic Parkinson's disease is manifest histologically by depigmentation of cells of the substantia nigra and locus ceruleus.

131–D. Myasthenia gravis is an autoimmune disorder caused by autoantibodies to acetylcholine receptors of the neuromuscular junction.

132–B. Huntington's disease is manifest anatomically by progressive degeneration and atrophy of the caudate nucleus, putamen, and frontal cortex.

133–B. Hypertrophic osteoarthropathy, manifest as clubbing of the fingers and associated periostitis of the distal radius and ulna, is associated with chronic lung disease, cyanotic heart disease, and other systemic disorders.

134–E. Felty's syndrome is splenomegaly and neutropenia associated with rheumatoid arthritis.

135–A. Androblastoma (Sertoli cell tumor), a non-germ cell tumor derived from the sex cord, is most often benign. The endodermal sinus tumor is a malignant germ cell tumor with peak incidence in infancy and early childhood. The mature teratoma of the testis is almost always malignant, in contrast to the corresponding tumor in the ovary (dermoid cyst). Mixed germ cell tumors include varying mixes of seminoma, embryonal carcinoma, teratoma, and choriocarcinoma. The seminoma is a malignant germ cell tumor accounting for 40% of germ cell tumors.

136–E. Seminoma, a germ cell tumor of the testis with peak incidence in the mid-30s age group, is analogous to, and closely resembles, dysgerminoma of the ovary.

137–F. The prototype of the nephritic syndrome is poststreptococcal glomerulonephritis.

138–F. As the name implies, poststreptococcal glomerulonephritis follows a streptococcal infection, most often tonsillitis or streptococcal impetigo of the skin.

139–C. Congenital infection with either cytomegalovirus or Toxoplasma is often associated with periventricular cerebral calcifications, often visible on X-ray.

140–C. Congenital infection with either cytomegalovirus or Toxoplasma is characterized by multisystem disease, often involving the brain, retina, liver, and other organ sites.

Index

Note: Page numbers in *italic* denote illustrations; those followed by (t) denote tables; those followed by Q indicate questions; and those followed by E indicate explanations.